Clinical Exercise Physiology

Clinical Exercise Physiology

Edited by

SCOTT M. HASSON, Ed.D., P.T., FACSM

Director of Advanced Studies,
School of Physical Therapy,
Texas Woman's University,
Houston, Texas

with 8 contributors
with 105 illustrations

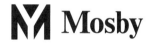 Mosby

St. Louis Baltimore Boston Chicago London Madrid Philadelphia Sydney Toronto

M **Mosby**

Dedicated to Publishing Excellence

Executive Editor: Martha Sasser
Developmental Editor: Barbara Menczer
Editorial Assistant: Kellie F. White
Project Manager: Patricia Tannian
Production Editor: Mary McAuley
Senior Book Designer: Gail Morey Hudson
Cover Designer: Teresa Breckwoldt
Manufacturing Supervisor: Betty Richmond
Copyright © 1994 by Mosby–Year Book, Inc.

Printed in the United States of America
Composition by Carlisle Communications, Ltd.
Printing/binding by Maple-Vail Book Mfg. Group

Mosby–Year Book, Inc.
11830 Westline Industrial Drive
St. Louis, Missouri 63146

Library of Congress Cataloging in Publication Data

Clinical exercise physiology / edited by Scott M. Hasson; with 8
    contributors.
        p.   cm.
    Includes bibiliographical references and index.
    ISBN 0-8151-4210-2
    1. Exercise therapy.   I. Hasson, Scott Mather, 1956-
    [DLNM: 1. Exercise—physiology. 2. Respiratory System—
physiology. 3. Cardiovascular System—physiology.
4. Musculoskeletal System—physiology. WE 103 C6407 1993]
RM725.C58 1993
615.8′2 — dc20
DNLM/DLC   93-34145
for Library of Congress   CIP

93 94 95 96 97 / 9 8 7 6 5 4 3 2 1

CONTRIBUTORS

ODED BAR-OR, MD

Professor of Pediatrics,
Director, Children's Exercise
and Nutrition Centre,
McMaster University,
Hamilton, Ontario,
Canada

LAWRENCE P. CAHALIN, PT, CCS

Cardiopulmonary Physical Therapy
Transplant Coordinator,
Massachusetts General Hospital,
Boston, Massachusetts

DONNA FROWNFELTER, MA, PT, RRT

Committed to Excellence
Physical Therapy Consultants,
Glenview, Illinois

LEWIS M. NASHNER, ScD

Chairman,
NeuroCom International, Inc.;
Adjunct Senior Scientist,
R.S. Dow Neurological Sciences Institute,
Portland, Oregon

ELIZABETH J. PROTAS, PT, PhD

Assistant Dean and Professor,
School of Physical Therapy,
Texas Woman's University,
Houston, Texas

ROY J. SHEPHARD, MD, PhD, DPE

Professor of Applied Physiology,
School of Physical and Health Education,
University of Toronto,
Toronto, Ontario,
Canada

KATHLEEN WESTPHAL, PhD, PT

Research Physiologist,
Occupational Physiology Division,
United States Army Research Institute of
Environmental Medicine,
Natick, Massachusetts

JAY H. WILLIAMS, PhD

Associate Professor,
Department of Health and Physical Education,
Virginia Polytechnic Institute and State University,
Blacksburg, Virginia

This text is dedicated to
my wife and best friend
Ellen

and my wonderful children
Karen, Annie, and Katie

In addition
this text is in memory of my son
Eric Scott
who died before birth but will never be forgotten

PREFACE

The purpose of *Clinical Exercise Physiology* is to show the student and seasoned clinical practitioner alike the physiologic basis for movement dysfunction and the impact of exercise on patients with diseases and disorders. Although the text is designed with the physical therapy student in mind, practicing physical therapists, physicians, and physical educators who work with patients will also benefit from the clinical knowledge presented in the text. The text is organized into five parts, each containing chapters that deal with normal physiology paired with "clinical" chapters that examine exercise tolerance and response to training for specific patients. A "preface" describes the objectives of each part, and in each chapter students are given a list of terms to focus on during their studies. In addition, "clinical pearls" emphasizing notable techniques and information are italicized throughout the text, case studies of authentic patient treatments and responses are presented in each "clinical" chapter, and each chapter ends with a short list of study questions. These questions will direct the student's thinking toward indications and contraindications for exercise and designs for exercise programs.

The text compares normal exercise tolerance, exercise prescription, and the effect of exercise training with exercise tolerance and prescription and the effect of training in patients with specific diseases. Topics include principles of exercise training, normal and abnormal metabolism, pulmonary and cardiovascular function and dysfunction, neuromuscular and musculoskeletal function and dysfunction, and specific implications of exercise for chronically ill children, adolescents, and elderly persons. Most physical therapy and medical curricula do not address the effect of exercise tolerance and training in patients with specific diseases, perhaps because data on exercise for specific patients is published in such a wide variety and number of journals. *Clinical Exercise Physiology* is unique in that it compiles and presents scientifically based exercise information on most common diseases and some rare disorders. Chapters providing the student with the physiologic basis of exercise are written by expert applied and basic scientists. The goal of these "physiology" chapters is to develop the structural and functional basis on which to compare exercise response and training in healthy persons and persons with specific diseases. In "clinical" chapters world-renowned physical therapists and physicians describe through exercise literature and personal experience how patients with specific diseases and disorders respond to exercise and training. Exercise prescriptions, including indications, contraindications, and precautions, are also described in these "clinical" chapters and are exemplified in case studies.

I would like to thank my contributors for providing such excellent work. I would also like to thank those many scientists who care for patients and whose work is cited throughout this text. For those academicians who have chosen to teach exercise physiology to their students, I congratulate you. I hope this text gives you a logical guideline and pertinent information. Finally, to the student, you are our future in the allied health and medical professions. I have written and edited this text with you in mind. Please feel free to contact my associates and me for questions, advice, and clarification; not all of our knowledge and clinical skills can be transcribed to the written word. Thus, speaking for my colleagues and myself, I assure you that our ultimate goal is to mentor as many of you as possible in the area of clinical exercise physiology. Enjoy the text, and I look forward to speaking with you in the future at meetings and gatherings of clinicians, educators, and scientists. Good luck in your endeavors.

Scott M. Hasson

CONTENTS

PART I

PRINCIPLES OF EXERCISE TRAINING

■ *KEEP IN MIND WHILE YOU READ* . . . *Roy Shephard sets the stage for the rest of the text by describing concepts of exercise and physical activity. Exercise training and the variables that influence normal physiologic changes in healthy persons are discussed at length. Please focus on these normal responses and the types of exercise prescription recommended for normal, healthy individuals. Throughout the text, use the normal adaptations and prescriptions as bases for comparison of healthy persons with individuals who have specific diseases or disorders.* ■

RESPONSES TO EXERCISE AND FACTORS IN EXERCISE TRAINING

Roy J. Shephard

This book provides physiotherapists, physicians, and other clinical practitioners with an understanding of the physiologic processes that occur as healthy individuals and patients in a variety of categories undertake progressive exercise with a view to improving both local and overall physical function. Chapter 1 defines the concepts of exercise and physical activity and explores the various factors that determine the body's responses to physical training, placing particular emphasis on the key variables that influence the training response (intensity, frequency, duration, and mode of exercise plus current level of fitness). Psychologic responses to training, including the processes of habituation and task learning, are also discussed.

EXERCISE, PHYSICAL ACTIVITY, AND FITNESS EXERCISE

The average person considers *exercise, physical activity,* and *fitness* synonymous terms. The term *exercise* implies, strictly speaking, the voluntary performance of one or more bouts of physical activity with the deliberate intention of improving physical performance, physical condition, or health.[19]

Physical Activity

Physical activity encompasses all forms of movement, whether undertaken voluntarily (exercise and sport) or unavoidably (during the performance of occupational and domestic chores). In the past a substantial part of the total daily physical activity of most adults was attributable to occupational and domestic responsibilities. With current trends to mechanization and automation, however, this stimulus has been lost, and in consequence the physical condition of most persons living in developed societies has deteriorated. Individuals now must turn increasingly to deliberate leisure-time exercise and sport to find sufficient physical activity to develop or sustain physical condition.[93]

Physical Fitness

Physical fitness remains a difficult term to define.[25] The development of physical fitness may imply a general improvement in cardiorespiratory or muscular condition or a specific gain in the ability to perform a particular task. After a week of vigorous debate the World Health Organization described physical fitness as "the ability to perform muscular work satisfactorily."[2] This definition avoids controversy but remains somewhat dissatisfying. Despite semantic difficulties, it is clear that exercise and physical fitness are related and that an increase in physical fitness is a potential consequence of regularly repeated bouts of exercise, given a training regimen that is appropriate to the needs of the individual.

If the exercise program is focused on aerobic fitness, the likely consequence of training is an increase in maximal oxygen intake, the ability to transport oxygen from the atmosphere to the working muscles. Traditionally, maximal oxygen intake has been regarded as one of the best measures of an individual's level of training. In the healthy adult the maximal oxygen intake is determined primarily by the maximal cardiac output (in other words, maximal oxygen intake is a measure of cardiovascular fitness), but in persons with various diseases other links in the chain of oxygen transport, such as ventilatory capacity, may become the determining factors. Reliance on maximal oxygen intake as the sole index of fitness has been increasingly questioned; a substantial portion of individual differences in maximal oxygen intake (30% to 40%) is attributable to a combination of social and genetic inheritance[87,101,102,126] rather than to a training response. Moreover, there is now evidence that, other factors being equal, the responses to a given training regimen are quite strongly influenced by genetic factors.[87] In addition, consensus is growing that levels of physical activity insufficient to augment maximal oxygen intake may, nevertheless, have a beneficial influence on various aspects of health, such as a reduction of cardiac risk factors.

Although the shift of emphasis from the results of training (cardiac function and muscular strength) to the process itself may be important for the epidemiologist, for the physiotherapist who is concerned with the restoration of function, it is difficult to dissociate fitness from improvement of the various determinants of physical function such as maximal oxygen intake, muscle strength, and flexibility.

EFFECTS OF TRAINING
General Considerations

When a patient repeats a given bout of exercise on a regular basis, as when meeting a normal training prescription, the various body systems undergo a progressive adaptation to the imposed stress, which is described by many exercise scientists as an "increase of fitness."

Details of the altered functional response depend on the type of exercise that has been prescribed, but in general the following gains are noted:

1. A higher peak rate of working becomes possible for the task that has been practiced.
2. The prescribed submaximal activity can be carried out more readily, with less subjective perception of effort.
3. The disturbances of body function initially associated with undertaking a prescribed activity of given intensity and duration are progressively reduced.
4. The rate of recovery for physiologic variables after a given bout of the prescribed exercise is speeded.
5. If the prescription is well-designed, similar benefits are experienced when the patient performs other types of physical activity.[125]

Nature of Training Responses

Generalized training responses can be functional or structural. Functional changes reflect a better coordination of the body responses; for example, a larger fraction of the total blood volume may be stored centrally, where it can augment cardiac output, or the firing of a number of motor units may be better synchronized, thereby increasing peak muscle force. The structural changes develop more slowly; for example, hypertrophy of the left ventricle might increase the peak stroke volume of the heart or hypertrophy of the skeletal muscles might increase the force of muscle contraction.

Although it is useful to distinguish functional and structural training responses, both lead to an enhanced maximal performance. It is also useful to distinguish cardiorespiratory training (in which the primary objectives are the development of aerobic endurance and the reduction of cardiac risk factors) from muscular training (in which the main focus is the strengthening of muscles, tendon, and bone).

Cardiorespiratory training. The most obvious manifestation of cardiorespiratory training is a decrease in heart rate both at rest and at a given

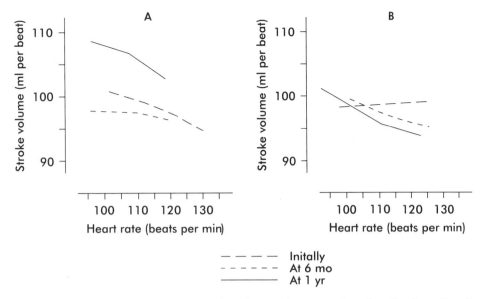

Fig. 1-1 The relationship of cardiac stroke volume to heart rate. Data from Southern Ontario Multicentre exercise–heart trial for patients given exercise programs, **A,** of high intensity and, **B,** of low intensity for 6 and 12 months. (From Shephard RJ: *Ischemic heart disease and exercise,* London, 1981, Croom Helm.)

intensity of submaximal exercise. Laboratory tests also show an increase in peak power output and an increase in maximal oxygen intake. Typically the gains are 10% to 20%, but they can be much larger when the initial training level is low (as in a person recovering from bed rest) and when the training stimulus is progressively increased.

Early functional responses to cardiorespiratory training include an alteration in the balance of sympathetic (accelerator) and parasympathetic (decelerator) drives to the cardiac pacemaker in the sinoatrial node, an increase in the total blood volume, and an increase in the tone of the peripheral veins. In consequence, central blood volume rises. The resting stroke volume is augmented, and the cardiac ejection fraction is better sustained during vigorous effort, allowing an increase of the prime determinant of oxygen transport, the peak cardiac output.[67] At the same time, a larger fraction of the available blood flow is directed to the active muscles (and to the skin in a hot climate), so the maximum arteriovenous oxygen difference is increased.[12,71,111,112,140]

When training is both protracted and vigorous, eventual structural adaptations occur in the heart, although, depending on genetic constitution, some individuals respond more readily than others to a given training load. A progressive hypertrophy of the left ventricular wall[25,63,82,113] reduces unit work per sarcomere of the heart wall,[57] facilitating maintenance of the cardiac stroke volume at high rates of working[145] and allowing the cardiac output to increase to a higher maximal level (Fig. 1-1).

After protracted, vigorous training the heart becomes more resistant to oxygen lack; any ST depression seen initially on the exercise electrocardiogram may be lessened or reversed and the ventricular fibrillation threshold is increased.[94] Structural changes, such as increases in the dimensions of the coronary arteries or the collateral blood supply to the myocardium, may contribute to these alterations.[65,74,149] However, the main explanations seem to be a reduction of cardiac work rate (the product of heart rate and blood pressure, both of which are reduced) and a facilitation of coronary perfusion by means of a relative lengthening of the diastolic phase of the heart cycle that occurs when the heart rate is reduced.

A strengthening of the respiratory muscles increases vital capacity and allows the patient to develop and sustain a larger maximum voluntary ventilation, which lessens the unpleasant breathlessness (dyspnea) that often limits effort in an older person. The changes in the strength of the chest muscles are likely to be small in a standard cardiac training program, but hypertrophy can be augmented by the addition of deliberate resistance exercises to develop the chest muscles. Such exercises may help overcome the respiratory fatigue that can limit prolonged exercise in an older person who has an increased respiratory work load as a result of chronic obstructive lung disease.

A further structural consequence of repeated, prolonged bouts of moderate endurance training is a progressive replacement of fat by lean tissue.[134,138] This alteration sometimes occurs without any net change in body mass, and the clinical emphasis on ''weight loss'' is evidently misplaced. Favorable changes in cardiac risk factors other than body fat also develop, particularly a 5- to 10-mm Hg decrease in systolic blood pressure both at rest and during exercise, an increase in insulin sensitivity, and a decrease of total serum cholesterol with an increase in the scavenging high-density lipoprotein (HDL) component. These various changes depend essentially on meeting a specific weekly energy expenditure (a walking or running distance of 18 to 20 km per week); the figure is sufficiently large that an effective prescription usually augments cardiorespiratory function. Nevertheless, in principle, body composition could undergo a favorable change as long as energy consumption were increased, without necessarily inducing any substantial increment of cardiac or respiratory fitness.

The flexibility of the exercised joints is increased, the tendons and articular cartilages that have been active are strengthened,[90] and osteoporosis is slowed or sometimes even reversed in weight-bearing bones.[22,143,158]

Hormonal reactions to a given absolute intensity of exercise are generally reduced by endurance training. For instance, secretion of catecholamines decreases at any given rate of working.[153] The person also perceives a given bout of exercise as less stressful,[16] and depending on initial reactions to the test work

rate, there may be either an increase or a decrease in the secretion of cortisol.[135] The tendency to tissue damage at any given intensity of vigorous exercise is also reduced, and in consequence there is a decrease in bloodstream accumulation of enzymes such as creatine kinase and lactate dehydrogenase during a prolonged bout of training.[4]

Muscle development. When the focus of training is on muscular development, functional changes are again responsible for early increases in maximal muscle force. An increased synchronization of neural firing, the mobilization of an increased fraction of the total pool of motoneurons, and possibly a greater relaxation of antagonists all contribute to greater peak forces without any change in muscle dimensions.[41]

As the individual continues with a muscle-building program, the activity of the sarcoplasmic enzymes increases, although the balance of change between aerobic and anaerobic enzyme systems depends on the type of exercise that has been pursued.[50,66] With aerobic, lightly resisted activity the main increase is in the oxidative enzymes, so in a well-trained person a higher proportion of fat is metabolized, conserving glycogen and extending his or her endurance capability. On the other hand, resistance exercise increases the activity of the enzymes involved in anaerobic metabolism.

Repeated bouts of prolonged isometric or resisted isotonic exercise lead to increase of muscle bulk in those body parts that have been active.[41] Muscle bulk is important to the health of an older person. As the muscles become stronger, a given task can be performed at a smaller fraction of maximal muscle force; there is less occlusion of the local blood supply, a smaller rise in blood pressure, and less danger that the development of a given muscle force will provoke a cardiovascular catastrophe.

Specificity of training responses. The adaptations of body function and structure that contribute to the previously mentioned changes are often relatively specific to the type of training that has been undertaken. For example, there is little cross-transfer of benefit between cardiorespiratory and muscular types of training. (Indeed, by leading to a high rate of protein metabolism, vigorous cardio-respiratory training may impede a strengthening of the skeletal muscles.) Likewise, endurance training that has been focused on the arm muscles does relatively little to improve cardiorespiratory performance when the patient must carry out an endurance activity using the legs.[86] In contrast, nearly 50% of the endurance training developed by means of regular leg ergometer exercise can be transferred to the subsequent performance of rhythmic endurance work by the arms,[24] and the generalization of the cardiorespiratory benefit resulting from treadmill or outdoor running to other forms of cardiorespiratory exercise is relatively complete.

Training benefits such as a strengthening of tendons and bones and an improvement in flexibility are particularly specific to the regions that have been exercised.

Time course of physiologic responses. The time course of the various training responses varies with the health of the individual, the pattern of the chosen training regimen (a progressively increasing load or a program of fixed intensity), and the precise intensity of training that has been adopted.

In clinical practice it is particularly important to stress that the gains in physical condition resulting from endurance training are largely lost after 2 to 3 weeks of inactivity (for instance, a period of enforced bed rest.[118,146] Conversely, much of the lost physical condition can be regained by a few weeks of renewed training.[118] Hickson et al.[62] suggested that the half-time for gains of maximal oxygen intake was as short as 10 days when subjects were given a constant training stimulus. However, critics of that study have pointed out that a well-designed training plan does not give a constant training stimulus but rather calls for a progressive increase in both the intensity and the duration of effort as the patient's physical condition improves.[75]

Given a progressive training plan, healthy 65-year-old patients can make quite large gains in maximal oxygen intake in as few as 7 weeks of training.[137] On the other hand, a person who has sustained a myocardial infarction finds difficulty in exercising strenuously during the first few months after the incident. In such patients early training

responses reflect peripheral rather than central circulatory adaptations.[99] After 12 months of training at progressively higher intensities, some increase in cardiac stroke volume is eventually seen,[99,55] although this increase could reflect a strengthening of the skeletal muscles and thus a reduction in the "afterload" opposing ventricular ejection rather than cardiac hypertrophy and a more forceful ventricular contraction. In "postcoronary" patients the increase in maximal oxygen intake can continue slowly over several years, provided that they continue to follow a progressive training program[127] (Fig. 1-2).

Not all elements of the body's training response develop in parallel. For instance, Saltin[116] drew attention to a discrepancy between the activity of muscle enzymes (which usually change in as few as 7 to 10 days of training[61]) and the increase in maximal oxygen intake (which may continue over many weeks or months). In Saltin's view the difference in time course for the increments of muscle enzyme activities and peak oxygen transport is good evidence that the rise in maximal oxygen intake reflects central changes (particularly an increase of maximal cardiac output) rather than peripheral adaptations such as the enzyme changes that might have allowed an increased extraction of oxygen in the working muscles).

Smith and O'Donnell[142] suggested further that changes in the ventilatory threshold developed faster than gains in maximal oxygen intake and that the latter in turn was modified more rapidly than was the heart rate response to submaximal exercise. In contrast, Rogers et al.[108] noted an improvement in submaximal exercise responses before gains in maximal oxygen intake had occurred. Possibly, such differences in results reflect discrepancies in the type or intensity of training that the patient has undertaken.

INTENSITY OF TRAINING
General Considerations

The intensity of a training program may be determined by physiologic considerations, although sometimes the optimal prescription has to give place to the clinically attainable. Physiologists

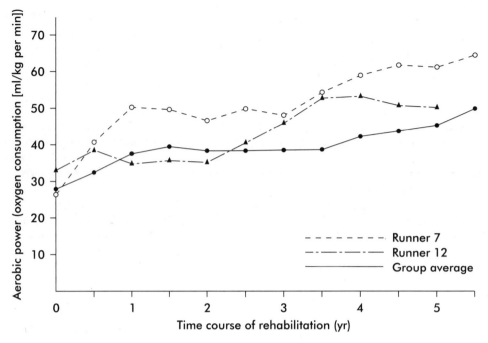

Fig. 1-2   Time courses of the increase in directly measured maximal oxygen intake with vigorous training. Data from study of 13 postcoronary runners who finally participated in marathon events. Group average and individual data for two runners who making particularly large gains are shown. (From Shephard RJ: *Ischemic heart disease and exercise,* London, 1981, Croom Helm.)

have argued that the rate of any type of adaptation is determined primarily by the intensity of the stimulus. Thus at first inspection the best training response might be anticipated with a high intensity of effort.

However, it is a little unfair to argue from the response to an external stimulus such as a hot environment to the internally generated exercise stimulus. Adoption of a high intensity of effort necessarily implies a brief bout of exercise, particularly in an older individual. The disturbance of normal physiologic function and thus the magnitude of the training "impulse" may be more profound and more long-lasting when the patient is persuaded to undertake a sustained period of activity of more moderate intensity.

Training Threshold

Whether the intent is to develop the cardiorespiratory performance or to enhance muscular strength, a certain critical threshold intensity of effort must be reached to initiate a training response.

Definition of this threshold is important to the international athlete who wishes to maximize the training response without causing "staleness" or the tissue damage associated with "overtraining," to the busy executive who wishes to minimize personal investment of both time and effort in exercise, and to the older patient adversely affected by a specific chronic disease process in which the margin between an effective and a dangerously intensive training program becomes much narrower than normal, with a corresponding need for greater sophistication in the prescription of exercise.

Concept of Overloading

If structural training such as skeletal muscle or ventricular hypertrophy is to occur, body systems

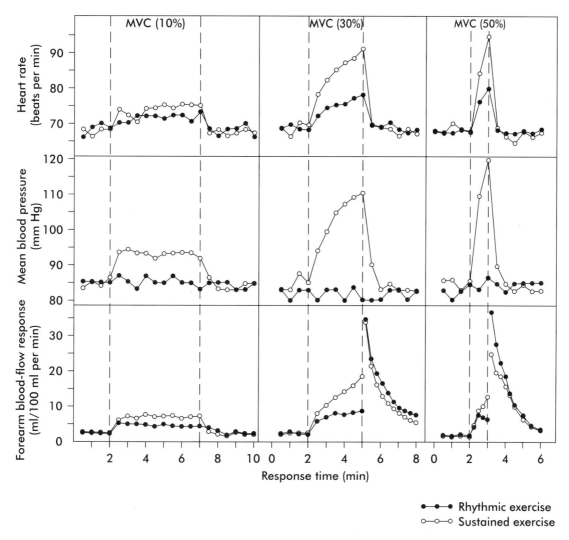

Fig. 1-3 Heart rate, arterial blood pressure, and forearm blood flow responses to isometric contractions at 10%, 30%, and 50% of maximum voluntary contraction (MVC), or force. (From Lind S, McNicol G: *Can Med Assoc J* 96:710, 1967.)

must be overloaded. For instance, if exercise is performed in an upright posture, the cardiac stroke volume is not maximized until the patient has developed 50% of maximal oxygen intake.[6,37,139,140] The accompanying rise in systolic blood pressure (which offers an increased afterload to the left ventricle) is a function of both the intensity and the duration of effort. Both isometric and isotonic muscular activity cause rapid rises in systemic blood pressure (Fig. 1-3) and thus have a greater likelihood than does aerobic activity of stimulating ventricular hypertrophy.

Overloading can be excessive. The problem of overtraining of the skeletal muscles has been discussed. The heart seems less vulnerable to overloading, although some reports indicate that prolonged, intensive cardiovascular effort such as participation in the Hawaiian triathlon can cause both cardiac fatigue (with a reduction of ejection fractions) and pulmonary edema, even in a healthy young adult. However, such levels of effort are not typical of the exercise that is prescribed for the average patient. More common cardiac dangers that result from an excessive intensity of effort are the provocation of myocardial ischemia, ventricular fibrillation, and cardiac failure.[98,127] The risks of such sequelae are greatest in the patient with known coronary atherosclerosis, but irregular, intense exercise can occasionally provoke a cardiac catastrophe in an older adult who is symptom free and has had a stress electrocardiogram with negative results. Heavy preloading or afterloading of the ventricles can also provoke cardiac decompensation in a patient with a tendency to myocardial ischemia and congestive heart failure.

To induce hypertrophy of skeletal muscle,[152] it is important to develop a moderate overload, but attempts to accelerate such training by excessive loading can cause microscopic or gross muscular damage. At the cellular level, overloading induces changes both in membrane permeability and in the rate of protein transcription. Booth and Watson[15] found that in rats, muscle protein synthesis decreased during the first 30 minutes of activity but when the exercise was continued for 7 hours, there was an increased rate of protein formation. Potential triggers to increased protein synthesis include an increased intracellular concentration of free amino acids brought about by a tension-induced degradation of muscle protein, an increased influx of amino acids from the blood stream via the stretched sarcolemma, and an impact of decreasing intracellular adenosine triphosphate (ATP) and pH levels on Ca^{2+}-mediated stimulation of RNA transcription.[15] Plainly, overly intensive exercise can induce local hypoxia and excessive changes in membrane permeability, a leakage of vital cellular constituents into the extracellular space, and the development of microtraumata.[8,26]

A moderate overload is desirable from a psychologic perspective. It is vital that the patient accept the prescribed intensity of effort as appropriate to personal training goals. Recruits sometimes drop out of exercise classes not because the effort is too

demanding, but because the prescription lacks sufficient challenge.

Cardiovascular Threshold

The concept of a threshold intensity of effort for cardiovascular training has been attributed to Karvonen, Kentala, and Mustala.[70] The original investigation studied the responses of young men. One group trained at an average heart rate of 135 beats per minute without significant change in physiologic responses to a given bout of exercise. A second group trained at a heart rate of 160 to 180 beats per minute. In the latter group the training response was sufficiently large that to maintain a consistent exercise heart rate, it was necessary to increase the treadmill speed by 25% to 30% over a 4-week period.

Subsequent authors have applied Karvonen's findings to persons of all ages, regardless of their initial physical condition. Some investigators have interpreted the results as showing a cardiovascular or cardiorespiratory training threshold at 60% of the difference between resting and maximum heart rates (145 beats per minute in a young adult). Others have suggested from the same data that the threshold for training the cardiovascular system or the overall cardiorespiratory transport of oxygen lies at 60% of maximal oxygen intake (a heart rate of about 135 beats per minute in a young adult), and a few authors have placed the training threshold at 60% of maximal heart rate (corresponding to about 117 beats per minute).

In fact, Karvonen and his associates did not define any precise universal threshold. Their experiments merely established that when the training stimulus was a relatively brief bout of tread mill exercise, a cardiovascular training response occurred at a heart rate of 170 beats per minute but not at 135 beats per minute.

The threshold intensity for cardiorespiratory training is probably modified both by the initial fitness of the individual and by the duration of the activity. Certainly there are circumstances in which oxygen transport can increase while the heart rate remains much below 160 to 180 beats per minute. For instance, Bouchard et al.[17] induced some training when patients performed cycle ergometer exercise at a heart rate of 130 beats per minute for no more than 10 minutes per day and Durnin, Brockway, and Whitcher[35] reported substantial improvement in the endurance fitness of young soldiers who marched 10 to 30 km per day at heart rates that are unlikely to have exceeded 120 beats per minute.

Older patients are often limited by unpleasant breathlessness, in addition to the cardiovascular risks discussed in the preceding paragraphs, and they may face orthopedic barriers to the performance of intensive exercise. Thus there is increasing interest in the training potential of fast walking. Oja[96] maintained that the physiologic responses to a walking program can match those obtained with a jogging regimen, and he has subsequently encouraged the population of Tampere, a medium-sized Finnish city, to walk to work. Certainly, fast walking can develop more than 70% of maximal oxygen intake in middle-aged and elderly patients.[107] Moreover, the threshold for cardiovascular training is unlikely to be identical in young and older adults: in older individuals it is probably biased downward by a sedentary life-style. Restriction of recent activity is particularly typical of patients who have recently been hospitalized for treatment of myocardial infarction, and such individuals may demonstrate a training response to exercise heart rates as low as 110 beats per minute.[72]

The importance of the intensity of training relative to the other potential variables in an exercise prescription has been much discussed. The author attempted to resolve this issue by carrying out a series of treadmill experiments in which young, healthy men were randomly allocated to training regimens differing in intensity, frequency, and duration.[123] A multiple regression analysis of the data demonstrated that the most important determinant of training in these individuals was the intensity of effort relative to their initial fitness. Subsequent experiments performed in other laboratories have not added greatly to this conclusion. Reports have claimed an effect of intensity,[38] of intensity but not initial fitness,[47] of both fitness and intensity,[122] the latter variable becoming insig-

nificant after equating the total amount of work performed,[121] of intensity despite matching of initial fitness and the total amount of work performed,[156] and of intensity and duration.[29] Wenger and Bell[155] further claimed that the impact of a training program continued to increase with intensity of exercise up to loads demanding 90% to 100% of maximal oxygen intake.

Initial physical condition and training intensity are important variables when comparing the training responses of young and elderly patients. If initial physical condition is matched based on the absolute performance of the two groups (for instance, in terms of maximal oxygen intake measured in liters per minute) rather than by reference to age-related norms, responses may be compared (inappropriately) between sedentary young adults and extremely fit senior citizens. Likewise, if the intensity of training is matched in terms of the absolute oxygen consumption demanded by a given exercise prescription,[119] the stimulus applied to an older patient may be much greater than that for a younger individual; in consequence, the elderly patients may be judged to have better training responses than the younger patients and, more important, the elderly patients may be asked to exercise too vigorously. In fact, the aerobic component of exercise prescriptions should demand a constant fraction of the individual's maximal oxygen intake, and if training is planned in such terms, the training response is relatively independent of the age of the participant.[133]

The optimal intensity of endurance training lies at or just below a work rate at which lactate begins to accumulate. As previously described, this rate amounts to 60% to 70% of personal maximal oxygen intake in the typical sedentary individual but may reach 75% to 80% of aerobic power in a serious endurance competitor.[1] An appropriate intensity of effort can be prescribed in terms of distance and pace.[72,73] Alternatively, patients may count the pulse rate immediately (5 to 15 seconds) after exercise,[14] they may seek an intensity of exercise that initiates sweating,[80] or they may look for what is perceived as moderate effort, an intensity of exercise that allows continuation of normal conversation.[13,16,21]

A person can reach much higher intensities of effort with brief interval training (for instance, 10- to 30-second bouts of activity, followed by 10- to 30-second recovery periods) than with continuous types of exercise. By appropriate adjustment of the length of exercise bouts and recovery periods, interval training can be used to enhance anaerobic power, anaerobic capacity, or aerobic power.[5,36] Training at an intensity above the ventilatory threshold is needed to increase lactate tolerance[59]; one way to train the anaerobic energy systems is to increase the body mass during exercise sessions by wearing a 9- to 10-kg vest.[114] Brief interval training increases both muscle glycogen stores and the reserve of buffering alkalies in the active limbs, with increased local intramuscular concentrations of ATP, myoglobin, and glycolytic enzymes[128]; anaerobic power and anaerobic capacity are increased by these changes. More prolonged interval training (1-minute bouts of exercise, followed by 1-minute recovery periods) can be used to enhance aerobic power in patients for whom sustained exercise would be halted by myocardial oxygen lack and anginal pain.[127]

Muscle-Training Threshold

The intensity of effort that is selected influences patterns of muscle-fiber recruitment and thus the site and extent of any local training responses within the skeletal muscles. Moderate aerobic activity recruits mainly slow-twitch (type 1) fibers. Over several weeks their function is selectively enhanced and a greater tolerance of fatiguing muscular activity develops. The cross-sectional area of the individual muscle fibers increases relatively little, but the size, number, and complexity of mitochondria within the active fibers are all increased, with a corresponding augmentation of aerobic enzyme activity.[66] The effect is to encourage the metabolism of fat rather than glycogen during prolonged exercise,[129] a development that improves fitness for sustained activity.

Heavy resistance and isometric training lead to a selective recruitment of fast-twitch (type 2) fibers. Hypertrophy occurs in the active muscle fibers[150] and sometimes a splitting of the muscle fibers can also be detected,[51] but it is not yet established that such exercise can stimulate the formation of new muscle fibers.[147] Because the trained muscle fibers contain more contractile protein than they contained before training, hypertrophy may decrease the volume density of the muscle mitochondria.[88]

The acute cellular response to resisted exercise is a slowing of protein synthesis, but within 24 hours of such a training session the muscle fibers show supranormal rates of protein formation. If the training overload has been too great, the muscles may become sore, with a disruption of connective tissue and an increase in the hydroxyproline-to-creatine ratio.[151] Swelling and destruction of cristae suggest that the mitochondria can be damaged by excessive overloading of muscles.[4,8,40]

Muscle training often changes the relative proportions of type 2a (fast oxidative glycolytic) and type 2b (fast glycolytic) fibers, and high-intensity intermittent training may also convert type 1 fibers into type 2 fibers.[32,68,141,148]

A muscle-building prescription is usually regulated in terms of the fraction of maximal voluntary force that is to be developed. For example, a patient may be asked to perform three ''sets,'' each requiring 10 repetitions of a particular procedure at a defined fraction of maximal effort for that movement. Muscle endurance in a young adult is developed by frequently repeated sets of contractions at around 60% of maximal voluntary force, whereas peak force is increased by high-intensity contractions with only a limited number of repetitions[3,53,58]; however, in elderly patients or in an individual who has recently sustained a myocardial infarction the muscles are weaker, and initially a training plan may begin at only 40% to 50% of maximal voluntary force. During isometric effort an interaction occurs between the intensity and the duration of contraction; again, in a healthy young adult training is likely to occur if maximal contractions are held for 1 to 2 seconds; at 67% of maximal force, however, the minimal effective duration of contraction is 4 to 6 seconds[60] and a further prolongation of individual contractions is needed if the peak force is reduced to 40% to 50% of maximal voluntary effort.

Psychologic Reactions

The optimal intensity of training from the psychologic viewpoint is that perceived as achievable yet effective in attaining the goals set by the physiotherapist in discussion with the patient.

FREQUENCY AND DURATION OF TRAINING

The optimal frequency and duration of training reflect the anticipated time course of acute exercise responses and the subsequent recovery process. Acute responses have already been discussed; a person reaches a steady state of aerobic effort within 1 to 2 minutes, so the training impulse for three 10-minute bouts of exercise is only a little less than that derived from a single 30-minute session. The speed of recovery varies with the type, intensity, and duration of training; cardiorespiratory responses are largely normalized within 15 minutes, but for some of the metabolic and hormonal reactions, including the restocking of glycogen reservoirs, repair of microtraumata, and maximization of protein synthesis, a period as long as 24 to 48 hours may be required.

Frequency

Muscle phosphagen stores (ATP and creatine phosphate) are both depleted and replenished extremely rapidly.[31] Interval work designed to train anaerobic power may thus allow recovery periods as short as 10 to 60 seconds.[161]

If lactate accumulates at maximal speed, muscle fibers may reach their limiting concentration within a minute. Muscle and blood concentrations are substantially reduced by 15 to 30 minutes of recovery, allowing several similar bouts of activity to be repeated on the same day. Such patterns of training tend to maximize anaerobic capacity.

Much longer recovery intervals than those for lactate breakdown are needed to permit increased protein synthesis, restoration of glycogen reserves, and repair of exercise-induced microtraumata. Glycogen stores reach their initial resting level within 24 hours but continue to rise thereafter, peaking about 2 days after a prolonged bout of exercise.[117] Muscle soreness and an attendant ab-normal blood accumulation of certain enzymes such as L-lactic dehydrogenase persist for several days after completion of a strenuous exercise bout.[26] Thus distance training is best limited to alternate days or arranged as alternating light and heavy daily training sessions.

Empirical data suggest that the response to endurance training is increased on moving from one to five exercise sessions per week.[104,123,137] One critical variable is the extent of any overtraining that may occur during individual sessions. Individuals also differ widely in responsiveness to a given training regimen. Some persons maintain their physical condition with only two training sessions per week, but others need daily exercise.[85] The effectiveness of an increase in the frequency of training is due in part to an increase in the total amount of exercise undertaken.[64] Many of the processes involved in training, such as an increase in protein synthesis and the greater metabolism of body fat, are related in a semiquantitative fashion to the number of times that a given stress is presented or to the total quantity of work performed, or to both.

One practical argument against prescribing a low frequency of exercise is that the required bout of physical activity is then easily overlooked by the patient; however, daily exercise, or alternating days of heavy and light exercise are less easily forgotten. If the sessions are to be infrequent, the intensity or the duration of individual bouts, or both, must also be increased to obtain an equivalent training response, with a danger that the participant will become excessively fatigued. In contrast, if sessions are incorporated into each day's routine (for instance, a regular walk to the bus or the subway station), they become relatively automatic. Habit is an important determinant of both general and specific exercise behavior.[48]

If formal training sessions are too frequent, the patient may perceive them as excessively time-consuming, complaining of lack of time, staleness, fatigue, or boredom, with a likelihood of poor compliance with the prescription. Such problems are particularly likely in a young, competitive athlete who is pursuing specific training to the exclusion of normal social contacts. However, complaints can also arise in older patients, perhaps because they are being asked to make long journeys to a physiotherapy department to obtain relatively brief bouts of exercise or perhaps because a further investment of time and effort is seen as yielding muscle soreness or pain rather than commensurate gains in physical condition. The ideal program is thus sufficiently frequent to become habitual but leaves the participant plenty of time for other pursuits. The intensity of individual sessions is carefully regulated to produce no more than pleasant tiredness on the following day, and the ''opportunity cost'' of travel is held to a minimum and is compatible with the severity of the condition and the intelligence of the patient.

Duration

The training response to an individual exercise bout is influenced by its duration. Two bursts of exercise of moderate duration may induce a somewhat smaller physiologic response than would a single training bout of equivalent total duration. However, psychologic adaptations, particularly the progressive decrease of exercise heart rate with habituation, depend more on the number of sessions that have been taken than on their duration.

Provided a patient does not increase his or her food intake, there is a roughly stoichiometric relationship between fat loss and the added energy expenditure induced by moderate endurance exercise plus any postexercise stimulation of metabolism. If the exercise bout is prolonged, however, the patient starts to move in a less coordinated fashion, which increases the metabolic cost of a given rate of external working.[20] Moreover, fat accounts for a larger proportion of total metabolism in prolonged bouts of low-intensity effort than in shorter bursts of high-intensity activity. For any given total energy expenditure, walking at a moderate pace is thus a more effective method of inducing fat loss than vigorous running. According to some studies, a threshold energy expenditure equivalent to a walking distance of 18 to 20 km per week is needed to optimize the blood lipid profile (Fig. 1-4).[77,159]

Some of the adverse physiologic reactions to overload, for instance, the progressive rise of blood pressure with isometric effort,[84] are proportional to the duration of an exercise bout. A short training session may thus provide a valuable stimulus both to the cardiovascular system and to the skeletal muscles, but a more prolonged bout of activity of similar intensity can give rise to acute myocardial ischemia or strain of the skeletal muscles; particular care is needed to restrict the duration of individual muscle contractions when inducing muscle hypertrophy in frail elderly persons and in patients who have sustained a myocardial-infarction.

Prolonged exercise or training sessions give biochemical,[26] humoral,[81] and immunologic[78] evidence of overstrain. The incidence of gross musculoskeletal injuries also rises when an excessive weekly jogging distance is attempted.[106] For the average middle-aged person a useful ceiling seems to be a weekly walking or jogging distance of about 50 km, perhaps 10 km per day if the person is exercising 5 days per week.

The duration of an individual exercise bout has less influence on training responses than does the intensity of effort.[29,123] Nevertheless, a prolonged bout of moderate exercise such as brisk walking is often a more practical prescription than short periods of intensive effort, both for a person who wishes to train while en route to a workplace that lacks shower facilities and for an older patient who might be endangered by more intensive activity.

MODE OF TRAINING
Cardiorespiratory Training

Assuming that training is undertaken regularly, how important is the mode of exercise? Beaudet[11] found no difference in the gains in maximal oxygen intake in response to swimming, running, and cycling programs. Likewise, Milburn and Butts[92] reported similar gains in oxygen transport with aerobic dance and a jogging program. The consensus is that any activity involving a large proportion of the skeletal muscle mass is effective. Nevertheless, specificity is evident with respect to habituation, task learning, local circulatory adaptations, and general

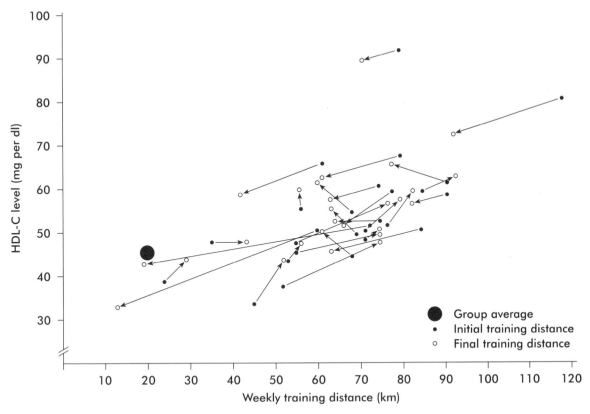

Fig. 1-4   Influence of weekly training distance on the blood levels of high-density lipoprotein–cholesterol (HDL-C). The large mark indicates the average training distance for the entire group studied. The lines pair data for persons within the group who modified their training distances in preparation for marathon participation. The correlation coefficient (r) between increased training and increased HDL-C, as well as decreased training and decreased HDL-C, was 0.89. (From Kavanagh T et al: *Arteriosclerosis* 3:249, 1983.)

adaptations. Other important issues are the volume of active muscle and postural effects.

Habituation. Habituation is a form of negative conditioning.[46] If a person is asked to undertake an unfamiliar form of exercise, anxiety initially causes an excessive increase in heart rate in about one patient in four. As the required task is repeated and is seen as less threatening, the heart rate, blood pressure, and ventilatory reactions all diminish toward a steady level determined by the metabolic cost of the task. Such adaptation reduces the work rate of the heart and thus myocardial oxygen demand; in patients for whom effort is initially symptom limited by angina, there may be a considerable increase in the peak rate of working.

The fastest habituation occurs during the course of the first two or three test sessions. Although some of the adaptation is task specific, there can also be a transfer of habituation to other, similar tasks, particularly if the test setting remains unchanged.

Task learning. Task learning transfers neural control of an activity from the motor cortex to the cerebellum. Movements become not only "automatic," but also mechanically more efficient, and in consequence the oxygen cost of the activity is decreased.[123] This decrease may substantially extend the performance of a near-maximal task both for an athlete and for an elderly person with limited physical reserves. However, there is usually little transfer of such learning from one type of exercise to another.

Local adaptations. Specific local circulatory adaptations occur when a chosen mode of aerobic exercise involves a relatively small group of muscles, for instance, the operation of an arm ergometer, a pulley system[54] or a swim bench.[44] After training, the peak oxygen intake is increased if the individual is using the exercised muscles, but little of the gain in power output is transferred to the performance of other types of exercise.[24,86,109]

During maximal effort, specificity of training is more marked for the cycle ergometer than for the treadmill (probably because the peak power output on the cycle depends heavily on quadriceps strength). During submaximal exercise, however, the adaptations induced on the treadmill (for example, a slowing of heart rate for a given oxygen consumption) are more specific than those developed on a cycle ergometer.[39]

The mechanisms contributing to specific local training include a local strengthening of the active muscles, which allows them to contract at a smaller fraction of their maximal voluntary force,[125] facilitating perfusion of the working limbs. There may also be a local increase of muscle capillarization[27,120,144] and an increased activity of aerobic enzymes in the muscle sarcoplasm. The latter changes facilitate local oxygen extraction for a given blood flow,[27] although the intramuscular extraction of oxygen during maximal exercise is usually fairly complete, even before training.[116] A further possible factor is that the training sessions in some way increase neural traffic to the medullary cardiovascular centers from local chemoreceptors in the exercised muscles, thus inducing a greater local vasodilatation in these muscles.

General adaptations. Repeated sessions of large-muscle exercise improve the function of the central circulation. Such gains are then generalizable to other modes of aerobic activity. Ultimately there may be some cardiac hypertrophy, but the immediate benefit is attributable to an increase in venous tone and thus an augmentation of central blood volume (a greater preloading of the heart), an increase in myocardial contractility, and a decrease in systemic blood pressure (decreased after-loading).

Wilmore et al.[160] found a transfer of training from cycling or jogging to treadmill performance, and White[157] found the trampoline to be as effective a method of improving cardiorespiratory function as cycling or treadmill exercise. On the other hand, Daub et al.[28] suggested that ice-hockey training (a more intermittent and "anaerobic" form of activity) did not improve peak performance in such activities as skating and cycling. Likewise, Wilmore et al.[160] found no gains in treadmill performance after 20 weeks of tennis.

Volume of active muscle. Effective central cardiovascular training requires the involvement of a substantial muscle mass. Appropriate activities to prescribe include walking, jogging, running, swimming, cycling, and cross-country skiing.[97] Little additional benefit is obtained by carrying hand-held weights.[7,23] Negative features of such deliberate arm loading include a greater impact stress when jogging, greater discomfort, and a larger rise in systemic blood pressure (particularly in hypertensive patients[52]). If the prescribed activity involves a small muscle mass (for example, the use of the arms or the forearms rather than the legs), the increments of heart rate and blood pressure for any given oxygen consumption are greater, with a corresponding increase in the cardiac work rate and associated risks of myocardial ischemia.[95] An intensive circuit-training program that involves heavy arm work can lead to a large secretion of epinephrine and norepinephrine.[100] The rise in blood pressure during exercise is generally proportional to the fraction of maximal muscle force that is exerted,[30,84] although when the active muscles are small (for example, a simple handgrip), the impact on systemic blood pressure is somewhat less than it would be during a corresponding contraction of the large leg muscles.[49] Other factors being equal, the rise in systemic blood pressure is also related to the proportion of fast-twitch fibers in the muscles that are activated.[42, 115]

The peak heart rate is generally lower with arm than with leg exercise[139] because effort is limited by peripheral muscular fatigue rather than cardiovascular performance. The muscular component of perceived effort is greater with small-muscle exercise than with large-muscle exercise.[136] Deliberate training of small muscles becomes necessary when weakness has developed during bed rest or plaster immobilization and when a patient's work demands either dynamic or isometric exercise using that particular group of muscles.

Postural effects. Most common modes of endurance exercise are performed standing or sitting. Adoption of an upright posture reduces preloading of the heart, at least until the muscle pump has overcome gravitational pooling in the veins of the legs. A somewhat greater cardiovascular response to training might thus be anticipated when exercising in a lying position, for example, during swimming of moderate intensity. A combination of the horizontal posture and a cooling of the superficial veins by the water increases the central blood volume and thus the stimulus to cardiovascular training.

Exercise with support of the body mass by immersion in water[83, 131] or sitting on a chair[91] can be particularly helpful to the patient with degenerative changes in the knee joints or the lower part of the spine. On the other hand, modes of exercise in which all or part of the body mass must be supported by prolonged isometric contraction (for example, a prolonged series of pushups or pullups) place an additional strain on the circulation. Both systemic blood pressure and heart rate rise, and if the contractions are maintained for more than a few seconds or the recovery interval between contractions is too short, there is a risk of causing significant myocardial ischemia.

Gravitational stimulation may be important in sustaining bone mass. If so, swimming would be a less desirable type of training than rapid walking, particularly for an older person. However, the forces needed to stimulate bone growth are still vigorously debated. It may be that muscle contraction can load the bones as effectively as gravity can. Thus some reports have found that swimming protects the participant against osteoporosis, and others have noted unusual bone development in the playing arm of tennis players.[103]

Muscular Training

As with endurance training, there is some commonality of response among different modes of muscle strengthening. For example, Gettman, Culter, and Strathman[45] found similar increments of lean tissue mass in response to isotonic and isokinetic circuit training. However, increments of peak force show some specificity in the velocity of contraction[56,69,110] and the joint angle adopted during training. Presumably because of differences in fiber recruitment, a training program that involves explosive movements or a rapid speed of contraction develops muscle power, whereas a prescription that relies on slower movements increases muscle strength. Isometric training is particularly liable to induce gains of strength only at the specific joint angle where exercise has been undertaken[60]; a portion of the apparent gains on isometric testing seems to be due to a learning of technique rather than to a true muscle hypertrophy.

Although a carefully designed training program can develop cardiovascular and muscular function simultaneously, an excess of endurance training is likely to hamper the development of muscular strength,[34] particularly in parts of the body that have not been involved in the aerobic activity.

Subjective Considerations

Subjective factors are too rarely considered when prescribing a training program. *If two modes of training theoretically yield essentially similar physiologic dividends, in practice the program that the individual prefers will be the most effective. No program will produce its intended effects unless the level of patient compliance is high.* Due account must be taken of the individual's motives for exercising, his or her available skills, and available resources.

Plainly, patient compliance can be enhanced by considering the individual's likely motives for participating. If the patient's prime goal is recovery from illness or injury, enhancement of personal health, ascetic challenge, or reduction of stress,[79] a solitary activity such as jogging may be an appropriate recommendation, but a different type of prescription is needed for a middle-aged adult who seeks the excitement of competition or an increase in social contacts. Much also depends on the need of the individual for supervision, either because of continuing medical concerns or because of poor self-motivation. Many patients respond better in a program that provides frequent encouragement and reassurance. Thus Bassey et al.[10] found only a limited training response when an unsupervised aerobics program was offered to factory workers, and Kavanagh and Shephard[75] noted smaller physiologic gains during a home exercise program than during standard training based in a rehabilitation center.

Discouragement often arises because the patient fails to reach a level of performance at which exercise becomes enjoyable. It is thus helpful to prescribe activities well suited to the patient's body build. Ideally the physiotherapist should seek to develop the patient's existing skills. Account should also be taken of equipment available to the patient, financial resources available for the purchase of other items that are still needed, and the opportunity costs such as travel that are involved in undertaking different modes of exercise.[132]

Musculoskeletal injuries can have a negative effect on motivation. Thus it is important to recognize that some modes of exercise are more likely to cause injury than others. For example, skipping is reputed to be worse than jogging,[18] which in turn is worse than fast walking. Aerobic dance also has à bad reputation as a result of a combination of poor program design, improper footwear, and hard floor surfaces.[43] The risk of injury increases with the intensity of exercise, the severity of any competition, and the volume of activity that is undertaken per week.[105]

CURRENT LEVELS OF FITNESS AND TRAINING RESPONSES

The potential to develop human physical condition is not limitless. Indeed, since the selection and training of male international athletes are now almost as rigorous as possible, highly characteristic sport-specific averages for variables such as maximal oxygen intake are emerging.[126] Attempts at further training are not going to yield any larger dividends for these athletes or, in a lesser sense, for the average patient. Whether cardiorespiratory function[125] or muscle strength[60] is being trained, the response to a given bout of training become progressively smaller as that person's potential is approached.

Not surprisingly, current fitness appears as an important variable in analyses of factors determining the response to either cardiorespiratory or muscular training.[123] Indeed, the prescription is normally related to the person's condition by expressing the recommended exercise as a percentage of aerobic power in cardiorespiratory training and as a fraction of maximal voluntary contraction in the various types of muscular training.

When advising exercise programs for an older person, it is important that both initial fitness and the intensity of training be gauged relative to standards of fitness for average patients of similar age. If standards of aerobic power or muscular strength are applied without reference to age, the elderly individual may be gauged as excessively unfit or may be asked to perform an exercise program of excessive intensity.

The potential to develop a training response is much greater in the person who is unfit or has been confined to bed. Nevertheless, it must be stressed that practical constraints often limit the ability of the sedentary person to realize this training potential. For example, if the muscles are weak or the patient is obese, or both, attempts at vigorous training may quickly lead to musculoskeletal problems ranging from muscle pulls to stress fractures. Further problems in the obese person result from an accumulation of heat, if training is attempted in a warm climate. Thus a frail or an obese individual needs to commence training at a much lower percentage of maximal oxygen intake than that appropriate for a person who begins training in moderate physical condition. Moreover, although the potential benefits of a sustained training session of 30 to 60 minutes are greater than for shorter sessions, the person who is unfit may find it necessary to break the bouts of exercise into segments of 10 to 15 minutes during the first few weeks of training.

A second practical issue in the development of a training response is that as training develops physical condition, a fixed prescription demands a lower relative intensity of effort from the patient and is thus ineffective in yielding further improvements in condition. If a person is to train to the ceiling of his or her potential, the prescription must be upgraded whenever the exercise heart rate falls consistently below the intended value, provided that the patient is filling the prescription comfortably, without symptoms of distress.[75]

Even when an exercise prescription is progressively increased, the patient eventually approaches an asymptote of physical condition. From the viewpoint of motivation the diminution of training response at this stage is important. During the first few weeks of conditioning, gains in performance during daily life and improvements in test score are readily appreciated by the participant, and such dividends provide a major encouragement to continued exercise. When ever-increasing training efforts apparently lead to nothing but discouraging muscle soreness and fatigue, however, the patient may become discouraged and cease exercising. Thus it is important that the physician warn the patient, while the performance is still improving, that a plateau of physical performance will eventually be reached but that a continuation of activity at this stage is vital to the maintenance of physical condition.

As performance begins to peak, one way of demonstrating continuing gains to the patient is to describe gains in endurance rather than improved speeds of performance. A second way of maximizing effects and thus encouraging the patient is to present changes as a slowing of the rate of aging. *If a patient has participated faithfully in a long-term training program, exercise capacity can be described truthfully as matching that of a sedentary individual 10 or 20 years younger, a benefit that can be claimed for few other types of therapy.*

PSYCHOLOGIC REACTIONS TO TRAINING

Psychologic reactions to training vary with the initial mental health of the patients. If the exerciser initially has a well-balanced personality, little change of mood is likely, despite prolonged, repeated bouts of exercise. However, if the patient is initially anxious or depressed (for instance, as a consequence of a life-threatening illness such as an acute myocardial infarction), the mood is often improved by participation in a program of endurance training.[76]

Immediate Psychologic Reactions to Exercise

The immediate psychologic response to a vigorous session of exercise is generally an increase in arousal.[89,162] If the exerciser initially feels bored or depressed, training may provide temporary relief of such sensations; indeed, many patients comment that they exercise to "feel better."[130] On the other hand, if a patient initially has pathologic anxiety or is overaroused, the acute effect of training may be to increase such anxiety.

Whether exercise serves to increase or to decrease an anxiety depends in part on the ambience of the exercise session and on the ability of the participant to meet the expectations of the physiotherapist. Success creates a helpful feeling of self-efficacy, but failure has a negative impact both on mood and on compliance with the prescribed activity. If relaxation is an important goal, a country walk of moderate intensity may be a much more effective prescription than a vigorous, overly competitive game of squash with an employer.[132] Those interested in the psychologic benefits of exercise are increasingly commending moderate, prolonged activity rather than brief sessions of all-out competitive effort.

If vigorous exercise is undertaken immediately before retiring for the evening, the immediate arousing effect may cause a loss of sleep.[154] On the other hand, when moderate activity is taken earlier in the evening, it facilitates sleep, enhancing the important slow-wave component of the electroencephalogram.[33]

Habituation

The earliest central nervous system adaptations to repeated bouts of exercise occur in the prefrontal cortex.[46] During the first few days the body becomes "habituated" or accustomed to a particular exercise situation, so the task gradually induces less arousal.[124] There is a parallel attenuation in such physiologic markers of arousal as the increment of heart rate and the rise in blood pressure observed at a given intensity of effort. Such changes are similar to the responses that might be anticipated with cardiorespiratory training and are often wrongly regarded as evidence of cardiovascular conditioning.

Individuals differ in the initial level of arousal and the rate of habituation. Patients who have consulted a physician concerning a major clinical disorder are particularly likely to be anxious at their first visit, showing an exaggerated response to a first bout of laboratory exercise. The same individuals show a correspondingly large attenuation of response as they become habituated to the doctor, the environment of the test laboratory, and the functional consequences of their clinical problem.

Test Learning

Learning of a given type of exercise leads to a transfer of movement control from the motor cortex to the cerebellum. In the course of this process, performance of the task becomes mechanically more efficient. Inevitably a corresponding decrease in cardiorespiratory demand occurs with the greater mechanical efficiency. The heart rate is thus reduced at any given intensity of submaximal effort, and although there has been no cardiovascular training response, a higher peak performance is possible. Task learning is particularly likely in elderly persons. Older patients often are poorly coordinated, have a bad posture, and adopt inefficient patterns of movement when they first perform a task as simple as walking on a treadmill or riding on a cycle ergometer. Further, they may show substantial gains in mechanical efficiency and thus functional capacity as faulty movement patterns are corrected by the physiotherapist.

Although not normally considered a form of training, the development of mechanically efficient movement patterns can make an important contribution to the quality of life for older patients. For example, a person with advanced chronic obstructive pulmonary disease may have extensive destruction of lung tissue. No physiotherapy program can regenerate the damaged alveolar tissue. If the mechanical efficiency of cycling can be increased from 20% to 23%, however, the patient is immediately able to work at a rate 15% greater than previously.

SUMMARY

Intensity, duration, frequency, and mode of exercise together with current fitness levels all influence both acute responses to exercise and the response to a training program. Whether training the cardiovascular system or the muscles, the fastest changes are induced by a high intensity of exercise relative to the individual's initial physical condition. However, weakness after illness, increasing age, and the onset of various diseases and disorders often preclude the use of a heavy overload in clinical situations. Thus it is important to recognize that more moderate intensities of exercise can lead to a gradual improvement in physical condition in those who begin training from a low level of fitness, provided that the training sessions are prolonged or frequent, or both. A program that exercises most of the large muscles and joints has the advantage that gains can be generalized to other types of physical activity. If a body part has been immobilized after surgery or there is a need to prepare a patient for return to a specific, heavy occupational task, however, more localized types of training may also be helpful.

REFERENCES

1. American College of Sports Medicine: *Guidelines for graded exercise testing and prescription,* ed 3, Philadelphia, 1986, Lea & Febiger.
2. Andersen KL et al: *Fundamentals of exercise testing,* Geneva, 1971, World Health Organization.
3. Anderson T, Kerney JT: Effects of three resistance training programs on muscular strength and absolute and relative endurance, *Res Q* 53:1, 1982.
4. Armstrong RB: Muscle damage and endurance events, *Sports Med* 3:370, 1986.
5. Åstrand I et al: Intermittent muscular work, *Acta Physiol Scand* 48:448, 1960.
6. Åstrand PO et al: Cardiac output during submaximal and maximal work, *J Appl Physiol* 19:268, 1964.

7. Auble TE, Schwartz L, Robertson J: Aerobic requirements for moving handweights through various ranges of motion while walking, *Phys Sportsmed* 15(6):133, 1987.

8. Banister EW: Energetics of muscular contraction. In Shephard RJ, editor: *Frontiers of fitness,* Springfield, Ill, 1971, Charles C Thomas.

9. Bartels R et al: American Association for Health, Physical Education and Recreation Convention (abstracts). (Cited in reference 104.)

10. Bassey EJ, et al: An unsupervised ''aerobics'' physical training programme in middle-aged factory workers: feasibility, validation and response, *Eur J Appl Physiol* 52:120, 1983.

11. Beaudet SM: Comparison of swimming with running as training stimuli, *Ergonomics* 27:955, 1984.

12. Besdine RW, Harris TB: Alteration in body temperature (hypothermia and hyperthermia). In Andres R, Bierman EL, Hazzard WR, editors: *Principles of geriatric medicine* New York, 1985, McGraw Hill.

13. Birk TJ, Birk CA: Use of ratings of perceived exertion for exercise prescription, *Sports Med* 4:1, 1987.

14. Boone T, Edwards CA: Effect of carotid palpation on post-exercise heart rate: validity of palpation recovery technique to estimate actual exercise heart rate, *Ann Sports Med* 4:29, 1988.

15. Booth FW, Watson PA: Control of adaptations in protein levels in response to exercise, *Fed Proc* 44:2293, 1985.

16. Borg G: The perception of physical performance. In Shephard RJ, editor: *Frontiers of fitness,* Springfield, Ill, 1971, Charles C Thomas.

17. Bouchard C et al: Minimalbelastungen zur Pravention kardiovaskularer Erkrankungen, *Sportarzt und Sportmedizin* 7:348, 1966.

18. Buyze MT et al: Comparative training responses to rope skipping and jogging, *Phys Sportsmed* 14(11):65, 1986.

19. Caspersen CJ, Powell KE, Christenson GM: Physical activity, exercise, and physical fitness: definitions and distinctions for health-related research, *Public Health Rep* 100:126, 1985.

20. Chad KE, Wenger HA: The effects of exercise duration on the exercise and post-exercise oxygen consumption, *Can J Sport Sci* 13:204, 1989.

21. Chow RJ, Wilmore JH: The regulation of exercise intensity by ratings of perceived exertion, *J Cardiac Rehab* 4:382, 1984.

22. Chow RK et al: The effect of exercise on bone mass of osteoporotic patients on fluoride treatment, *Clin Invest Med* 10(2):59, 1987.

23. Claremont AD, Hall SJ: Effects of extremity loading upon energy expenditures and running mechanics, *Med Sci Sports Exerc* 20:167, 1988.

24. Clausen JP: Effects of physical training on cardiovascular adjustments to exercise in man, *Physiol Rev* 57:779, 1977.

25. Cox ML, Bennett JB, Dudley GA: Exercise training-induced alterations of cardiac morphology, *J Appl Physiol* 61:926, 1986.

26. Cummins P et al: Comparison of serum cardiac specific troponin-I with creatine kinase, creatine kinase MB isoenzyme, tropomyosin, myoglobin and C-reactive protein release in marathon runners: cardiac or skeletal muscle trauma? *Eur J Clin Invest* 17:317, 1987.

27. Daub WD et al: Cross-adaptive responses to different forms of leg training: skeletal muscle biochemistry and histochemistry, *Can J Physiol* 60:628, 1982.

28. Daub WD et al: Specificity of physiological adaptations resulting from ice-hockey training, *Med Sci Sports Exerc* 15:290, 1983.

29. Davies CTM, Knibbs AV: The training stimulus: the effects of intensity, duration and frequency of effort on maximum aerobic power output, *Int Z Angew Physiol* 29:299, 1971.

30. Davies CTM, Starkie DW: The pressor response to voluntary and electrically evoked isometric contractions in man, *Eur J Appl Physiol* 53:359, 1985.

31. di Prampero PE: Anaerobic capacity and power. In Shephard RJ, editor: *Frontiers of fitness,* Springfield, Ill, 1971, Charles C Thomas.

32. Donselaar Y et al: Fibre sizes and histochemical staining characteristics in normal and chronically stimulated motoneurons of the cat's spinal cord, *J Physiol* (*Lond*) 382:237, 1987.

33. Driver HS et al: Submaximal exercise effects on sleep patterns in young women before and after an aerobic training programme, *Acta Physiol Scand* 133 (suppl 574):8, 1988.

34. Dudley GA, Fleck SJ: Strength training and endurance training, *Sports Med* 4:79, 1987.

35. Durnin JVGA, Brockway JM, Whitcher HW: Effects of a short period of training of varying severity on some measurements of physical fitness, *J Appl Physiol* 15:161, 1960.

36. Edwards RHT et al: Cardio-respiratory and metabolic costs of continuous and intermittent exercise in man, *J Physiol* 234:481, 1968.

37. Ekblom B, Hermansen L: Cardiac output in athletes, *J Appl Physiol* 25:619, 1968.

38. Faria IE: Cardiovascular responses to exercise as influenced by training of various intensities, *Res Q* 41:44, 1970.

39. Fernhall B, Kohrt W: The effect of training specificity on maximal and submaximal physiological responses to treadmill and bicycle ergometry, *Med Sci Sports Exerc* 17:225, 1985.

40. Friden J: Muscle soreness after exercise: implications of morphological changes, *Int J Sports Med* 5:57, 1984.

41. Fried T, Shephard RJ: Assessment of a lower extremity training programme, *Can Med Assoc J* 103:260, 1970.

42. Frisk-Holmberg M et al: Muscle fibre composition in relation to blood pressure response to isometric exercise in normotensive and hypertensive subjects, *Acta Med Scand* 213:21, 1983.

43. Garrick JG, Gillien DM, Whiteside P: The epidemiology of aerobic dance injuries, *Am J Sports Med* 14:67, 1986.

44. Gergley T et al: Specificity of arm training on aerobic power during swimming and running, *Med Sci Sports Exerc* 16:125, 1984.

45. Gettman LR, Culter LA, Strathman TA: Physiologic changes after 20 weeks of isotonic vs isokinetic circuit training, *J Sports Med Phys Fitness* 20:265, 1980.

46. Glaser EM: *The physiological basis of habituation,* London, 1966, Oxford University.

47. Gledhill N, Eynon RB: The intensity of training. In Taylor AW, editor: *Training: scientific basis and application,* Springfield, Ill, 1972, Charles C Thomas.

48. Godin G, Shephard RJ: Use of attitude-behaviour models in health promotion, *Sports Med* 10:103, 1990.

49. Going SB, Ball TE, Massey BM: Cardiovascular response in men and women to maximum voluntary isometric contractions by three muscle groups, *Med Sci Sports Exerc* 15:163(abstract), 1983.

50. Gollnick PD, Hermansen L: Biochemical adaptations to exercise: Anaerobic metabolism, *Exerc Sport Sci Rev* 1:1, 1983.

51. Gonyea W, Ericson GC, Bonde-Peterson F: Skeletal muscle fiber splitting induced by weight-lifting exercise in cats, *Acta Physiol Scand* 99:105, 1977.

52. Graves JE et al: The effect of hand-held weights on the physiological responses to walking exercise, *Med Sci Sports Exerc* 19:260, 1987.

53. Grimby G: Progressive resistance exercises for injury rehabilitation: special emphasis upon isokinetic training, *Sports Med* 2:309, 1985.

54. Grogan JW, Kelly JM: Metabolic responses of upper body training on arm, leg and combined arm-leg exercise, *Med Sci Sports Exerc* 17:268, 1985.

55. Hagberg JM, Ehsani AA, Holloszy JO: Effect of 12 months of intense exercise on stroke volume in patients with coronary artery disease, *Circulation* 67:1194, 1983.

56. Hakkinen K, Komi PV: Training-induced changes in neuromuscular performance under voluntary and reflex conditions, *Eur J Appl Physiol* 55:147, 1986.

57. Hamrell BB, Hultgren PB: Sarcomere shortening in pressure load hypertrophy, *Fed Proc* 45:2591, 1986.

58. Hansen JW: Effect of dynamic training on the isometric endurance of the elbow flexors, *Int Z Angew Physiol* 23:367, 1967.

59. Heinritze J et al: Effects of training at and above the lactate threshold on the lactate threshold and maximal oxygen uptake, *Eur J Appl Physiol* 54:84, 1985.

60. Hettinger T: *Physiology of strength,* Springfield, Ill, 1961, Charles C Thomas.

61. Hickson RC, Rosenkoetter MA: Separate turnover of cyctochrome c and myoglobin in the red types of skeletal muscle, *Am J Physiol* 241:C140, 1981.

62. Hickson RC et al: Time course of the adaptive responses of aerobic power and heart rate to training, *Med Sci Sport Exerc* 13:17, 1981.

63. Hickson RC et al: Reduced training duration effects on aerobic power, endurance and cardiac growth, *J Appl Physiol* 53:225, 1982.

64. Hill JS, Wearing GA, Eynon RB: Effect of frequency of exercise on adult fitness, *Med Sci Sports* 3:k, 1971.

65. Ho KW et al: Differential effects of running and weightlifting on the rat coronary arterial tree, *Med Sci Sports Exerc* 15:472, 1983.

66. Holloszy JO, Booth FW: Biochemical adaptations to endurance exercise in muscle, *Ann Rev Physiol* 38:273, 1976.

67. Holmgren A: Cardio-respiratory determinants of cardiovascular fitness, *Can Med Assoc J* 96:697, 1967.

68. Howald H: Training induced morphological and functional changes in skeletal muscle, *Int J Sports Med* 3:1, 1982.

69. Kanehisa H, Miyashita M: Specificity of velocity in strength training, *Eur J Appl Physiol* 52:104, 1983.

70. Karvonen MJ, Kentala E, Mustala O: The effects of training on heart rate: a "longitudinal" study, *Ann Med Exp Fenn* 35:307, 1957.

71. Katz A et al: Oxygen tension in antecubital vein blood of trained and untrained males after maximal leg exercise, *Can J Appl Sport Sci* 9:11, 1984.

72. Kavanagh T: *Heart attack? counter attack!* Toronto, 1976, Van Nostrand Reinhold.

73. Kavanagh T: *The healthy heart programme,* Toronto, 1980, Van Nostrand Reinhold.

74. Kavanagh T: Does exercise training improve coronary collateralization? a new look at an old belief, *Phys Sportsmed* 17(1):96, 1988.

75. Kavanagh T, Shephard RJ: Exercise for post-coronary patients: an assessment of infrequent supervision, *Arch Phys Med Rehab* 61(3):114, 1980.

76. Kavanagh T et al: Depression following myocardial infarction: the effects of distance running, *Ann NY Acad Sci* 301:1029, 1977.

77. Kavanagh T et al: Influence of exercise and lifestyle variables upon high density lipoprotein cholesterol after myocardial infarction, *Arteriosclerosis* 3:249, 1983.

78. Keast D, Cameron K, Morton AR: Exercise and the immune response, *Sports Med* 5:248, 1988.

79. Kenyon GS: Six scales for assessing attitudes towards physical activity, *Res Q* 39:566, 1968.

80. Kohl HW et al: A mail survey of physical activity habits as related to measured physical fitness, *Am J Epidemiol* 127:1228, 1988.

81. Kuipers H, Keizer HA: Over-training in elite athletes: review and directions for the future, *Sports Med* 6:79, 1988.

82. Landry F, Bouchard C, Dumesnil J: Cardiac dimension changes with endurance training: indications of a genotype dependency, *JAMA* 254:77, 1985.

83. Lawrence G: *Aqua-fitness for women,* Toronto, 1981, Personal Library.

84. Lind AR, McNicol GW: Muscular factors which determine the cardiovascular responses to sustained rhythmic exercise, *Can Med Assoc J* 96:706, 1967.

85. Linden RJ, Mary DASG, Winter C: The frequency of exercise required for the maintenance of cardiorespiratory fitness, *J Physiol* 357:100P, 1984.

86. Loftin M et al: Effect of arm training on central and peripheral circulatory function, *Med Sci Sports Exerc* 20:136, 1988.

87. Lortie G et al: Familial similarity in aerobic power, *Hum Biol* 54:801, 1982.

88. MacDougall JD et al: Mitochondrial volume density in human skeletal muscle following resistance training, *Med Sci Sports* 11:164, 1979.

89. Martens R: Arousal and motor performance, *Exerc Sport Sci Rev* 2:155, 1974.

90. Matsuda JJ, Vailas AC: The selective response of connective tissue to moderate exercise, *Med Sci Sports Exerc* 16:120, 1984.

91. McNamara PS, Otto RM, Smith TK: The acute response of simulated bicycle and rowing exercise on the elderly population, *Med Sci Sports Exerc* 17:266(abstract), 1985.

92. Milburn S, Butts NK: A comparison of the training responses to aerobic dance and jogging in college females, *Med Sci Sports Exerc* 15:510, 1983.

93. Montoye HJ: *Physical activity and health: an epidemiological study of an entire community,* Englewood Cliffs, NJ, 1975, Prentice Hall.

94. Noakes TD, Higginson L, Opie LH: Physical training increases ventricular fibrillation threshold of isolated rat hearts during normoxia, hypoxia and regional ischemia, *Circulation* 67:24, 1983.

95. Noble BJ et al: Stress response to high-intensity circuit weight training in experienced weight trainers, *Med Sci Sports Exerc* 16:146, 1984.

96. Oja P: Comparison of the physiological effects of different forms of physical activity, *Finn Sports Exerc Med* 2:62, 1983.

97. Oja P et al: Effects of running and cross-country skiing on cardio-respiratory responses to exercise, *Med Sci Sports Exerc* 17:270, 1985.

98. Parker JO, DiGiorgi S, West RO: A hemodynamic study of acute coronary insufficiency precipitated by exercise: with observations on the effects of nitroglycerin, *Am J Cardiol* 17:470, 1966.

99. Paterson DH et al: Effects of physical training upon cardiovascular function following myocardial infarction, *J Appl Physiol* 47:482, 1979.

100. Pels AE et al: Effects of leg press training on cycling, leg press and running peak cardiorespiratory measures, *Med Sci Sports Exerc* 19:66, 1987.

101. Pérusse L, LeBlanc C, Bouchard C: Inter-generation transmission of physical fitness in the Canadian population, *Can J Sport Sci* 13:8, 1988.

102. Pérusse L et al: Genetic and environmental sources of variation in physical fitness, *Ann Hum Biol* 14:425, 1988.

103. Pirnay F et al: Bone mineral content and physical activity, *Int J Sports Med* 8:331, 1987.

104. Pollock M: The quantification of endurance training programs, *Exerc Sport Sci Rev* 1:155, 1973.

105. Pollock ML: How much exercise is enough? *Phys Sportsmed* 6(6):50, 1979.

106. Pollock ML et al: Frequency of training as a determinant for improvement in cardiovascular function and body composition of middle-aged men, *Arch Phys Med Rehab* 56:141, 1975.

107. Porcari J et al: Is fast walking an adequate aerobic training stimulus for 30- to 69-year-old men and women? *Phys Sportsmed* 15(2):119, 1987.

108. Rogers MA et al: Effect of 6d of exercise training on responses to maximal and submaximal exercise in middle-aged men, *Med Sci Sports Exerc* 20:260, 1988.

109. Rösler K et al: Transfer effects in endurance exercise: adaptations in trained and untrained muscles, *Eur J Appl Physiol* 54:355, 1985.

110. Rösler K et al: Specificity of leg power changes to velocities used in bicycle endurance training, *J Appl Physiol* 61:30, 1986.

111. Rowell LB: Human cardiovascular adjustments to exercise and thermal stress, *Physiol Rev* 54:75, 1974.

112. Rowell LB: Cardiovascular adjustments to thermal stress. In American Physiological Society: *Handbook of physiology,* vol 27, Washington, DC, 1985, The Society.

113. Rubal BJ, Al Muhailani AR, Rosentswieg J: Effects of physical conditioning on the heart size and wall thickness of college women, *Med Sci Sports Exerc* 19:423, 1987.

114. Rusko H, Bosco C: Metabolic responses of endurance athletes to training with added load, *Eur J Appl Physiol* 56:412, 1987.

115. Rusko H, Rahkila P: Effect of training on aerobic capacity of female athletes differing in muscle fibre composition, *J Sports Sci* 1:185, 1983.

116. Saltin B: Oxygen transport in the circulatory system during exercise in man. In Keul J, editor: *Limiting factors of physical performance,* Stuttgart, 1973, G. Thieme.

117. Saltin B, Hermansen L: Glycogen stores and prolonged severe exercise, In Blix G, editor: *Nutrition and physical activity,* Uppsala, 1967, Almqvist and Wiksell.

118. Saltin B et al: Response to exercise after bedrest and after training, *Am Heart Assoc Monogr* 23:1, 1968.

119. Saltin B et al: Physical training in sedentary middle-aged and older men. II. Oxygen uptake, heart rate and blood lactate concentration at submaximal and maximal exercise, *Scand J Clin Lab Invest* 24:323, 1969.

120. Sexton WL, Korthuis RJ, Laughlin MH: High-intensity exercise training increases vascular transport capacity of rat hind quarters, *Am J Physiol* 254:H274, 1988.

121. Sharkey BJ: Intensity and duration of training and the development of cardio-respiratory endurance, *Med Sci Sports* 2:197, 1970.

122. Sharkey BJ, Holleman JP: Cardio-respiratory adaptations to training at specified intensities, *Res Q* 38:698, 1967.

123. Shephard RJ: Intensity, duration and frequency of exercise as determinants of the response to a training regime, *Int Z Angew Physiol* 26:272, 1968.

124. Shephard RJ: Learning, habituation and training, *Int Z Angew Physiol* 28:38, 1969.

125. Shephard RJ: *Endurance fitness,* ed 2, Toronto, 1977, University of Toronto.

126. Shephard RJ: *Human physiological work capacity,* London, 1978, Cambridge University.

127. Shephard RJ: *Ischemic heart disease and exercise,* London, 1981, Croom Helm.

128. Shephard RJ: *Physiology and biochemistry of exercise,* New York, 1982, Praeger.

129. Shephard RJ: *Biochemistry of exercise,* Springfield, Ill, 1983, Charles C Thomas.

130. Shephard RJ: Physical activity and the healthy mind, *Can Med Assoc J* 128:525, 1983.

131. Shephard RJ: Physical activity for the senior: a role for pool exercises? *CAHPER J* 50(6):2, 20, 1985.

132. Shephard RJ: *Economic benefits of enhanced fitness,* Champaign, Ill, 1986, Human Kinetics.

133. Shephard RJ: Physical activity and aging, London, 1987, Croom Helm.

134. Shephard RJ: *The determination of body composition in biological anthropology,* London, 1989, Cambridge University.

135. Shephard RJ, Sidney KH: Effects of physical exercise on plasma growth hormone and cortisol levels in human subjects, *Exerc Sport Sci Rev* 3:1, 1975.

136. Shephard RJ et al: Muscle mass as a factor limiting physical work, *J Appl Physiol* 64:1472, 1988.

137. Sidney KH, Shephard RJ: Frequency and intensity of training for elderly subjects, *Med Sci Sports Exerc* 10:125, 1978.

138. Sidney KH, Shephard RJ, Harrison J: Endurance training and body composition of the elderly, *Am J Clin Nutr* 30:326, 1978.

139. Simmons R, Shephard RJ: Effects of physical conditioning upon the central and peripheral circulatory responses to arm work, *Int Z Angew Physiol* 30:73, 1971.

140. Simmons R, Shephard RJ: Measurement of cardiac output in maximum exercise: application of an acetylene rebreathing method to arm and leg exercise, *Int Z Angew Physiol* 29:159, 1971.

141. Simoneau JA et al: Human skeletal muscle fiber type alteration with high-intensity intermittent training, *Eur J Appl Physiol* 54:250, 1985.

142. Smith DA, O'Donnell TV: The time course during 36 weeks' endurance training of changes in VO_2 max and anaerobic threshold as determined with a new computerized method, *Clin Sci* 67:229, 1984.

143. Stillman RJ et al: Physical activity and bone mineral content in women aged 30 to 85 years, *Med Sci Sports Exerc* 18:576, 1986.

144. Tamaki N: Effect of endurance training on muscle fiber type, composition and capillary supply in rat diaphragm, *Eur J Appl Physiol* 56:127, 1987.

145. Tanaka K et al: Transient responses in cardiac function below, at and above anaerobic threshold, *Eur J Appl Physiol* 55:356, 1986.

146. Taylor HL et al: The effect of bed rest on cardiovascular function and work performance, *J Appl Physiol* 2:223, 1949.

147. Taylor NAS, Wilkinson JG: Exercise-induced skeletal muscle growth: hypertrophy or hyperplasia? *Sports Med* 3:190, 1986.

148. Tesch P, Karlsson J, Sjödin B: Muscle fiber type distribution in trained and untrained muscles of athletes. In Komi PV, editor: *Exercise and sport biology,* Champaign, Ill, 1982, Human Kinetics.

149. Thomas DP: Effects of acute and chronic exercise on myocardial ultrastructure, *Med Sci Sports Exerc* 17:546, 1985.

150. Thorstensson A: Muscle strength, fibre types and enzyme activities in man, *Acta Physiol Scand Suppl* 443:1, 1976.

151. Turto H, Lindy S, Haline J: Protocollagen proline hydroxylase activity in work-induced hypertrophy of rat muscle, *Am J Physiol* 226:63, 1974.

152. Vandenburgh HH: Motion into mass: how does tension stimulate muscle growth? *Med Sci Sports Exerc* 19:S142, 1987.

153. Von Euler US: Sympatho-adrenal activity in physical exercise, *Med Sci Sport* 6:165, 1974.

154. Vuori I et al: Epidemiology of exercise effects on sleep, *Acta Physiol Scand* 133(suppl 574):3, 1988.

155. Wenger HA, Bell GJ: The interactions of intensity, frequency and duration of exercise training in altering cardiorespiratory fitness, *Sports Medicine* 3:346, 1986.

156. Wenger HA, MacNab RBJ: Total work intensity and duration of a training program as determinants of endurance fitness. In Taylor AW, editor: *Application of science and medicine to sport,* Springfield, Ill, 1972, Charles C Thomas.

157. White JR: Changes following ten weeks of exercise using a minitrampoline in overweight women, *Med Sci Sports* 12:103, 1980.

158. Williams JA et al: The effect of long-distance running upon appendicular bone mineral content, *Med Sci Sports Exerc* 16:223, 1984.

159. Williams PT et al: The effects of running mileage and duration on plasma lipoprotein levels, *J Am Med Assoc* 247:2672, 1982.

160. Wilmore JH et al: Physiological alterations consequent to 20-week conditioning programs of bicycling, tennis and jogging, *Med Sci Sports* 12:1, 1980.

161. Wilt F: Training for competitive running. In Falls H, editor: *Exercise physiology,* New York, 1968, Academic.

162. Yerkes RM, Dodson JD: The relation of strength of stimulus to rapidity of habit formation, *J Comp Neurol Psychol* 18:459, 1908.

STUDY QUESTIONS

- Describe the factors that must be considered when prescribing an exercise program.
- Describe differences in mode and intensity of exercise when training the cardiorespiratory system for endurance and for skeletal muscle development.
- Relate the overload principle and the concept of threshold of exercise intensity for training of cardiorespiratory endurance and skeletal muscle development.
- Describe why frequency and duration of exercise might vary in exercise program prescriptions for a fit individual and for a patient with poor endurance and muscle weakness.
- Describe potential psychologic benefits and risks that may occur as results of exercise training.

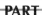

EXERCISE AND METABOLISM

■ *KEEP IN MIND WHILE YOU READ . . . In Chapter 2 Scott Hasson describes transportation, storage, and utilization of fuel sources in normal metabolism at rest and during exercise and the impact of exercise training on these processes. In addition, possible causes of fatigue at varying intensities of exercise are explored, and measurement techniques for assessment of aerobic and anaerobic metabolism are described. Acute exercise tolerance and trainability in patients with metabolic disorders, including diabetes and obesity, are described in Chapter 3. Please focus on indications and contraindications for exercise in these patients.* ■

CHAPTER 2

METABOLIC RESPONSES DURING EXERCISE AND NORMAL EFFECTS OF TRAINING

Scott M. Hasson

BIOCHEMICAL ENERGETICS

Utilization of energy is essential for all cellular activity and thus for life itself. To perform energy consuming-activities such as mechanical movement, synthesis of cellular compounds, creation of concentration gradients, and storage of fuels energy must be available or produced. To contract muscles adenosine triphosphate (ATP) must be available to the cell. Adenosine triphosphate is the "currency" that most enzymes recognize and utilize to initiate and sustain activity. Inherent or immediate muscle ATP stores are small, and it is estimated that these immediate stores normally can sustain maximal muscle activity for only a few seconds.[32] The breakdown or hydrolysis of ATP is illustrated in Fig. 2-1. Hydrolysis of ATP to adenosine diphosphate (ADP) and ADP to adenosine monophosphate (AMP) results in the liberation of relatively large amounts of free energy that allows for enzymatic reactions to occur. Adenosine triphosphate is not the only nucleotide that can be hydrolyzed to give free energy. Guanosine triphosphate (GTP), cytidine triphosphate (CTP), and uridine triphosphate (UTP) all have specific, albeit small, roles in providing energy for specific enzyme reactions. Adenosine triphosphate, however, is the most prevalent energy-rich nucleotide and is recognized as the critical energy link for functioning enzymes that run the human organism.

An intermediate high-energy phosphate compound (phosphocreatine [PCr]) allows a muscle to extend the duration of maximal contraction for an additional 10 to 20 seconds before ATP production is dominated by oxidation of endogenous and exogenous fuel sources.[50,51] Phosphocreatine maintains a relatively constant concentration of ATP until a muscle nears exhaustion. The process of PCr breakdown, which produces more ATP, is illustrated in Fig. 2-2. Once the muscle activity has ceased, the process is reversed and ATP is hydrolyzed to rebuild the muscle PCr stores (Fig. 2-2).

Of the many dietary requirements essential for adequate nutrition, only proteins, carbohydrates, and fats are able to provide energy for muscular contractions. Proteins are not considered a primary fuel source at rest or during exercise at any intensity of work load unless the individual's nutritional status is thoroughly impaired.[38] Thus a person's ATP production is primarily achieved by means of the oxidation of the two remaining major fuels, carbohydrate and fat. Early pioneering work of Krogh

1. $ATP + H_2O \longrightarrow ADP + P_i +$ **Energy**

2. $ADP + H_2O \longrightarrow AMP + P_i +$ **Energy**

Fig. 2-1 Reactions during hydrolysis of adenosine triphosphate. P_i, Inorganic phosphate.

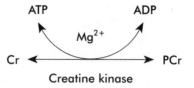

Fig. 2-2 Phosphocreatine (PCr) used to produce adenosine triphosphate (ATP). *ADP,* Adenosine diphosphate; *Cr,* creatine; *Mg,* magnesium.

and Lindhard[38] and Christensen and Hansen[14] clearly established that both fats and carbohydrates are metabolized during exercise. The relative contributions of each fuel type to overall energy production is influenced by such factors as physical condition and training practices,[26,27] nutritional state and dietary practices,[58] and intensity and duration of the exercise performed.[10,14]

Transport and storage of fuel sources, utilization of fuel sources, hormonal control of fuel storage and utilization, fuel source selection during exercise and possible causes of fatigue, effect of chronic exercise training on fuel storage, use, and regulation, and measurement techniques for assessing aerobic metabolism and anaerobic power are further explored in this chapter.

TRANSPORT AND STORAGE OF FUEL SOURCES
Endogenous and Exogenous Fuel Sources

Endogenous fuel sources are those that are already within the body. The two major endogenous fuel sources are fats and glycogen. Fat is a fuel deposited for long-term storage. Most fat is stored in adipose tissue around organs and in well-defined subcutaneous areas. However, a small portion of fat is also stored within the skeletal muscle. Glycogen is a fuel deposited for short-term storage. Glycogen is primarily stored within the liver and the skeletal muscle. Glycogen is a complex compound made up of many glucose molecules that have been chained together.

Exogenous fuels are those transported via the circulation to metabolically active tissues. The major exogenous fuel sources are, like endogenous fuel sources, free fatty acids and glucose. The stored fat in adipose tissue is hydrolyzed so that it can be mobilized for use as fuel. Hydrolysis of fat results in isolation of triglycerides (three chains of

fatty acids held together by a glycerol molecule). Triglycerides are further hydrolized, yielding blood-borne free fatty acids (FFAs). Glycerol cannot be further used in the adipose tissue and is released into the circulation. Glycerol is taken up by the liver and used as a fuel source or converted into glucose or fatty acid. Glucose can come directly from the diet, when foods rich in carbohydrates are eaten, or from the liver glycogen stores. Liver glycogen can be catalyzed, resulting in a stripping of glucose molecules from the multichained glycogen stores. The result of liver glycogenolysis is the release of glucose into the circulatory system.

Glucose Transportation and Storage

Glucose is stored in the form of multiple polymers that are called *glycogen* in animals and *starch* in plants. Glucose is obtained from consumption of dietary carbohydrates. Carbohydrates are composed mainly of polysaccharides (starch) but also include glycogen and disaccharides. Polysaccharides (complex sugars) come from plant matter; glycogen is of animal origin. The disaccharides are sucrose and lactose. Sucrose is also known as "table sugar" and contains one molecule of glucose bound to one molecule of fructose. Lactose, commonly called "milk sugar," contains one molecule of glucose and one molecule of galactose. So that absorption can take place from the small intestine, all carbohydrates are converted to monosaccharides (glucose, fructose and galactose), which are six-carbon compounds. Carbohydrates are reduced to monosaccharides by enzymes from the salivary gland and the pancreas. The most common

Table 2-1 Transport of fats by plasma lipoproteins

Lipoprotein	Composition (%)				Function
	Fat	Phospholipid	Cholesterol	Protein	
Chylomicron	87	8	3	2	Transports triglyceride from small bowel to adipocyte
VLDL	55	20	15	10	Transports triglyceride from liver to adipocyte
LDL	8	24	43	25	Transports cholesterol from small bowel to many sites
HDL	0.6	21	20	55	Transports cholesterol from small bowel to many sites

HDL, High-density lipoprotein; *LDL*, low-density lipoprotein; *VLDL*, very-low-density lipoprotein.

enzyme, amylase, is produced by both organs. Most fructose and galactose molecules are immediately converted to glucose at the small intestine.[12] Once in the circulation, most glucose is transported to the liver (if the individual is at rest).[44] In addition, the central nervous system preferentially uses glucose as a fuel source. The control of glucose uptake by tissues is regulated by insulin. Normal hormonal control at rest and during exercise is discussed later in this chapter.

As mentioned earlier, the two main storage depots for glycogen are the liver and skeletal muscle. The liver has a higher concentration of glycogen (65 g per kg of tissue) than does skeletal muscle (15 g per kg of tissue).[30,52] In total quantity, however, the majority of stored glycogen is within the skeletal muscle because the summed mass of skeletal muscle in the body is much greater than the total mass of the liver. The process of glycogen formation is the same at the liver and at the site of the skeletal muscle. Glycogen is made by the addition of one glucose molecule at a time to an existing glycogen molecule. The enzyme that allows for linear expansion of the glycogen molecule is glycogen synthase. Glycogen formation is not all linear, however, but includes multiple branching, which maximizes storage capacity. Branching within the glycogen molecule takes place because of an enzyme called *glycosyl-4:6-transferase*. The amount of glycogen storage in the liver is most closely related to diet. The amount of muscle glycogen stored depends not only on the diet but also on exercise activity.

Fat Transportation and Storage

Fat is stored by all advanced vertebrates in discrete adipose tissue. Individual adipocytes store large amounts of triglycerides, potentially constituting 90% of the cell mass. For the body to store fat, foods rich in fats or carbohydrates, or both, must be ingested. On ingestion, fatty acids are converted to triglycerides for transport and deposition into the adipocyte. The formation of triglycerides occurs when three molecules of FFA are placed on a glycerol backbone. The triglyceride is then transported to the adipose tissue via the circulation in the form of small droplets coated with cholesterol and phospholipids. These blood-borne droplets are called *lipoproteins* (if small) or *chylomicrons* (if large). Blood lipoproteins differ in the amount of lipid or fat that is transported. The fat content ranges from low (high-density lipoproteins [HDL]) to high (very-low-density lipoproteins [VLDL]). In most cases the transport of dietary FFAs in the form of triglycerides from the small bowel to adipose tissue is by means of chylomicrons (the largest of the lipoprotein molecules). Transport of fats by plasma lipoproteins is summarized in Table 2-1.

Carbohydrates can be stored as fats. The process of glucose conversion to fatty acids occurs primarily in the liver but can be performed directly by the adipocyte. Glucose is transported to the liver from the small bowel via the circulation. The first step in the conversion process is the oxidation of glucose to the two-carbon compound, acetylcoenzyme A (acetyl-CoA).

The terms *oxidation* and *reduction* must be defined here. There are three kinds of oxidation. Originally the term referred to the first kind, which occurs when elemental oxygen is combined to a compound. The second type of oxidation is a dehydrogenation, which is a removal of hydrogen, including both the proton and its associated electron, from a compound. The third type of oxidation occurs when an electron is removed from a compound. A reduction of a compound occurs when an electron is accepted, as in the second and third types of oxidation.

The process of glucose oxidation is described in greater detail later in this chapter. Each glucose molecule is oxidized to form two acetyl-CoA molecules. In the next step a chain of these acetyl-CoA molecules is developed. This occurs initially by attachment of an acetyl-CoA molecule onto an enzyme called fatty acid synthase. Subsequent acetyl-CoA molecules are added until a chain of 16 carbons is formed. All the acetyl-CoA molecules are reduced to acyl coenzyme A (acyl-CoA) molecules. Three fatty acid chains are then attached to a glyceryl backbone and ready for transport to the adipocyte. The triglyceride carrier molecules from the liver are the VLDLs (Table 2-1).

Fat and glycogen storage depends on diet, activity, and normally functioning "metabolic" hormones. Hormonal control of fuel storage is discussed later in this chapter.

UTILIZATION OF FUEL SOURCES
Anaerobic and Aerobic Processes

When ATP and PCr are utilized as the major fuel sources during activity, the activity is considered *anaerobic*. This simply means that fuel sources are not oxidized for ATP production and that an oxygen molecule is not the final acceptor of an electron and a proton (hydrogen ion [H^+]) liberated from the oxidative process.

Recall from the earlier discussion of the terms *oxidation* and *reduction* that "oxidation" could mean that an electron and a proton (H^+) are removed from a molecule and that ultimately some other molecule accepts the electron and is reduced. Many molecules can participate in removal and acceptance of electrons. However, the dominant electron transfer molecules in human metabolic pathways are (1) the oxidized form of nicotinamide adenine dinucleotide phosphate ($NADP^+$) and reduced nicotinamide adenine dinucleotide phosphate (NADPH), (2) the oxidized form of nicotinamide adenine dinucleotide (NAD^+) and re-

duced nicotinamide adenine dinucleotide (NADH) and (3) the oxidized form of flavin adenine dinucleotide ($FADH^+$) and reduced flavin adenine dinucleotide ($FADH_2$). As can be seen, the first of each pair is the form of the molecule that will accept an electron and a proton. The second of each pair is the reduced version, which always has an additional electron and proton. During aerobic metabolism electrons and paired protons are exchanged from one molecule to another (fuel source molecule to electron transfer molecule).

If enough oxygen is present, the electrons and protons are transferred again. This next exchange of electrons and protons occurs inside the mitochondria (electron transfer molecule to electron transport system [ETS] cytochromes). In the ETS all electrons that were removed during oxidation of fuel sources are processed, and the electrons' energy is captured to add a high-energy phosphate bond to ADP, thus producing ATP. The protons and the energy-depleted electrons are finally accepted by oxygen. The result is production of metabolic water. When oxygen is the final acceptor, the total process is called *aerobic metabolism*.

When oxygen supply does not meet the demand, however, both anaerobic and aerobic production of ATP occur. The dominant process (aerobic or anaerobic) depends on oxygen content of the muscle mitochondria and therefore is ultimately related to the fitness level of the person and the intensity of the activity performed.

Glucose Utilization

Glucose can be used to produce ATP aerobically and anaerobically. The oxidation of glucose begins either with the removal of a glucose molecule from muscle glycogen or with the removal of glucose from the circulation. The glucose molecule is phosphorylated (phosphate group added to the glucose from breakdown of ATP to ADP). Glucose that is coming from muscle glycogen is already phosphorylated, and only exogenous glucose undergoes the process. The six-carbon phosphorylated glucose molecule is then converted to two three-carbon phosphorylated molecules (triose phosphate). Each triose phosphate molecule is converted to pyruvate, an unphosphorylated three-

Circulating glucose into muscle
(from breakdown of liver glycogen or carbohydrate foodstuffs from digestive tract)

↓

Glucose 6-phosphate
(from breakdown of muscle glycogen or phosphorylation of circulating glucose [uses ATP])

↓

Fructose 6-phosphate
(formation as an isomerization of glucose-P or phosphorylation of circulating fructose [uses ATP])

A

↓

Fructose 1,6-biphosphate
(additional phosphorylation of fructose-P [uses ATP])

↓

Two molecules of triose phosphates formed
(from cleavage of hexose-2P)

↓

Two molecules of pyruvate formed
(formation as oxidation occurs of triose phosphates [Net two electrons removed] and generation of four
ATP molecules [substrate-level phosphorylation of ADP])

B   Glucose + 2 NAD$^+$ + 2 (ADP + P$_i$) $\longrightarrow$ 2 Pyruvate$^-$ + 2 NADH + 2 ATP

Fig. 2-3   A, Anaerobic glycolysis. **B,** Complete Embden-Meyerhof (glycolytic) pathway.

$$\text{Pyruvate} + \text{NADH} + \text{H}^+ \xrightarrow{\text{Lactate dehydrogenase}} \textbf{Lactate} + \text{NAD}^+$$

Fig. 2-4   Lactate production from reduction of pyruvate, which occurs when O$_2$ demand exceeds O$_2$ supply (completion of anaerobic glycolysis pathway).

carbon compound. As the triose phosphate molecules are converted to pyruvate, ATP is produced when energy is released from the removal of the phosphate group. The entire process of glucose conversion to two molecules of pyruvate occurs in the cytoplasm of the cell. This process is called *glycolysis* or *anaerobic glycolysis* (Fig. 2-3) and results in the net production of two ATP molecules and the transfer of two electrons to NAD$^+$. The total process has been described as anaerobic metabolism resulting in production of energy from

glucose without oxygen. Therefore, if oxygen is not readily available, pyruvate is reduced to form lactate and H$^+$ (lactic acid) (Fig. 2-4).

If oxygen is readily available, pyruvate is shuttled into the mitochondria, further oxidation of the pyruvate molecule takes place, and acetyl-CoA (a two-carbon compound) is produced (Fig. 2-5). During this step of acetyl-CoA production, two electrons are transferred to carriers and two molecules of carbon-dioxide are released. Acetyl-CoA enters into the Krebs cycle (citric acid cycle) and is completely

$$\text{Pyruvate} + \text{NAD}^+ \xrightarrow{\text{Pyruvate dehydrogenase}} \text{Acetyl-CoA} + \text{NADH} + \text{CO}_2$$

Fig. 2-5 Acetyl-CoA production from oxidation of pyruvate, which occurs when O_2 supply is abundant.

A

Formation of citrate
(from combining acetyl-CoA [two-carbon compound] and oxaloacetate [four-carbon compound])

↓

α-Ketoglutarate
(formation after citrate is converted to isocitrate and then oxidized and decarboxylated [net two electrons removed and two CO_2 molecules produced])

↓

Succinate
(formation after α-ketoglutarate is oxidized and decarboxylated [net two electrons removed and two CO_2 molecules produced] and generation of two GTP molecules [substrate-level phosphorylation of GDP])

↓

Oxaloacetate regeneration
(formation as oxidation of succinate to fumarate [net two electrons removed]; fumarate is converted to malate, which undergoes a final oxidation to become oxaloacetate [net two more electrons removed])

B $\text{Acetyl-CoA} + 3\,\text{NAD}^+ + \text{FADH}^+ + \text{GDP} + P_i + H_2O \longrightarrow 2\,CO_2 + \text{CoA} + 3\,\text{NADH} + \text{FADH}_2 + \text{GTP}$

Fig. 2-6 **A** and **B,** Schemata of the citric acid (Krebs) cycle, which occurs for each of the two acetyl-CoA molecules formed during glycolysis when O_2 supply is abundant. *FADH$^+$,* oxidized form of flavin adenine dinucleotide; *FADH$_2$,* reduced form of flavin adenine dinucleotide; *GDP,* guanosine diphosphate; *GTP,* guanosine triphosphate; *NAD,* nicotinamide adenine dinucleotide; *NAD$^+$,* oxidized form of NAD; *NADH,* reduced NAD; *P$_i$,* inorganic phosphate.

oxidized, transferring eight electrons to carriers (Fig. 2-6). In addition, four more molecules of carbon dioxide are released into the circulatory system from the muscle. At this time all the electron carriers transfer their electrons and protons to the cytochromes of the ETS (Fig. 2-7). The result of "aerobic glycolysis" or aerobic production of energy from glucose is the production of 36 ATP molecules from one molecule of glucose.

Fat Utilization

Fats cannot be utilized anaerobically. Fatty acids are oxidized for energy production through the process of β oxidation. Each fatty acid, which is a chain of carbon molecules with saturated or unsaturated oxygen bonds, is broken down into pairs of carbons that enter the Krebs cycle as acyl-CoA (Fig. 2-8). Each pair of carbons resulting from the breakdown of fatty acid is oxidized during the Krebs cycle, and pairs of electrons are transported to the ETS in the same fashion as in glucose oxidation. The results are production of ATP and metabolic water and the release of carbon dioxide. For one 16-carbon fatty acid molecule the yield may be as high as 130 ATP molecules requiring 23 molecules of oxygen. Fats cannot be used anaerobically because

Substrate oxidized and carriers reduced
(In glycolytic pathway and formation of acetyl-CoA from pyruvate and
during citric acid cycle, NAD^+ is reduced to NADH and $FADH^+$ is reduced to $FADH_2$.)

A

↓

Carriers reoxidized in three steps
Occurs in the mitochondria via (1) ubiquinone, (2) cytochrome C oxidase, and (3) molecular oxygen;
each electron transfer after NADH involves phosphorylation of ADP to ATP [net three ATP molecules
produced from reoxidation of NADH to NAD^+])

1. **Glucose** oxidized to acetyl-CoA

B   2. **Acetyl-CoA** oxidized via the **citric acid cycle**

3. **Electron carriers** reoxidized via the **ETS**, with O_2 as final acceptor of
electrons and protons to form CO_2, H_2O, and **ATP**

Fig. 2-7   **A** and **B,** Schemata of the electron transport system (ETS) and aerobic glycolysis.
B, Complete "aerobic" glycolysis of glucose. *ADP,* Adenosine diphosphate; *ATP,* adenosine
triphosphate; *FADH*$^+$, oxidized form of flavin adenine dinucleotide; *FADH²,* reduced form of
flavin adenine dinucleotide; *NAD,* nicotinamide adenine dinucleotide; *NADH,* reduced form
of NAD; *NAD*$^+$, oxidized form of NAD.

the acyl-CoA cannot be transformed into pyruvate
and therefore cannot be reduced to lactic acid or
transformed into a compound further up the glycolytic chain. The transforming of pyruvate to acyl-
CoA or acetyl-CoA is a one-way chemical reaction
and is not reversible. In addition, fatty acids are used
primarily as a fuel source only when oxygen is in
abundance at the mitochondrial site. When oxygen is
abundant, fatty acids are the predominant fuel
source, since more ATP can be produced by oxidation of a fat molecule than by oxidation of a glucose
molecule. When oxygen begins to get scarce, such as
when an exercise event is initiated or when the intensity is higher than normal and more ATP is
needed, glucose is preferentially used. Glucose is
used because its oxidation requires less oxygen per
mole than does the oxidation of fatty acids. In other
words, because glucose is a more efficient fuel than
fats are, glucose tends to be spared until oxygen
availability becomes threatened (oxygen demand approaches oxygen availability).

The use of fatty acids and glucose is duration- and
intensity-dependent during exercise. Fuel utilization,
however, is ultimately controlled by metabolic hormones, which are discussed in the following section.

HORMONAL CONTROL OF FUEL STORAGE AND UTILIZATION
Fuel Storage

During times of relative inactivity fuels are
stored. The most active hormone in the storage of
fats and glucose is insulin. Insulin is a relatively
small protein produced by the β cells of the pancreatic islets of Langerhans. A rise in the concentration of blood glucose is the primary stimulus for
secretion of insulin. This response is extremely
rapid, beginning within the first minute after detection of an elevation in blood glucose concentration. Insulin initiates the rapid uptake of glucose
into skeletal muscle and adipose tissue. Liver cell
uptake of circulating glucose is insulin independent. The exact mechanism of the action of insulin
is still in question; however, it is believed to initiate
an inhibitory effect on cyclic AMP pro-
duction.[43] When insulin is present, the enzymes
necessary for glycogenolysis (breakdown of glycogen), gluconeogenesis (production of glucose),
and lipolysis (fat breakdown) are inactivated and
the activity of enzymes for glycogenesis (glycogen
synthesis and storage) and lipoprotein lipase activity of adipose and muscle tissue is increased,

FFA into muscle
(mobilized from adipocytes into circulation or already stored in muscle)

↓

Formation of acyl-CoA
(from FFA at outer mitochondrial border via acyl-CoA synthetase,
requiring phosphorylation of **GTP**)

↓

**Transport of acyl-CoA into inner
mitochondrial membrane**
(transfer to carnitine via enzyme carnitine palmitoyl transferase)

↓

Cleavage into multiple acetyl-CoA
(acyl-CoA is oxidized by acyl-CoA dehydrogenase
[chain length–specific enzmyes] and then cleaved)

↓

Enter into citric acid cycle
(from combining acetyl-CoA [two-carbon compound] and
oxaloacetate [four-carbon compound])

A

B

$$\text{Palmitate fatty acid} + \text{CoA} + \text{GTP} \longrightarrow \text{Palmitate acyl-CoA} + \text{GDP} + P_i$$

$$\text{Palmitate acyl-CoA} + 23\ O_2 + 129\ (\text{ADP} + P_i) \longrightarrow 16\ CO_2 + 129\ \text{ATP}$$

Fig. 2-8 **A** and **B,** Free fatty acid (FFA) oxidation, which occurs when O_2 supply is abundant. *ADP,* Adenosine diphosphate; *ATP,* adenosine triphosphate; *GDP,* guanosine diphosphate; *GTP,* guanosine triphosphate; *P_i,* inorganic phosphate.

thus enhancing fat storage. The insulin plasma concentration required to inhibit or promote the previously mentioned activities varies. Inhibition of glycogenolysis and lipolysis and enhancement of glycogenesis require only small changes in insulin plasma concentration.[55] The processes of inhibiting production of glucose and promoting fat storage require higher or more prolonged concentrations of the hormone.

Fuel Utilization

Endogenous fuels are utilized when activity level increases. The effect of initiating exercise on metabolic hormones is explored in more detail in this section. The hormones that initiate fuel mobilization and enhance use of fuels are catecholamines and glucagon. In addition, inhibition of insulin release during exercise enhances the reverse of the described hormonal functions.[60]

Many studies have demonstrated that insulin concentration does not increase and in most cases decreases after glucose consumption if exercise of low (50%) maximum oxygen consumption (Vo_2max), moderate (50% to 75%) Vo_2max, or high (75% to 100%) Vo_2max intensity is initiated.[1,2,11,23] Two hypotheses are advanced to explain plasma insulin decline after an initial rise in response to a glucose challenge. First, once exercise is initiated, blood flow to the contracting muscle increases. As the circulation increases, a greater amount of plasma insulin is bound and absorbed by subcutaneous and muscle tissue.* The second hypothesis suggests that an exercise is initiated, there is an accompanying increase in sympathetic tone. Sympathetic stimulation inhibits the β-cell insulin

---

*References 7, 21, 36, 37, 46, and 54.

production and secretion.[15,24] Regardless of the cause of insulin decline, the result is an increase in blood glucose concentration from the liver via glycogenolysis and gluconeogenesis. It is possible that the increase in blood glucose concentration may overshadow muscle tissue utilization, resulting in hyperglycemia (high blood-glucose concentration).

A metabolic hormone other than insulin that is produced in the pancreas is glucagon. Glucagon is produced by the α cells of the islets of Langerhans. Release of glucagon is stimulated by a decrease in blood glucose concentrations. The effect of glucagon is to stimulate liver glycogenolysis and gluconeogenesis and to mobilize fatty acids from the adipose tissue triglyceride stores.[2,34] The mechanism for glucagon action is mediated through cyclic AMP, which as a secondary messenger activates the phosphorylation of the enzymes necessary for glycogenolysis.

When exercise is initiated and the blood glucose level is low, glucagon plasma concentration is increased, resulting in a release of hepatic glucose. If use exceeds the demand, however, which may occur during prolonged exercise of moderate to high intensity, blood glucose concentration eventually falls and fatigue may occur.[57]

As is evident in the preceding discussion of insulin and glucagon, they have opposite effects. When the level of blood fuel is high (for example, after a meal), insulin is released and storage of fuel is promoted. When the blood fuel level is low (such as after fasting or during exercise), glucagon is released and liberation of fuel from deposits is promoted.

The catecholamines are a group of hormones that affect fuel utilization during exercise. Epinephrine and norepinephrine are produced in the adrenal medulla in response to sympathetic stimulation and are released directly into the circulatory system. The effect of epinephrine and norepinephrine on the blood glucose and fatty acid concentrations is equivalent to the effect of glucagon because all three hormones activate the same secondary messenger, cyclic AMP. However, the catecholamines are active in skeletal muscle, adipose tissue, and liver, whereas glucagon is effective only in the liver and adipose tissue.[60] By interfering with insulin action,[59] catecholamines

have an effect not only on the mobilization of fuels but also on the uptake of circulatory fuels by the active skeletal muscle. Catecholamine levels are low when an individual is at rest and in a calm state. The plasma concentration increases when the individual is in a state of movement or nervous tension. Norepinephrine concentration increases during low-intensity exercise of 50% Vo_2max or less and increases dramatically when heavier work loads are approached. Epinephrine levels, however, do not increase during low-intensity exercise but do increase during high-intensity exercise.[49] Catecholamine plasma concentrations are independent of blood glucose concentration and are therefore regulated by a totally different mechanism than that for insulin and glucagon regulation.

Glucagon-insulin interaction mainly controls the liver and adipose stores (glucose and FFA mobilization or uptake), whereas catecholamine-insulin interaction controls glucose uptake at the skeletal muscle via presently unknown indirect mechanisms.

FUEL SOURCE SELECTION DURING EXERCISE

The selection of a predominantly utilized fuel, fat or carbohydrate, is closely related to both intensity and duration of the exercise. Low-intensity exercise of long duration (less than 50% Vo_2max) is characterized by oxidation of both FFA and carbohydrate to supply ATP for contracting skeletal muscle. As exercise duration increases or when exercise is at a lower intensity of work load, a greater percentage of FFA oxidation for ATP production occurs.[14,45,47] This enhanced utilization of FFA as the predominant fuel source is linked to adequacy of the oxygen supply, which is abundant in persons with moderate and high levels of fitness who are exercising at 50% or less Vo_2max.

Conversely, when exercise is performed at work loads of moderate to heavy intensity (greater than 50% Vo_2max), FFA oxidation contributes less to ATP production. At high-intensity work loads (75% to 90% Vo_2max), FFA oxidation accounts for approximately 25% of the fuel,[27,31,47] and during maximal and supermaximal exercising conditions (greater than 100% Vo_2max) little if any energy is derived from FFA metabolism.[16] Supermaximal exercise (greater than 100% Vo_2max) is exercise performed at an intensity beyond the individual's maximal oxygen consumption and thus is anaerobic and cannot be sustained beyond a short period. For example, during sprinting, although the oxygen consumed is not greater than maximal, the required energy demand is. The work of sprinting can be performed, but the energy required cannot be wholly supplied by the oxygen delivered. Other anaerobic fuel sources must be used anaerobically, such as high-energy phosphates (ATP and PCr) and glycogen.

Possible Causes of Fatigue During Exercise of Varying Intensity

Physical fatigue, defined as a state of disturbed homeostasis resulting from work and work environment,[13] would appear to be closely related to availability of fuel sources. This does not appear to be the case, however, in low-intensity exercise (less than 50% Vo_2max) of long duration, when subjective fatigue does occur without accumulation of lactate within the blood or depletion of carbohydrate and fat stores.[4,19] Asmussen and Mazin[3] have demonstrated a central neural component rather than a metabolic component in fatigue that occurs during low-intensity exercise.

Fatigue resulting from exercise performed at moderate to high intensity (greater than 50% Vo_2max) appears to be highly correlated to available carbohydrate supply or lactate accumulation, or both. Decrease in performance during exercise of moderate intensity (50% to 75% Vo_2max) in highly trained individuals appears to be related closely to depletion of hepatic glycogen,[57] muscle glycogen,[8,27] and eventually blood glucose.[40] The depletion of liver glycogen is accompanied by a great dependence on metabolic precursors for hepatic glucose production. After 4 hours of exercise, gluconeogenesis may account for as much as 45% of hepatic glucose output.[57] Despite the progressive decline in liver glycogen stores, blood glucose levels remain essentially unchanged until liver glycogen content is depleted by approximately 75%.[20,56] When this level of depletion is reached, an imbalance between muscle glucose uptake and hepatic glucose

output develops.[57] The result is an unavoidable decline in blood glucose and muscle glycogen concentrations. When hypoglycemia does occur, fatigue may result, and the inability to adequately supply glucose to nonexercising areas of the body (for example, brain) may result in nausea and extreme discomfort.[5] Individuals with low fitness levels may be unable to exercise at 50% to 75% Vo_2max for a prolonged period, primarily because of a more rapid depletion of muscle glycogen and possible accumulation of H^+ within the muscle.[28] Thus the mechanism that results in fatigue during moderate-intensity exercise of long duration appears to be highly dependent on the individual's fitness level.

Decrease in performance during high-intensity exercise (75% to 90% Vo_2max) in highly trained individuals appears to be related primarily to depletion of muscle glycogen stores[8] and possible H^+ accumulation within the muscle as the intensity of the exercise becomes greater.[25] Under these exercise conditions hepatic glycogen and blood glucose concentrations do not decline, whereas during exercise of moderate intensity and longer duration they do decline.[30] Duration of exercise is also limited to 90 minutes at most for highly trained individuals. Individuals with low fitness levels can tolerate high intensity of exercise only for a relatively short period because of accumulation of high levels of muscle H^+.[18] Exercise at supermaximal intensity (greater than 100% Vo_2max) can be tolerated only for a short time, since the energy source is anaerobic (that is, glycolysis or dependence on high-energy phosphates).

Activity that depends on liver glycogen, muscle glycogen, and blood glucose concentrations usually is influenced by diet before or during exercise training. Thus for the untrained or active individual diet normally influences exercise at an intensity classified as (1) moderate (50% to 75% Vo_2max) with a duration of 30 minutes to 1 hour, not exceeding 1½ hours, (2) high (75% to 90% Vo_2max) for much shorter durations, from one tenth to three tenths of an hour, not exceeding 30 minutes, or (3) a combination of the two, in which the intensity of exercise oscillates between the two categories.

EFFECT OF REGULAR EXERCISE TRAINING ON FUEL AND HORMONAL CONTROL
Fuel Storage

The effect of regular exercise training is to reduce adipose tissue and subsequent triglyceride stores within the adipocytes.[61] In addition, the trained individual has a much lower plasma FFA concentration than normal at rest and during a brief bout of exercise.[61] The decrease in FFA plasma concentration during exercise is believed to be primarily due to slower lipolysis, probably as a result of the marked blunting of the catecholamine response observed in trained individuals.[61] Despite the decreased availability and oxidation of plasma FFA concentration, the rate of fat oxidation observed in trained individuals actually increases.[29] The source of the additional fatty acid oxidation in the trained state appears to result from an increased utilization of intramuscular triglycerides.[33]

In addition to increased oxidation of intramuscular triglycerides, an increase in muscle glycogen stores is evident after chronic endurance training.[22] However, both liver and muscle glycogen stores are less affected by training than by dietary activity.[58]

Fuel Utilization

As mentioned earlier, plasma concentrations of FFAs are the primary fuel source in persons at rest and in untrained individuals in good health who are performing exercise at a low intensity. Also, availability of plasma FFA decreases after training. The individual who is in a highly trained state uses FFA from plasma and intramuscular sources as the primary fuel during exercise of moderate intensity.[33] Recall that FFA availability is much greater than glycogen availability and that use of fuel depends on oxygen availability. The highly trained individual uses FFA at a higher exercise intensity than do untrained individuals (1) because more oxygen is available as a result of improved delivery and extraction of oxygen at the muscle site and (2) because oxidation of muscle FFA concentration is greater. Therefore muscle glycogen stores are spared until muscle FFA concentration decreases or exercise intensity increases. As exercise intensity increases, the need for oxygen increases and oxygen availability becomes threatened.[48] In addition to improved oxygen muscle efficiency resulting from an increase in muscle mitochondrial content and oxidative capacity, the highly trained individual also has an increase in the number of enzymes and their activity associated with fatty acid oxidation.[42]

Muscle glycogen and plasma glucose use is also improved in the trained state. The "normal untrained" individual is unable to compete with the highly trained endurance athlete. The endurance athlete is able to exercise for more than 3 hours at moderate intensity and for as long as 1½ hours at high intensity. This improved performance primarily results from the ability of the muscle to extract more oxygen,[35] an increase in mitochondrial content and oxidative capacity,[17] and an increase in the ability to oxidize pyruvate to acetyl-CoA.[6] With training, therefore, fuel sources within the muscle increase and the ability to deliver and extract more oxygen and improve oxidative capacity improves dramatically. The result is the ability to use fats for fuel at much higher intensities of exercise than normal and to spare muscle glycogen. The sparing of muscle glycogen greatly improves the ability to perform exercise at high intensities, since fatigue is no longer the result of H^+ accumulation but instead depends on glycogen and blood glucose availability.

Fuel Regulation

Hormones that control fuel regulation—insulin, catecholamine, and glucagon—are affected by regular exercise training. With regular training, an increase in the sensitivity of muscle tissue to insulin-stimulated carbohydrate metabolism occurs[7,36,39] and is coupled with a decrease in the response of insulin release for any given load of glucose.[9,41,53] In other words, it appears that an adaptation occurs with insulin and associated adipose and muscle insulin receptors, since less insulin is required to cause glucose uptake at rest or during exercise, either because the number of insulin receptors are increased or because their sensitivity or activity is improved. The results are a much improved glucose tolerance and tighter control of plasma glucose levels at rest and during exercise.

Catecholamine responses are affected by regular physical training. Catecholamine release from the adrenal medulla is lower at any given work load for trained individuals than for untrained persons.[49] The total amount of catecholamine release, however, is greater in the trained individual. The metabolic response to catecholamines at low exercise intensity is greater in the trained individual. As with insulin receptors, the catecholamine receptors (increased either in number or in activity) appear to be much more sensitive than normal to the presence of the hormone. Thus greater fuel mobilization and uptake occur with the release of less catecholamine.[49] The increased catecholamine concentration causes an increase in glucagon release and insulin inhibition,[60] resulting in enhanced mobilization of FFA from the adipose tissue, glucose release (glycogenolysis) from the liver, and glucose and FFA uptake at the skeletal muscle site during exercise.

As a result of regular training there is an increase in the sensitivity of liver tissue to glucagon-stimulated glucose release.[60] In other words, the adaptation that appears to occur with glucagon and associated liver cell receptors is that less glucagon is required to cause glucose release at rest or during exercise because either the number of glucagon receptors are increased or their sensitivity or activity is improved. Like the training effect for insulin, the result is a much improved glucose tolerance and tighter control of plasma glucose levels at rest and during exercise.

TECHNIQUES FOR ASSESSING AEROBIC CAPACITY AND ANAEROBIC POWER

This chapter would be incomplete without a discussion of techniques for assessing aerobic capacity and anaerobic power. Techniques for evaluating aerobic capacity and tests for anaerobic power are presented in the following sections.

Aerobic Capacity

Aerobic capacity, or the ability to deliver and utilize oxygen, can be assessed by direct and indirect measures. The "gold standard" is evaluation of oxygen consumption per unit time (Vo_2) by means of inspiratory and expiratory volume measures and expired oxygen and carbon dioxide concentrations. The preceding gas measures are direct measures of oxygen consumption. The treadmill, cycle ergometer, and upper body ergometer are often used to assess a patient's aerobic capacity. *With the advent of telemetry oxygen-consumption systems, aerobic capacity can be assessed during functional activities like gardening, industrial work, and unrestricted gait.*

Indirect measures of aerobic capacity can be performed on ergometers when the clinician has an accurate assessment of work load on the device. When indirect measures are used, ventilatory volumes and expired gas concentrations are not measured. Instead, the method of assessing aerobic capacity is to determine heart rate response. Heart rate has a strong linear correlation to oxygen consumption. Thus if the work load is known and a measure of heart rate can be obtained, aerobic capacity can be estimated. Nomograms and predictive equations exist for treadmill and cycle ergometer protocols.

Aerobic capacity can be predicted indirectly by evaluating the results of field tests of running, stepping and walking. A field test is one that can be conducted outside the laboratory or clinical setting. The predictions of oxygen consumption are determined by means of statistical equations that correlate direct measures and field test measures in the same individual: the larger the population evaluated in this fashion, the stronger the predictive ability of the field test. Although field tests are the least accurate method of determining aerobic capacity, for large groups of individuals they can be performed easily and quickly.

Anaerobic Power

Anaerobic power, or the ability to move the body or a body segment rapidly with great force, can be assessed by means of direct and indirect measures. The "gold standard" is evaluation of power by means of dynamometry or ergometry, in which force and velocity of movement can be assessed simultaneously. As with aerobic capacity, however, direct measures are for the most part restricted to nonfunctional activities. A telemetry system for the simultaneous evaluation of force production and velocity does not yet exist.

Indirect measures of anaerobic power are currently based on field tests of stair running, running the 40-yard dash, and vertical jumping. The equations used multiply *displacement* and *mass* to get *work;* work is then divided by the *elapsed time* required to complete the event. Advantages of field tests are that these activities are function oriented and can be tested easily.

REFERENCES

1. Ahlborg G, Felig P: Influence of glucose ingestion on fuel-hormone response during prolonged exercise, *J Appl Physiol* 41:683, 1976.
2. Ahlborg BJ, Felig P: Substrate utilization during prolonged exercise preceded by ingestion of glucose, *Am J Physiol* 233:E188, 1977.
3. Asmussen E, Mazin B: A central nervous system component in local muscular fatigue, *Eur J Appl Physiol* 38:9, 1978.
4. Astrand I: Aerobic work capacity in men and women with special reference to age, *Acta Physiol Scand Suppl* 169:1, 1960.
5. Astrand PO, Rodahl K: *Textbook of work physiology,* New York, 1986, McGraw-Hill.
6. Baldwin KM et al: Respiratory capacity of white, red and intermediate muscle: adaptive response to exercise, *Am J Physiol* 222:373, 1972.
7. Berger M et al: Effect of physical training on glucose tolerance and on glucose metabolism of skeletal muscle in anaesthetized normal rats, *Diabetologia* 16:179, 1979.
8. Bergstrom J et al: Diet, muscle glycogen and physical performance, *Acta Physiol Scand* 71:140, 1967.
9. Bjorntorp P et al: Carbohydrate and lipid metabolism in middle-aged physically well-trained men, *Metabolism* 21:1037, 1972.
10. Bock AV et al: Studies in muscular activity. IV. "Steady state" and the respiratory quotient during work, *J Physiol (Lond)* 66:162, 1928.
11. Bonen A et al: Glucose ingestion before and during intense exercise, *J Appl Physiol* 50:766, 1981.
12. Chen M, Whistler RL: Metabolism of D-fructose, *Adv Carbo Chem Biochem* 34:265, 1977.
13. Christensen EH: Muscular work and fatigue. In Rodahl K, Horvath SM, editors: *Muscle as a tissue,* New York, 1960, McGraw-Hill.
14. Christensen EH, Hansen O: Zur methodik der respiratorischen quotient: bestimmungen in ruhe und arbeit, *Scand Arch Physiol* 81:137, 1939.
15. Christensen N et al: Catecholamines and exercise, *Diabetes* 28(suppl 1):58, 1979.
16. Davies CTM, Barnes C: Plasma FFA in relation to maximum power output in man, *Int Z Agnew Physiol* 30:247, 1972.
17. Davies KJA, Packer L, Brooks GA: Biochemical adaptations of mitochondria, muscle, and whole animal respiration to endurance training, *Arch Biochem Biophys* 209:538, 1981.
18. Ekblom B et al: Effect of training on circulatory response to exercise, *J Appl Physiol* 24:518, 1968.
19. Essen B, Hagenfeldt L, Kaijser L: Utilization of blood-borne and intramuscular substrates during continuous and intermittent exercise in man, *J Physiol* 265:489, 1977.
20. Felig P: The glucose-alanine cycle, *Metabolism* 22:179, 1973.
21. Felig P, Wahren J: Role of insulin and glucagon in the regulation of hepatic glucose production during exercise, *Diabetes* 28(suppl 1):71, 1979.
22. Fitts RH et al: Skeletal muscle respiratory capacity, endurance, and glycogen utilization, *Am J Physiol* 228:1029, 1975.
23. Galbo H, Holst JJ, Christensen NJ: The effect of different diets and of insulin on the hormonal response to prolonged exercise, *Acta Physiol Scand* 107:19, 1979.
24. Galbo H et al: Glucagon and plasma catecholamines during beta-receptor blockade in exercising man, *J Appl Physiol* 40:855, 1976.
25. Gollnick PD, Bayly W, Hodgson D: Exercise intensity, training, diet, and lactate concentration in muscle and blood, *Med Sci Sports Exerc* 18:334, 1986.
26. Henriksson J: Training-induced adaptation of skeletal muscle and metabolism during submaximal exercise, *J Physiol* 270:661, 1977.
27. Hermansen L, Hultman E, Saltin B: Muscle glycogen during prolonged severe exercise, *Acta Physiol Scand* 71:129, 1967.
28. Holloszy JO, Coyle EF: Adaptations of skeletal muscle to endurance exercise and their metabolic consequences, *J Appl Physiol* 56:831, 1984.
29. Holloszy JO et al: Utilization of fat as substrate during exercise: effect of training, *Biochem Exerc* 16:183, 1986.
30. Hultman E: Studies on muscle metabolism of glycogen and active phosphate in man with special reference to exercise and diet, *Scand J Clin Invest* 19(suppl 94):1, 1967.
31. Hultman E: Muscle glycogen stores and prolonged exercise. In Shephard RJ, editor: *Frontiers of fitness,* Springfield, Ill, 1971, Charles C Thomas.
32. Hultman E, Bergstrom J, McLeanan-Anderson N: Breakdown and resynthesis of adenosine triphosphate in connection with muscular work in man, *Scand J Clin Lab Invest* 19:56, 1967.
33. Hurley BF et al: Muscle triglyceride utilization during exercise: effect of training, *J Appl Physiol* 60:562, 1986.
34. Issekutz B, Vranic M: Significance of glucagon in the control of glucose production during exercise in dogs, *Am J Physiol* 238:E13, 1980.
35. Karlsson J, Nordesjo LO, Saltin B: Muscle glycogen utilization during exercise after physical training, *Acta Phys Scand* 90:210, 1974.

36. Koivisto V, Soman V, Felig P: Effects of acute exercise on insulin binding to monocytes in trained athletes: changes in the resting state and after exercise, *J Clin Invest* 64:1011, 1979.

37. Koivisto V, Soman V, Felig P: Effects of acute exercise on insulin binding to monocytes in obesity, *Metabolism* 39:168, 1980.

38. Krogh A, Lindhard J: Relative value of fat and carbohydrate as source of muscular energy, *Biochem J* 14:290, 1920.

39. LeBlanc J et al: Effects of physical training and adiposity in glucose metabolism and ^{125}I-insulin binding, *J Appl Physiol* 46:235, 1979.

40. Levin SA, Gordon B, Drick CL: Some changes in the chemical constituents of the blood following a marathon race, *JAMA* 82:1778, 1924.

41. Lohmann DF et al: Diminished insulin response in highly trained athletes, *Metabolism* 27:521, 1978.

42. Mole PA, Oscai LB, Holloszy JO: Adaptation of muscle to exercise: increase in levels of palmityl CoAsynthetase, carnitine palmityltransferase, and palmitylCoA dehydrogenase and in the capacity to oxidize fatty acids, *J Clin Invest* 50:2323, 1971.

43. Naveri H et al: Muscle metabolism during and after strenuous intermittent running, *Scand J Clin Lab Invest* 38:329, 1978.

44. Nilsson LH, Hultman E: Liver and muscle glycogen in man after glucose and fructose infusion, *Scand J Clin Lab Invest* 33:5, 1974.

45. Paul P: Effects of long-lasting physical exercise and training on lipid metabolism. In Howald H, Poortmans JR, editors: *Metabolic adaptation to prolonged physical exercise,* Basel, 1975, Birkhauser Verlag.

46. Pederson O, Beck-Nielson H, Heding L: Increased insulin receptors after exercise in patients with insulin dependent diabetes mellitus, *New Engl J Med* 302:886, 1980.

47. Pruett EDR: Glucose and insulin during prolonged work stress in men living on different diets, *J Appl Physiol* 28:199, 1970.

48. Rennie MJ, Holloszy JO: Inhibition of glucose uptake and glycogenolysis by availability of oleate in well-oxygenated perfused skeletal muscle, *Biochem J* 168:161, 1977.

49. Richter EA et al: Regulation of carbohydrate metabolism in exercise, *Biochem Exerc* 16:151, 1986.

50. Sahlin K, Harris RC, Hultman E: Creatine kinase equilibrium and lactate content compared with muscle pH in tissue samples obtained after isometric contraction, *Biochem J* 152:173, 1975.

51. Sahlin K et al: Lactate content and pH in muscle samples obtained after dynamic exercise, *Pflugers Arch* 367:143, 1976.

52. Saltin B, Karlsson J: Muscle glycogen utilization during work of different intensities. In Pernow B, Saltin B, editors: *Muscle metabolism during exercise,* New York, 1971, Plenum.

53. Seals DR et al: Effects of endurance training on glucose tolerance and plasma lipid levels in older men and women, *JAMA* 252:645, 1984.

54. Vranic M, Kawamori R: Essential roles of insulin and glucagon in regulating glucose fluxes during exercise in dogs, *Diabetes* 28(suppl 1):45, 1979.

55. Vranic M, Lickley H: Hormonal mechanisms that act to preserve glucose homeostasis during exercise: two controversial issues, *Biochem Exerc* 21:279, 1989.

56. Wahren J: Quantitative aspects of blood flow and oxygen uptake in the forearm during rhythmic exercise, *Acta Physiol Scand* 67(suppl 269):1, 1966.

57. Wahren J: Glucose turnover during exercise in man, *Ann N Y Acad Sci* 301:45, 1977.

58. Wahren J, Felig P, Ahlborg G: Glucose metabolism during exercise in man, *J Clin Invest* 50:2715, 1971.

59. Wasserman DH, Lickley H, Vranic M: Interactions between glucagon and other counter-regulatory hormones during normoglycemic and hypoglycemic exercise, *J Clin Invest* 74:1404, 1984.

60. Wasserman DH, Vranic M: Interaction between insulin, glucagon and catecholamines in the regulation of glucose production and uptake during exercise: physiology and diabetes, *Biochem Exerc* 16:167, 1986.

61. Winder WW et al: Training-induced changes in hormonal and metabolic responses to submaximal exercise, *J Appl Physiol* 46:766, 1979.

SUGGESTED READINGS

Baldwin KM et al: Glycolytic enzymes in different types of skeletal muscle: adaptation to exercise, *Am J Physiol* 225:962, 1973.

Costill DL et al: Effects of elevated plasma FFA and insulin on muscle glycogen usage during exercise, *J Appl Physiol* 43:695, 1977.

Costill DL et al: Adaptations in skeletal muscle following strength training, *J Appl Physiol* 46:96, 1979.

Coyle EF et al: Carbohydrate feeding during prolonged exercise can delay fatigue, *J Appl Physiol* 55:230, 1983.

Coyle EF et al: Substrate usage during prolonged exercise following a preexercise meal, *J Appl Physiol* 59:429, 1985.

Coyle EF et al: Muscle glycogen utilization during prolonged strenuous exercise when fed carbohydrate, *J Appl Physiol* 61:165, 1986.

Davies KJA, Packer L, Brooks GA: Exercise bioenergetics following sprint training, *Arch Biochem Biophys* 215:260, 1982.

Foster C, Costill DL, Fink WJ: Effects of preexercise feedings on endurance performance, *Med Sci Sports Exerc* 11:1, 1979.

Galbo H, Holst JJ, Christensen NJ: Glucagon and plasma catecholamine responses to graded and prolonged exercise in man, *J Appl Physiol* 38:70, 1975.

Hargreaves M et al: Effect of preexercise carbohydrate feedings on endurance cycling performance, *Med Sci Sports Exerc* 19:33, 1987.

Hickson RC, Heusner WW, Venttuss YD: Skeletal muscle enzyme alterations after sprint and endurance training, *J Appl Physiol* 40:868, 1976.

Holloszy JO: Biochemical adaptations in muscle: effect of exercise on mitochondrial oxygen uptake and respiratory enzyme activity in skeletal muscle, *J Biol Chem* 242:2278, 1967.

Jandrain B et al: Metabolic availability of glucose ingested 3 hours before prolonged exercise in humans, *J Appl Physiol* 56:1314, 1984.

Karlsson J: Muscle lactate, ATP, and CP levels during exercise after physical training in man, *J Appl Physiol* 33:199, 1972.

MacDonald I, Keywer A, Pacy D: Some effect in man of varying the load of glucose, sucrose, fructose or sorbitol on various metabolites in blood, *Am J Clin Nutr* 31:1305, 1978.

MacDougall JD et al: Biochemical adaptation of human skeletal muscle to heavy resistance training and immobilization, *J Appl Physiol* 43:700, 1977.

Neufer PD et al: Improvements in exercise performance: effects of carbohydrate feedings and diet, *J Appl Physiol* 62:983, 1987.

STUDY QUESTIONS

- Describe the production of ATP via the breakdown of food.

- Describe the processes of aerobic and anaerobic metabolism at rest and during low-intensity and high-intensity exercise.

- Describe the restoration of depleted energy stores, including replenishment of ATP, PCr, muscle, and liver glycogen concentrations.

- Describe causes of fatigue at varying exercise intensities for fit and unfit individuals.

- Describe the interaction of insulin, glucagon, and catecholamine response in the control of glucose and fatty acid concentrations in the circulation. What is the effect of exercise training on hormonal control?

EXERCISE TOLERANCE AND TRAINING FOR PATIENTS WITH GENETIC METABOLIC DISORDERS, DIABETES, AND OBESITY

Scott M. Hasson

Proper utilization of energy sources is critical for individuals, especially when energy demands increase, such as during exercise or many work activities. Dysfunction of metabolism can occur when there is a problem with storage and utilization of fuels or hormonal regulation of fuels, or both. In Chapter 2 the framework is established to further explore the results of metabolic disorders in humans. The major emphases in Chapter 3 are to briefly describe rare muscle diseases and disorders that affect storage or use of fuels during exercise, or both, and the effect of exercise training in persons with these diseases; to describe types 1 and 2 diabetes and discuss the responses during exercise (that is, exercise tolerance) and the effect of training in these patients; and to describe the current theory concerning why obesity occurs and discuss responses during exercise and the effect of training in individuals with obesity.

MUSCLE DISEASES AND DISORDERS: EXERCISE TOLERANCE AND EFFECT OF TRAINING

Optimal metabolism ultimately depends on the ability to deliver, store, and use (oxidize) carbo-hydrates and fats. If deficiencies exist in any of these processes, the individual does not respond normally during exercise.

The diseases that affect storage and oxidation of the fuels within the muscle are quite rare. These diseases and their implications for exercise tolerance and the effect of exercise training are briefly described in this section.

Disorders of Lipid Metabolism

The first disorders described are those associated with lipid metabolism within the muscle. As discussed in the previous chapter, fatty acids are preferentially used by skeletal muscle during rest and activity of low to moderate intensity (30% to 60% of maximal oxygen consumption [Vo_2max]).[58,63] Free fatty acids (FFAs) are a major fuel source and are either transported from adipose tissue or stored directly within the muscle. FFAs can be used only in the presence of oxygen and are oxidized through the processes of β oxidation, the Krebs cycle, and the electron transport system within the mitochondria.

The major disorders of lipid metabolism are associated with carnitine and carnitine palmitoyl-

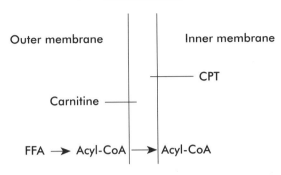

Fig. 3-1   Free fatty acid (FFA) transport within the mitochondria. *CPT,* Carnitine palmityl transferase.

transferase (CPT) enzyme deficiency. Free fatty acids from adipose tissue or diet enter muscle by diffusion, and intramuscular triglycerides are degraded to FFA. Free fatty acids are taken within the muscle to the mitochondria for oxidation. The FFAs are converted to long-chain acyl-coenzyme A (acyl-CoA) compounds and transported from the outer to the inner mitochondrial membrane by CPT (Fig. 3-1). To allow this transport from the outer to the inner mitochondrial membrane to take place, carnitine, a small amine molecule, is required. Carnitine is acquired from diet (red meat and dairy products) or synthesized from amino acids in the liver and kidney. Myopathic carnitine deficiency may result from insufficient diet but also may occur as a result of the inability to transport the carnitine to the muscle. The clinical findings in persons with carnitine deficiency include proximal muscle weakness,[13] severe muscle fatigability,[27] fat accumulation within the muscle, and occasionally, hypertrophic cardiomyopathy.[21] Carnitine replacement therapy, administered intravenously or orally, is usually beneficial.[65] If the enzyme CPT is deficient, similar findings of muscle weakness and fatigability are present.[19] There is no cure or replacement therapy for CPT deficiency.

A disorder of lipid metabolism other than CPT enzyme deficiency and carnitine deficiency is abnormal oxidation. Once the long-chain acyl-CoA compound is in the inner mitochondrial membrane, the process of β oxidation takes place. The rare defects of abnormal β oxidation are usually associated with acyl-CoA dehydrogenase enzymes that catalyze the first step in β oxidation, which is removal of two hydrogen atoms and electrons. The acyl-CoA dehydrogenases are chain-length specific, with one isoenzyme active on short acyl-CoA chains (four to eight carbons), one on chains of intermediate length (six to sixteen carbons), and one on long acyl-CoA chains (six to eighteen carbons). If this initial dehydrogenation does not occur, β oxidation does not take place. The clinical findings are muscle fatigability, pain with exercise, and general hypotonia.[83] There is no cure for these disorders.

In all three disorders—carnitine deficiency, CPT deficiency, and both oxidation enzyme deficiencies—a low-fat, high-carbohydrate diet is recommended.[65] Individuals with carnitine deficiency, CPT enzyme deficiency, or β oxidation disorders or a combination of these do not tolerate any intensity of exercise well.[49] This feature may be due in part to preferential weakness of the large proximal muscles of the pelvic girdle and trunk and accessory ventilatory muscles.[65] During exercise testing patients with CPT enzyme deficiency demonstrated normal cardiac outputs, oxygen distraction at the muscle site, and $\dot{V}o_2max$, as long as carbohydrate fuel was available.[12,28] However, patients deficient in acyl-CoA dehydrogenase have much lower $\dot{V}o_2max$ levels, although cardiac output is within the normal range. In these patients there appears to be a decreased ability to extract and use oxygen efficiently.[15,27] Dietary therapy incorporating riboflavin and medium-chain triglycerides increases $\dot{V}o_2max$ by 200% to 300% in these acyl-CoA dehydrogenase–deficient patients, from 10 ml/kg per min up to 25 ml/kg per min.[15,27]

Individuals with lipid metabolism disorders do not appear to perceive difficulty during exercise, which has resulted in myoglobinuria (release of myoglobin into the circulation and ultimately the urine). The severe muscle damage may be related to hydrogen ion accumulation,[15,27,72,83] but defects of the muscle and mitochondrial membrane have not been ruled out.[90] In addition to decreased aerobic performance, anaerobic performance is negatively affected, with decreased power production, particularly after fasting.[5,14] This decrease may be due to muscle weakness and the high levels of lactic acid produced, which have been observed in these patients during intense exercise.

The effect of exercise training for patients with lipid disorders is unknown. It appears unlikely that a specific enzyme deficiency could be modified as a result of the stimulus of repeated exercise. In fact, as mentioned earlier, the severe muscle cramping and myoglobinuria observed during high-intensity exercise in patients with CPT enzyme and β oxidation deficiencies leads the practitioner away from the prescription of a frequent high-intensity training regimen. Low-intensity exercise appears to be better tolerated, but the duration of the exercise must be monitored closely so that muscle glycogen depletion does not occur. The effect of low- to moderate-intensity exercise on the values that constitute improved endurance in these individuals (cardiac output, oxygen consumption, and muscle and liver glycogen storage) are unknown.

A patient with a disorder in lipid metabolism does not tolerate exercise of moderate to high intensity well. In some cases nutrient replacement therapy is useful (for example, in cases of carnitine deficiency). Diets high in carbohydrate and low in fat are also recommended. Fasting is not recommended, since this may result in liver and muscle glycogen depletion. Data on exercise training is not available, but low-intensity activity of moderate duration may improve cardiopulmonary function and decrease risk factors associated with cardiovascular disease. To prevent acidosis and muscle damage, low-intensity, moderate-duration exercise should neither compromise nor overtax the glycogenolytic pathways. Glycogenolysis and glycolysis disorders are discussed in the following section.

Disorders of Glucose and Glycogen Metabolism

Circulating glucose and stored glycogen are the major fuel sources other than fats. As discussed in Chapter 2, glucose is stored as glycogen in the liver and muscle tissue. Muscle glycogen is used preferentially when exercise intensity becomes high, that is, at more than 75% of Vo_2max,[34,37,63] and during anaerobic activities that result in the production of lactate and hydrogen ion. Several rare genetic diseases result in the lack of enzymes that permit glycogenolysis or glycolysis to occur.

The most common glycogen disorder is McArdle's disease, a condition in which the enzyme glycogen phosphorylase is absent in the skeletal muscle. The utilization of glycogen that is already stored is the primary role of glycogen phosphorylase. The enzyme is responsible for the cleaving of single units of glucose and in the process phosphorylates these molecules (Fig. 3-2). In addition, glycogen phosphorylase catalyzes the reverse reaction. Thus glycogen storage is also affected but to a lesser degree than utilization. Other pathways using uridine diphosphate glucose are available for the formation and storage of glycogen. The result of glycogen phosphorylase deficiency is an accumulation of glycogen in the muscle, since glycogen cannot be used as a fuel source.[54] The individual is susceptible to severe muscle fatigue, muscle pain, and muscle damage during and after strenuous exercise.[47,67] Mild exercise is better tolerated, since FFA and circulatory glucose can be used as fuel.[61] Lactate and hydrogen ion are not produced during exercise. Therefore the severe fatigue observed in patients with McArdle's disease has been postulated to occur from other sources, which are discussed later.

As previously described, circulatory glucose (from diet or liver glycogenolysis) and FFAs (from adipose tissue stores) can be used as fuel sources during activity. Free fatty acids are predominantly used, and their utilization has been shown to occur at a greater level than normal.[30] This pronounced use of FFA has been associated with a "second wind" phenomenon in these patients, resulting in a spontaneous increase in exercise capacity at a point of severe fatigue.[60,61] This increase in FFA use has been linked to increased cardiac output (200% to 300%) at any given oxygen uptake at a submaximal exercise work load,[50] resulting in markedly increased local blood flow to the muscle.[2,51]

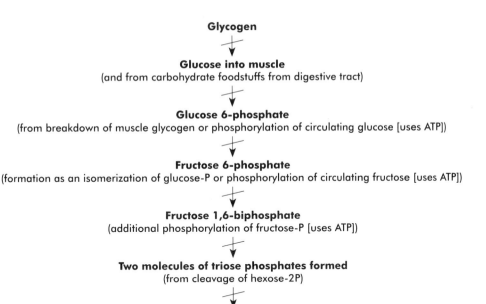

Fig. 3-2 **A** and **B,** Schemata depicting McArdle's disease. **B,** Complete Embden-Meyerhof (glycolytic) pathway. *ADP,* Adenosine diphosphate; *ATP,* adenosine triphosphate; *NAD,* nicotinamide adenine dinucleotide; *NADH,* reduced NAD; P_i, inorganic phosphate.

Coupled with increased blood flow is an increase in FFA mobilization from the adipocytes.[61] Dietary modifications and intravenous infusions of FFA and glucose have been shown to enhance muscle oxidative metabolism, improve Vo_2max, and decrease symptoms of muscle fatigue during activity.[29] However, there is no cure for this disease.

Without dietary manipulation, Vo_2max is severely reduced in the patient with McArdle's disease (35% to 50% of normal).[25,30,32,50] Maximal cardiac output appears to be normal, but the ability to extract and use oxygen at the muscle site is severely restricted.[29,48] Anaerobic performance is also reduced in these patients. Maximal isometric hand grip endurance is only 30% to 50% of normal. The muscle is less efficient than normal, since only adenosine triphosphate (ATP) and phosphocreatine stores can be used for this type of activity. Anaerobic glycogenolysis does not occur, thus the lack of high-intensity muscle endurance.[49]

A rare glycogen disorder is an absence of the enzyme phosphofructokinase (PFK). Phosphofructokinase is one of the enzymes responsible for the process of glycogen and glucose oxidation. The reaction PFK catalyzes is a nonreversible phosphorylation of fructose 6-phosphate to fructose

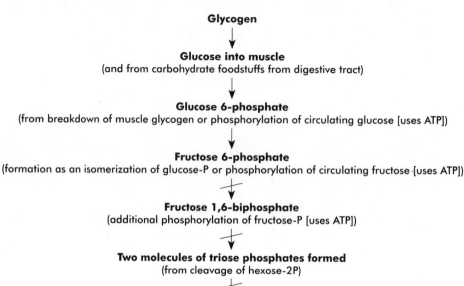

Glycogen

↓

Glucose into muscle
(and from carbohydrate foodstuffs from digestive tract)

↓

Glucose 6-phosphate
(from breakdown of muscle glycogen or phosphorylation of circulating glucose [uses ATP])

↓

Fructose 6-phosphate
(formation as an isomerization of glucose-P or phosphorylation of circulating fructose [uses ATP])

↓

Fructose 1,6-biphosphate
(additional phosphorylation of fructose-P [uses ATP])

↓

Two molecules of triose phosphates formed
(from cleavage of hexose-2P)

↓

Two molecules of pyruvate formed
(formation as oxidation occurs of triose phosphates [net two electrons removed] and generation of four ATP molecules [substrate-level phosphorylation of ADP])

B   Glucose + 2 NAD$^+$ + 2 (ADP + P$_i$) $\longrightarrow$ 2 pyruvate$^-$ + 2 NADH + 2 ATP

Fig. 3-3   **A** and **B,** Schemata depicting phosphofructokinase deficiency disease. **B,** Complete Embden-Meyerhof (glycolytic) pathway. *ADP,* Adenosine diphosphate; *ATP,* adenosine triphosphate; *NAD,* nicotinamide adenine dinucleotide; *NADH,* reduced NAD; *P$_i$,* inorganic phosphate.

1,6-biphosphate (Fig. 3-3), a critical step in the glycolytic pathway. The result of PFK deficiency is that glucose is unavailable for use as a fuel source.[79] Therefore in this condition circulatory glucose is not a viable fuel source, nor is glucose provided by muscle glycogen breakdown. This circumstance leads to an accumulation of glycogen in the muscle and a complete dependence on FFA for fuel during all activities, regardless of intensity.[31] As with McArdle's disease, patients deficient in PFK have severe fatigue when performing activity of moderate to high intensity.[89] Milder exercise is better tolerated, since FFA is used as a fuel

source.[31] Accumulation of lactate and hydrogen ion does not occur in PFK deficiency, since glycolysis is inactivated. Yet the patient is susceptible to fatigue, muscle contractures, pain, and muscle damage during strenuous ischemic exercise.[41]

Lipid oxidation is the only means of energy production in patients with PFK deficiency. These patients also have the phenomenon of "second wind" (similar to that in patients with McArdle's disease), which is related to increased FFA use, that follows near-exhaustion during exercise.[49] The mechanisms for increased FFA use appear to be the same as for patients with McArdle's disease (that is, increased cardiac output at any given level of oxygen uptake during submaximal exercise, increased local blood flow to skeletal muscle, and increased mobilization of FFA from adipocytes.[48] Infusion of FFA and dietary modifications appear to improve oxygen consumption and exercise performance and decrease the severity of fatigue.[48] Infusion of glucose in these patients appears to retard the process of FFA mobilization, and performance during exercise is actually poorer than without infusion of glucose, with markedly reduced oxygen consumption and earlier fatigability.[31] Haller et al.[31] coined the term "out-of-wind effect" to describe this response. As with McArdle's disease, there is no cure for PFK deficiency.

When PFK-deficient patients do not receive FFA manipulation, Vo_2max is severely reduced (30% to 40% of normal).[52] Maximal cardiac output is normal in these patients, but the ability to extract and use oxygen is severely restricted.[52] Anaerobic performance and power production are also severely affected, at only 10% to 20% of normal age-matched performance.[52] Maximal work loads during cycle ergometry were between 15 and 25 watts, whereas matched women in normal health achieved maximal work loads of 110 to 150 watts before the onset of fatigue.

As previously described, in patients with diseases that affect glycogenolysis and glycolysis, exercise of moderate to high intensity is not well tolerated. There is an increase in blood flow to the muscle (two to three times greater than normal) and an increase in cardiac output. These reactions may result in an increased substrate delivery, but during exercise of moderate to high intensity the demand for fuel exceeds the availability and the result is a severe fatiguing of the muscle. The fatigue in McArdle's disease and PFK deficiency is not caused by ATP depletion or hydrogen ion accumulation but might be due to accumulation of adenosine diphosphate (ADP), which would inhibit the production of ATP by the mitochondria.[48]

Other values are also affected in McArdle's disease and PFK deficiency. These patients have Vo_2max levels that are only one third of normal levels. The patients have normal cardiac output, but the ability to use oxygen within the mitochon-

dria is the limiting factor. This lack of oxygen use may be due to a decrease in the production of reduced molecules (primarily, reduced nicotinamide adenine dinucleotide [NADH]) during the Krebs cycle, since there is a lack of muscle pyruvate from glycolysis and subsequently a decreased formation of acetyl-CoA. These data appear to be supported by experiments performed to increase oxidative fuels by means of dietary manipulation or infusion therapy of FFA,[31,49] or both. Therefore an increase in dietary FFA in patients with either condition and the addition of glucose in patients with McArdle's disease may be beneficial but have not been thoroughly studied.

The effect of exercise training may be to decrease dependence on glycogen and to increase FFA use, thereby increasing oxygen extraction.[26,49] Muscle damage, swelling, and soreness during and after high-intensity exercise have been reported in these patients and appear to be related to ischemia.[81] Therefore, once again, high-intensity, isometric, and ischemic exercise should be avoided by individuals with these conditions. Low-intensity exercise appears to be better tolerated. The effect of low-intensity exercise training on FFA oxidation, work capacity, and fitness appears to be beneficial for patients with glycogenolysis and glycolysis disorders.[26]

If a patient has a disorder in glucose and glycogen metabolism, high-intensity exercise is not well tolerated. Diets high in FFA and glucose (for McArdle's disease only) may be beneficial. Fasting to increase FFA availability has been shown to be effective but in long-term practice may not be practical. Low-intensity exercise training appears beneficial and results in improved FFA use and increased work capacity; such training might decrease risk factors associated with cardiovascular disease and with the diets high in fat content that may be recommended for these patients.

Disorders of fuel use have been described. These disorders are rare, and many practitioners may never work with these patients. However, diseases of hormonal regulation and energy imbalance are much more common and are seen daily by many practitioners. Diabetes mellitus and obesity are discussed in the following section.

DIABETES AND OBESITY: EXERCISE TOLERANCE AND EFFECT OF EXERCISE TRAINING

Disorders of fuel use are described in the previous section. The control of fuel mobilization and the uptake of fuel are also critical processes that must be fine-tuned to optimize metabolism. In this section type 1 diabetes mellitus (insulin-dependent or juvenile-onset) and type 2 diabetes mellitus (non–insulin-dependent or adult-onset) are described. In addition, the implication of the disease for exercise tolerance and the effect of exercise training on the symptoms of the disease process are discussed.

Type 1 Diabetes

Type 1 diabetes is believed to be a genetic disease in which a lack of hormone production from the pancreas results in an absence of or low concentrations of insulin and glucagon. Insulin is released in response to increases in blood glucose concentration. The result is rapid uptake of glucose into skeletal muscle and adipose tissue. The processes of glucose storage (as glycogen) and fat storage are enhanced, and the processes of stored fuel breakdown and fuel mobilization are inhibited. Glucagon is a hormone that acts in direct opposition to insulin and works in close association with blood-borne catecholamines to promote stored fuel breakdown and mobilization and inhibit fuel storage. In the treatment of type 1 diabetes, insulin, not glucagon, is the hormone that is manipulated. In addition to insulin therapy, diet and exercise have been considered cornerstones for successful treatment of this disease. Dietary recommendations for the person with type 1 diabetes have shifted from a high-protein diet to a diet that is lower in protein and fat and includes complex carbohydrates from grains, vegetables, and fruits.[9] In the next section the response to exercise in individuals with type 1 diabetes is discussed in detail.

Exercise tolerance. How patients with type 1 diabetes respond to a bout of exercise depends on when and how an insulin dose is given and when food was ingested.

First, the response is described to a standard treatment of insulin injected into one or two sites subcutaneously 30 to 45 minutes after a meal and 15 minutes before exercise. This method of insulin replacement does not mimic the normal secretion of insulin from the pancreas. The result may be insulin deficiency or, more commonly, insulin excess.[92]

Insulin deficiency simply means that not enough insulin is present to cause glucose uptake from the circulatory system and to retard hepatic glycogenolysis and FFA mobilization. When insulin deficiency is present, exercise results in an increase in the already elevated plasma glucose level and an accelerated ketone body formation.[3] The stimulus of exercise in the presence of insulin is to increase uptake of glucose from the circulatory system. If insulin is not present or is in low concentrations, the uptake at the skeletal muscle can be slower than the release of glucose from the liver and mediated by increased catecholamine activity.[87] In addition, catecholamine-stimulated FFA release from adipose tissue results in accelerated ketone body formation in the liver. The result can be mental confusion and further deterioration in metabolic control.[92] Therefore under conditions of insulin deficiency in type 1 diabetes, exercise after feeding is not well tolerated. To reduce the hyperglycemic condition, exercise must be stopped and insulin given.

More commonly resulting from a standard form of insulin delivery than insulin deficiency is insulin excess. In this scenario the exercising muscles are taking up large amounts of blood glucose, yet there is an insulin-caused inhibition of hepatic glycogenolysis.[84] The catecholamine response has been placed in check by the hyperinsulinemic state. The result is a low blood glucose level (hypoglycemia), mental confusion, and occasionally nausea and coma.[39,93,94] Under conditions of insulin excess and hypoglycemia, therefore, exercise is not well tolerated. To increase blood glucose concentration, exercise must be stopped and glucose given. Hyperinsulinemia can be precipitated by the rapid absorption of an insulin depot in an exercising limb, which results in the insulin being absorbed too quickly into the circulatory system.[39,93] It is clear that the standard insulin injection method makes a normal metabolic response to exercise difficult to achieve.

Research into the use of moderate-intensity (60% to 70% Vo_2max) exercise of moderate duration (30 to 45 minutes) without insulin injection was undertaken to determine whether a more predictable, less hazardous method of controlling blood glucose levels could be established.[11] The reasoning behind the use of exercise alone to control blood glucose levels is that during exercise blood glucose is removed from the circulation by the active muscles. As discussed earlier, if insulin is present, this uptake is enhanced, but without insulin, uptake does occur. To achieve a lowered glucose level, however, hepatic glycogenolysis must not be overly stimulated by the catecholamine response observed during exercise. This type of research has shown that some patients are able to nicely lower the blood glucose level, whereas others are not.[11] These results may have occurred because some patients require a specific exercise intensity so that glucose, not FFA, is the preferential fuel and so that catecholamine is not overly stimulated. If the proper intensity were found (high enough to stimulate glucose preferentially, yet not so high as to cause an overstimulation of catecholamine), better glycemic control might be the result.[57] This adjustment of exercise intensity appears to be a case-by-case phenomenon and would require that the individual patient undergo different trials of varying exercise intensity while the blood glucose level is being monitored. Finding a proper intensity of exercise would be beneficial for the patient, since oscillating insulin concentrations make exercise a potentially hazardous activity and insulin use over time appears to have negative side effects. One recent intervention that has been tried and appears to be effective is the use of insulin infusion pumps.

Insulin infusion pumps can administer insulin subcutaneously or intravenously. The difference between injected insulin and insulin infused by pump is that the insulin delivered via the pump is not in a bolus ejected all at one time. The subcutaneous infusion pump has been used successfully with patients during exercise in both postabsorptive (overnight fasted) and postprandial conditions. Steady-state glucose concentrations have been maintained much like in normal controls.[62,93] In addition to the advantage of slow, controlled delivery of insulin, the overall insulin amount can be decreased by as much as 30%. The subcutaneous infusion pump has a distinct advantage over insulin injection but is not as "physiologically normal" as the pancreas's release of insulin directly into the circulatory system. This limitation has led to trial use of intravenous insulin infusion pumps. This type of technology, the delivery of insulin in a manner similar to that from the pancreas, may eventually result in the elimination of insulin injection therapy. The advantage of the IV pump is that less insulin is required than when injected, to achieve "normal" blood glucose responses at rest and during exercise.[62] The responses during exercise with and without insulin therapy have been discussed. Whether an exercise training regimen has a positive effect on patients with type 1 diabetes is discussed in the next section.

Effect of exercise training. As described earlier, there appears to be a positive effect on blood glucose concentration during exercise in some patients, even without insulin therapy. Can exercise training result in consistently lowered blood glucose concentrations for these patients? A well-controlled study failed to demonstrate a change in glycosylated hemoglobin as the measurement of blood glucose concentration.[86] However, this investigation appeared to study persons with diabetes who were already in moderate to good fitness condition. These individuals further improved fitness, as measured by Vo_2max, by an additional 20% to 25% after 12 weeks of training. These results of no change in glucose level control may have been different in nontrained sedentary persons with type 1 diabetes. Although there was no long-term effect of exercise training on control of blood glucose level, patients with type 1 diabetes should be encouraged to exercise for the same reasons that apply to persons in good health. The benefits of exercise training are improved endurance and, possibly, decreased atherosclerotic diseases (that is, cardiovascular, peripheral, and renal) and risk factors (cholesterol and lipid profiles)[44,86] that are common in in type 1 diabetes.[38] Although the reduced

Case Study 1 was designed to evaluate the effectiveness of an exercise training program on endurance and glycemic control in a physical therapy student, an active 22-year-old woman with type 1 diabetes. The woman had no history of retinopathy or kidney dysfunction.

Before treatment was initiated, baseline data were obtained, including body weight, body composition, and Vo_2max. The woman maintained normal drug therapy, which was injected insulin. Diet was not manipulated but was between 1800 and 2200 calories daily, comprising approximately 70% complex carbohydrate, 20% fat, and 10% protein. The woman was physically active, jogging two or three times per week for as long as 30 minutes at a pace of 11 minutes per mile. Her eventual goal was to run competitive races of 10 km and longer. Her best mile time to date was 8:12, with a 10-km time of 60:45.

The performance-enhancing exercise training program was 12 weeks in duration (five times per week) and consisted of endurance and power components. The endurance component was performed three times per week and consisted of jogging, cycling, and stationary cycling. The power component was performed two times per week and consisted of sprinting and sprint bouts of stationary cycling. During the initial week of training the following regimen was performed:

Monday (endurance day): Jogging at a 10-minute-per-mile pace for 35 minutes (3.5 miles, total)

Tuesday (power day): Stationary sprint cycling (ten repetitions of a 30-second sprint at 250 watts, with 60 seconds of recovery time between repetitions and 2 minutes of rest between the first five and the last five repetitions), resulting in nearly complete fatigue

Wednesday (day off)

Thursday (power day): Sprinting (nine 200-meter repetitions, with 90 seconds of recovery time between repetitions and 3 minutes of rest after every three repetitions, resulting in nearly complete fatigue

Friday (endurance day): Stationary cycling (30 minutes at 100 watts, attaining a heart rate of 170 to 175 beats per min)

Saturday (endurance day): Jogging at a 10-minute-per-mile pace for 35 minutes

Sunday (day off)

The final week of training was similar, with the same endurance and power days but different intensity and duration, as follows:

Monday (endurance day): Jogging at an 8.5-minute-per-mile pace for 60 minutes (7 miles, total)

Tuesday (power day): Stationary sprint cycling (twenty repetitions of a 30-second sprint at 350 watts, with 60 seconds of recovery time between repetitions and 2 minutes of rest after every five repetitions), resulting in nearly complete fatigue

Wednesday (day off)

Thursday (power day): Sprinting (eighteen 200-meter repetitions, with 90 seconds of recovery time between repetitions and 3 minutes of rest after every three repetitions), resulting in nearly complete fatigue

Friday (endurance day): Stationary cycling (60 minutes at 125 watts, attaining a heart rate of 170 to 175 beats per min)

Saturday (endurance day): Jogging at an 8.5-minute-per-mile pace for 60 minutes

Sunday (day off)

The woman ate fruit or bread, or both, approximately 60 minutes before exercise and received an insulin injection subcutaneously 30 minutes later, that is, thus 30 minutes before exercise. Blood glucose levels were monitored by the finger stick method before each exercise bout and measured with a portable glucometer to ensure euglycemic levels.

Initially the woman had a Vo_2max of 37.2 ml/kg per min, which was determined by means of a graded exercise treadmill test (Balke protocol) with metabolic measures from open circuitry (Gould 9000 metabolic cart). Her initial body weight was 56.8 kg, with an estimated body fat of 19.2% (skinfold measures).

After the 12-week training program her Vo_2max was increased by 27% (up to 47.2 ml/kg per min). Her body weight was reduced by 12 pounds (5.5kg), down to 51.4 kg, with a final estimated body fat of 14.2%. Two weeks later, after a tapering program, she ran a 10-km race, setting a personal best time of 45:22. The patient did not have hypoglycemia or hyperglycemia during the exercise training program.

incidence of morbidity and mortality have not yet been unequivocally proven, the possibility that daily exercise of low to moderate intensity may affect the prognosis of this condition should be further investigated.

Exercise appears to be beneficial in reducing blood glucose concentration with or without insulin therapy. The advent of insulin infusion pumps should further improve the control of insulin delivery and blood glucose concentrations at rest and during exercise for persons with type 1 diabetes. Regular exercise training has not been shown to give improved metabolic control of blood glucose concentration. However, the benefits of exercise training for these patients appear to be the same as for the normal population. *Exercise training and close monitoring of blood glucose concentration should be encouraged in these patients. Contraindications to certain types of exercise should be noted if autonomic neuropathy, kidney disease, or retinopathies exist. Exercise that may lead to dehydration (long duration, such as marathons and cycling events) and intense exercise that includes the possibility of increasing blood pressure (heavy resistance, such as weight lifting) should be avoided.[3]*

Type 2 Diabetes

Type 2 diabetes usually does not result from a deficiency in insulin but from a resistance or insensitivity to insulin. Many persons with type 2 diabetes are obese and actually have higher plasma insulin levels than do individuals of normal weight without diabetes.[6,17,71] In addition to obesity and metabolic abnormalities, the person with type 2 diabetes has a much higher risk for hyperlipidemia, atherosclerosis (vascular and peripheral), and hypertension than does the nondiabetic.[23,38,56,68] The treatment of type 2 diabetes is centered around diet, exercise, and modification of poor life-style habits (smoking, drinking, alcohol, and inactivity). Insulin therapy or drugs that stimulate insulin secretion (such as sulfonylurea) are rarely used in these patients, except when insulin secretion from the pancreas is low. Hormones other than insulin that control metabolic function appear normal in these patients. Why an insensitivity to insulin develops is presently unknown, but

in some cases it is reversible (to a degree) after dietary and life-style modifications and exercise. In the following section the response during exercise in individuals with type 2 diabetes is discussed.

Exercise tolerance. The person with uncontrolled type 2 diabetes has hyperglycemia (elevated blood glucose levels) and normal to elevated blood insulin levels. During a single 45-minute bout of exercise (moderate intensity, at 60% to 70% Vo_2max) blood glucose concentration can be substantially reduced.[55,91] Insulin levels do not appear to change much during exercise in these patients, since they have chronic hyperglycemia. A decline in blood glucose concentration, then, would appear to be primarily the result of peripheral utilization of the fuel at the skeletal muscle site with only minimal hepatic glycogenolysis and glucose release into the circulation. In other words, blood glucose is used at a faster rate than the rate at which it is being produced from the liver. However, the individuals do not become hypoglycemic. The findings of substantially lowered blood glucose levels in response to exercise,[55,91] coupled with results in normal individuals of improved insulin sensitivity after regular training,[4,40,45] have given rise to further scientific exploration to evaluate the effect of an exercise training regimen on long-term blood glucose and insulin concentration control in persons with type 2 diabetes.

Effect of exercise training. Exercise can control blood glucose levels in many persons with type 2 diabetes by significantly lowering the levels without drug intervention. Can a regular exercise training regimen result in consistently lowered blood glucose concentration and improve insulin sensitivity in type 2 diabetics? Unlike persons with type 1 diabetes, who do not show improved glycemic control, persons with type 2 diabetes demonstrate a significant decrease in glycosylated hemoglobin levels after just 6 weeks or more of training.[17,68,73] In addition, glucose tolerance test results are improved after training. The largest improvements in glucose tolerance test results appear to be in diabetics who have a milder than usual form of the disease (that is, blood glucose concentrations of less than 200 mg/dl).[73]

CASE STUDY 2

Case Study 2 was designed to evaluate the effect of a supervised diet and an exercise training program on endurance and glycemic control in a 72-year-old man with mild type 2 diabetes. Before treatment was initiated, baseline data were obtained, including body weight, body composition, estimated Vo_2max, and blood glucose levels. The patient was not placed on a drug therapy regimen during the diet and exercise intervention program.

The supervised exercise training program was 16 weeks in duration (five times per week) and consisted of an endurance component. The mode was walking; the goal was to achieve a heart rate response of 60% to 65% Vo_2max (125 to 130 beats per min), which did correspond to increased ventilation. Walking speed was progressively increased every 2 weeks approximately, when the ventilatory response decreased and the heart rate response was lowered by more than 5 beats per minute. The duration of exercise initially was 15 minutes, with final duration of 45 minutes.

The dietary plan was primarily a restriction of caloric intake to 1600 calories per day, comprising approximately 70% carbohydrate, 20% fat, and 10% protein.

Initially the man had a Vo_2max of 22.2 ml/kg per min, which was estimated from heart rate response during a submaximal treadmill test. Initial body weight was 86.7 kg, and estimated body fat was 24.2% (skinfold measures). Resting blood glucose level was 205 mg/dl (normal values are between 80 and 100 mg/dl).

After the 16-week diet and exercise program of paced walking, the man's estimated Vo_2max increased by 46% (up to 32.4 ml/kg per min). His body weight was reduced by 27 pounds (12.3 kg), down to 74.4 kg, with a final estimated body fat of 15.9%. Resting blood glucose level after the 16-week trial was reduced to 115 mg/dl, which is still a slightly hyperglycemic level. Subjectively the patient noted vast improvements in energy levels and endurance and a much improved self-image of his body.

However, exercise training of 6 to 24 weeks' duration does not appear to result in long-term glycemic control. Once exercise training is stopped, values of glucose tolerance quickly (within a week) reverts to pretraining levels.[68] In addition to glycemic control, oxygen consumption (fitness) is improved by 10% to 20% after 6 to 12 weeks of training at moderate to high intensities (60% to 75% Vo_2max) in persons with type 2 diabetes.[9,66,82] Oxygen consumption improvements tend to last much longer than do glucose tolerance improvements. Other health benefits that are derived from exercise training in persons with type 2 diabetes are weight loss (if a diet is observed),[9] improved lipid profile,[43] and decreased hypertension.[3] However, lipid profile and blood pressure improvements are, again, short-lived phenomena that quickly revert to pretraining levels once exercise is stopped. With continued exercise training, endurance substantially improves and factors affecting atherosclerosis are lowered.

In the studies performed on persons with type 2 diabetes moderate-intensity exercise (60% to 75% Vo_2max) appears to improve glycemic control and fitness levels. Lower-intensity exercise (40% to 60% Vo_2max) improves fitness (since many of these patients are in poor condition), lowers blood pressure, and decreases lipid profiles but does not appear to be as effective in controlling blood glucose levels during exercise, perhaps because at lower exercise intensities FFAs are preferentially used instead of blood glucose, as described in Chapter 2. Daily exercise of moderate intensity (fit patients) or low intensity (sedentary patients) is highly recommended for these patients. Exercise is well tolerated unless preexisting conditions of coronary artery disease, retinopathy, or sensory neuropathy exist; exercise should not be initiated in patients with these conditions until the patients are well evaluated.

Further recommendations can be made for the use of exercise, diet, and healthy life-style in the prevention of type 2 diabetes. *Usually a diagnosis of type 2 diabetes is made in persons older than 40 years of age, after the individual already has significant atherosclerotic disease. Exercise and diet appear to be useful in retarding further atherosclerosis; however, many of these patients are hesitant to embark on lifelong exercise and dietary regimens. Also, some have severe enough symptoms that only exercise of the lowest intensity can be tolerated. Therefore exercise and diet ultimately appear to be most beneficial for younger individuals before the onset of major macrovascular disease. Such individuals include the offspring of persons with type 2 diabetes and individuals with premature atherosclerotic disease.*[53]

It appears that exercise is beneficial in significantly reducing blood glucose concentration and that an exercise regimen results in improved glycemic control (although this improvement may be short-lived, if exercise ceases). Individuals with mild disease and minimal atherosclerosis improve most. Therefore early screening for diabetes, consultation, and the initiation of early intervention programs for offspring of persons with type 2 diabetes are highly recommended.

Obesity

Most scientific evidence has demonstrated that obese individuals have resting metabolic rates similar to those in persons of normal weight, when lean mass is equalized.[64,76] However, when matched by body weight with an individual who has a higher percentage of lean mass and a greater total of lean mass, the resting metabolic rate is less in the obese individual.[77]

When obese and normal individuals are placed on highly restrictive diets, both groups initially lose weight but the resting metabolic rate is substantially reduced in both groups as a result of loss of lean body mass.[75,88] Another common finding when normal and obese individuals are compared

is that obese individuals tend to be less active.[74,80] Decreased lean mass in relation to body weight, increased caloric consumption, and decreased activity might explain most cases of obesity.

The obese individual is at higher risk than the lean individual for diabetes, hyperlipidemia, atherosclerosis (vascular and peripheral), and hypertension.[36] The treatment of obesity has been centered around diet and exercise. As described briefly in the preceding paragraph, diet alone, when of extremely low caloric intake, has been successful in causing weight loss. Yet with this drastic dietary manipulation, resting and exercising metabolic rates appear to be negatively affected, since lean mass can be significantly reduced. It has been reported that some individuals who lose weight rapidly as a result of low-calorie diets regain lost weight after completion of the dietary effort and that in some cases the weight gain exceeds the amount initially lost.[22,75] In the following sections the responses to exercise and to exercise training regimens in obese individuals is further discussed.

Exercise tolerance. Exercise causes an increase in metabolic activity in obese individuals that is similar to the response in lean individuals.[78] The type of exercise does not appear to be a factor, since both weight bearing (walking or jogging) and non–weight bearing (cycle ergometry) produced similar energy expenditure in obese and lean individuals.[77] Another response during an exercise bout in the individual with obesity is an increase in insulin sensitivity. This improved insulin sensitivity results in an increase in total glucose uptake and glucose oxidation by active muscles.[7,18]

During exercise there is no difference in energy expenditure in obese and lean individuals. Postexercise energy expenditure is elevated in both groups but not for any extended period. Elevated energy expenditure usually lasts for only 2 to 3 hours after exercise, regardless of the individual's body composition. Lean individuals have greater energy expenditure than obese individuals[77] after exercise. Lean individuals have the greatest energy expenditure after exercise when they eat before the exercise event. Obese individuals, however, have the greatest energy expenditure after exercise when they eat immediately after exercise. Regardless of eating pattern, energy expenditure is greater in lean individuals than in obese individuals.[76] There appears to be a subtle metabolic defect in the obese individual that favors conservation of energy after activity. This conservation results in 50% less energy use after exercise than in lean individuals of comparable lean mass. The cause of this metabolic defect is unknown.

As described previously, the beneficial effects of exercise are improved metabolism and energy utilization. The question remains, can an exercise training regimen with or without dietary intervention result in sustained higher metabolic rates, lowered body weight, elevated lean mass, improved muscle strength and endurance, and decreased risk factors for cardiovascular disease?

Effect of exercise training. Before the effect of exercise training on the obese individual is discussed, the clinician must realize that many obese persons may not be able to participate initially in traditional exercise modes or to participate at durations and intensities that result in adaptations. Clinicians who are extremely active in working with obese patients have noted that individuals with body mass indexes (W divided by H^2, that is, W = body weight [kg] and H = body height [m]) greater than 40 and elevated body fat percentages have extremely low exercise tolerance.[22] In many cases these patients have extreme difficulty walking or riding a cycle ergometer. In these morbidly obese individuals initial weight loss might best be accomplished by a combination of dietary means and nontraditional exercise such as swimming pool therapy performed at low intensity with increased frequency of sessions at shorter duration. For individuals who are only slightly obese (body mass index of 20 to 25) weight reduction programs should almost exclusively emphasize exercise. It has been recommended that emphasis on exercise versus restrictive diet be related to this continuum of body mass index during initial intervention. However, practitioners should always evaluate nontraditional exercise modes that can be performed by morbidly obese individuals. Factors

in a successful exercise program include the following:

Promotion of cardiovascular and musculoskeletal fitness

Limited potential for increasing the incidences of orthopedic and cardiovascular diseases or disorders

Appeal to participants

Availability within the community

If these issues of effectiveness, safety, enjoyment, and practicality can be met, the chance for success in working with these patients is greatly improved.

As described in earlier sections, an exercise bout results in an elevation of the metabolic rate and increased energy consumption, at least for several hours after the activity. However, can metabolic rate, body weight, and lean mass in the obese patient be altered with training?

The major determinant of the resting metabolic rate is the individual's lean body mass. The major determinant of weight loss is negative energy balance (fewer calories consumed than used). With traditional aerobic training programs incorporating walking and cycling lean mass remains unchanged,[16] whereas in most studies of aerobic training with unaltered diet body weight does not change.[78] A few studies that incorporated daily exercise of long duration (90 to 120 minutes) without incorporating dietary restriction[24,46] did show significant loss of body weight. These two protocols are probably impractical for most individuals and certainly impractical for the morbidly obese patient.

Most studies have indicated that when aerobic training is coupled with caloric restriction, lean body mass decreases and resting metabolic rate is concurrently lowered but body weight is significantly reduced.[33] When compared to dietary restriction alone, aerobic exercise coupled with caloric restriction, although not lean-mass sparing, does not enhance loss of lean mass.[10,35]

Few studies have evaluated the effect of resistance training on metabolic rate, lean mass, and body weight changes in the obese individual. One problem that arises with resistance training

CASE STUDY 3

Case Study 3 was designed to evaluate the effect of an exercise training program on weight loss, endurance, and strength in a 48-year-old woman with morbid obesity (body mass index, 47.4; weight, 131 kg; and body fat, 47%).

Before treatment was initiated, baseline data were obtained, including body weight, body composition, estimated Vo_2 max, and strength in the upper and lower body. The patient was not placed on a restrictive diet during the exercise intervention program.

The supervised exercise training program was 16 weeks in duration (four times per week) and consisted of endurance and resistive training components, both performed during each training session. The mode for the endurance program was cycle ergometry, and the goal was to achieve a heart rate response of 70% Vo_2 max (140 to 160 beats per min). Initially the woman needed a resistance of only 60 watts to attain this high heart rate. Cycling resistance was progressively increased in 5- 10-watt increments approximately every 2 weeks, when the heart rate response was lowered by at least 5 beats per minute. The duration of exercise initially was 10 minutes, with final duration of 45 minutes.

The mode for the resistance program was a regimen of hydraulically resisted quadricep and hamstring curls, bicep and tricep curls, and bench press (Omnitron, Hydrafitness Industries, Belton, Texas). Each exercise bout consisted of four sets of six repetitions at most for each individual exercise. The duration for the resistance program was approximately 30 minutes.

Initially the woman had a Vo_2max of 14.2 ml/kg per min, which was estimated from heart rate response during a submaximal cycle ergometry test. Maximal muscle-strength measurements for one repetition each were obtained during knee flexion and extension, elbow flexion and extension, and the bench press.

After the 16-week exercise program of cycle ergometry and resistance training, the woman's estimated Vo_2max increased by 79% (up to 25.4 ml/kg per min). Her body weight was reduced by 48 pounds, down to 109.1 kg, with a final estimated body fat of 40.8% and a body mass index of 39.6. Her muscle strength increased by 42%, 36%, and 48% in the lower extremity and upper extremity and during the bench press, respectively. Subjectively the patient was enthusiastic about her appearance and physical accomplishments.

---

exercise protocols is that total energy use is usually much lower than in aerobic training exercise protocols.[20] In two studies that incorporated resistance training, total body fat and weight were unaltered.[1,42] Ballor et al.,[1] however, did find increases in lean mass in a group of obese individuals who weight trained without dietary intervention. When resistance training is coupled with a restricted diet, weight loss is accomplished and it appears that lean mass is not merely spared but increased.[1] However, the previously cited study incorporated data for only a few individuals (eight in each of four groups) and is the only study found to evaluate resistance training in combination with dietary restriction.

Since it is possible that weight reduction accomplished primarily by means of caloric restriction can reduce lean mass, the effect on performance must be discussed. It appears that a restricted diet does not result in decreased Vo_2max. Yet, submaximal aerobic endurance does appear to be decreased in obese individuals undergoing dietary restriction.[8] This decline in endurance appears to be related directly to a decrease in muscle glycogen stores. When dietary restriction is coupled with aerobic endurance training, the results of measurement of outcome are mixed for endurance performance. It appears that if the training intensity is moderate to high (greater than 70% Vo$_2$max), endurance performance is enhanced.[59] If the training intensity is low (less than 50% Vo$_2$max), endurance performance declines, as when dietary restriction alone is used.[85]

During severe dietary restriction in obese patients muscle strength declines,[69] resulting in muscle tissue atrophy and necrosis.[70] When dietary restriction is coupled with resistance training or high-intensity aerobic activity, strength is spared and hypertrophy of muscle may result.[1,59]

Further recommendations can be made for the use of exercise and diet in the prevention of obesity. As described in the earlier section on type 2 diabetes, exercise and diet appear to be useful in retarding atherosclerosis and cardiovascular disease. Yet, as with persons with type 2 diabetes, many obese patients are hesitant to embark on lifelong exercise and dietary regimens. Also, some obese patients are so large and deconditioned that only the lowest intensity of exercise can be tolerated for only brief duration. Again as for those with diabetes, exercise and diet appear to be most beneficial ultimately for younger individuals with obesity, especially obese adolescents (see Chapter 12).

It appears that exercise is beneficial in increasing metabolic rate, whereas an aerobic exercise training regimen does not appear to result in a sustained metabolic rate or elevation in lean mass. Aerobic training coupled with diet does result in lowered body weight, but lean mass may be decreased significantly. Resistance training alone or coupled with a restricted diet may increase lean mass, although total body weight is decreased. However, resistance training generally results in the utilization of fewer calories than do aerobic activities. *Generally exercise is the recommended intervention when the patient is slightly obese. For morbid obesity dietary intervention is recommended initially, since exercise tolerance is low. As with diabetes, the atherosclerotic process might be altered. Therefore dietary, exercise, and education interventions should be focused at the youngest population, the children.*

SUMMARY

Relatively few studies of the response to exercise and exercise training in patients with metabolic disorders have been published. It does appear that patients with diabetes and obesity can improve muscle strength and endurance and reduce cardiovascular risk factors by means of exercise training. Specific concerns and precautions for each patient group have been discussed, and strategies for improving cardiovascular condition and muscle strength have been provided in individual sections and in the case studies in this chapter.

REFERENCES

1. Ballor DL et al: Resistance weight training during caloric restriction enhances lean body weight maintenance, *Am J Clin Nutr* 47:19, 1988.
2. Barcroft H et al: The effect of exercise on forearm blood flow and on venous blood flow in a subject with phosphorylase deficiency in skeletal muscle (McArdle's syndrome), *J Physiol (Lond)* 184:44P, 1966.
3. Berger M: Exercise as therapy in diabetic and cardiac patients, *Biochem Exerc* 16:311, 1986.
4. Berger M et al: Effect of physical training on glucose tolerance and on glucose metabolism of skeletal muscle in anaesthetized normal rats, *Diabetologia* 16:179, 1979.
5. Bertorini TE et al: ATP degradation products after ischemic exercise: hereditary lack of phosphorylase or carnitine palmityltransferase, *Neurology* 35:1355, 1985.
6. Bjorntorp P: Effects of exercise on plasma insulin, *Int J Sports Med* 2:125, 1981.
7. Bjorntorp P et al: The effect of physical training on insulin production in obesity, *Metabolism* 19:631, 1970.
8. Bogardus C et al: Comparison of carbohydrate containing and carbohydrate restricted diets in the treatment of obesity, *J Clin Invest* 58:399, 1981.
9. Bogardus C et al: Effects of physical training and diet therapy on carbohydrate metabolism in patients with glucose intolerance and non–insulin-dependent diabetes mellitus, *Diabetes* 33:311, 1984.
10. Bosello O et al: Semistarvation and physical exercise in the treatment of obesity. In Enzi et al, editors: *Seron Symposium 28. Obesity: pathogenesis and treatment,* New York, 1981, Academic.
11. Caron D et al: The effect of postprandial exercise on meal-related glucose tolerance in insulin-dependent diabetic individuals, *Diabetes Care* 5:364, 1982.
12. Carroll JE et al: Biochemical and physiologic consequences of carnitine palmityltransferase deficiency, *Muscle Nerve* 1:103, 1978.
13. Carroll JE et al: Bicycle ergometry and gas exchange measurements in neuromuscular diseases, *Arch Neurol* 36:457, 1979.

14. Carroll JE et al: Fasting as a provocative test in neuromuscular diseases, *Metabolism* 28:683, 1979.

15. Carroll JE et al: Riboflavin-responsive lipid myopathy and carnitine deficiency, *Neurology* 31:1557, 1981.

16. Davis JR, Tagliaferro AR, Kertzer R: Variations of dietary-induced thermogenesis and body fatness with aerobic capacity, *Eur J Appl Physiol Occup Physiol* 509:319, 1983.

17. DeFronzo RA, Ferrannini E, Koivisto V: New concepts in the pathogenesis and treatment of non–insulin-dependent diabetes, *Am J Med* 74:52, 1983.

18. Devlin JT, Horton ES: Effects of prior high-intensity exercise on glucose metabolism in normal and insulin-resistant men, *Diabetes* 34:973, 1985.

19. DiMauro S, Melis-DiMauro PM: Muscle carnitine palmityltransferase deficiency and myoglobinuria, *Science* 182:929, 1973.

20. Dudley GA: Metabolic consequences of resistive-type exercise, *Med Sci Sports Exerc* 20:S158, 1988.

21. Engel AG, Angelini C: Carnitine deficiency of human skeletal muscle with associated lipid storage myopathy: a new syndrome, *Science* 179:899, 1973.

22. Garrow JS: Effect of exercise on obesity, *Acta Med Scand Suppl* 711:67, 1986.

23. Greenfield M et al: Mechanism of hypertriglyceridaemia in diabetic patients with fasting hyperglycaemia, *Diabetologia* 18:441, 1980.

24. Gwinup G: Effect of exercise alone on the weight of obese women, *Arch Intern Med* 135:676, 1975.

25. Hagberg JM et al: Exercise hyperventilation in patients with McArdle's disease, *J Appl Physiol* 52:991, 1982.

26. Haller RG, Lewis SF: Physical conditioning: a rational treatment of muscle phosphofructokinase deficiency, *Neurology* 38(suppl 1):341, 1988.

27. Haller RG et al: A lipid myopathy associated with a hyperkinetic circulatory response to exercise, *Trans Am Neurol Assoc* 104:117, 1979.

28. Haller RG et al: Hyperkinetic circulation during exercise in neuromuscular disease, *Neurology* 33:1283, 1983.

29. Haller RG et al: Myophosphorylase deficiency impairs muscle oxidative metabolism, *Ann Neurol* 17:196, 1985.

30. Haller RG et al: Ammonia production during exercise in McArdle's syndrome: an index of muscle energy supply and demand, *Neurology* 35:207, 1985.

31. Haller RG et al: Glucose impairs exercise performance in muscle phosphofructokinase deficiency: the ''out of wind'' effect, *Neurology* 39(suppl 1):270, 1988.

32. Heller SL et al: McArdle's disease with myoadenylate deaminase deficiency: observations in a combined enzyme deficiency, *Neurology* 37:1039, 1987.

33. Henson LC et al: Effects of exercise training on resting energy expenditure during caloric restriction, *Am J Clin Nutr* 46:893, 1987.

34. Hermansen L, Hultman E, Saltin B: Muscle glycogen during prolonged severe exercise, *Acta Physiol Scand* 71:129, 1967.

35. Hill JO et al: Effects of exercise and food restriction on body composition and metabolic rate in obese women, *Am J Clin Nutr* 46:622, 1987.

36. Hubert HB, Feinleib M, McNamara PM: Obesity as an independent risk factor for cardiovascular disease: a 26-year follow-up of participants in the Framingham study, *Circulation* 67:968, 1983.

37. Hultman E: Studies on muscle metabolism of glycogen and active phosphate in man with special reference to exercise and diet, *Scand J Clin Invest* 19(suppl 94):1, 1967.

38. Kannel WB, McGee DL: Diabetes and cardiovascular disease: the Framingham study, *JAMA* 241:2035, 1979.

39. Koivisto V, Felig P: Effects of leg exercise on insulin absorption in diabetic patients, *New Engl J Med* 298:77, 1978.

40. Koivisto V, Soman V, Felig P: Effects of acute exercise on insulin binding to monocytes in trained athletes: changes in the resting state and after exercise, *J Clin Invest* 64:1011, 1979.

41. Kono N et al: Increased plasma uric acid after exercise in muscle phosphofructokinase deficiency, *Neurology* 36:106, 1986.

42. Krotkiewski M et al: The effect of unilateral isokinetic strength training on local adipose and muscle tissue morphology, thickness, and enzymes, *Eur J Appl Physiol* 42:271, 1979.

43. Lampman RM, Schteingart DE: Effects of exercise training on glucose control, lipid metabolism, and insulin sensitivity in hypertriglyceridemia and non–insulin-dependent diabetes mellitus, *Med Sci Sports Exerc* 23:703, 1991.

44. Larsson Y et al: Effect of exercise on blood lipids in juvenile diabetes, *Lancet* 1:350, 1964.

45. LeBlanc J et al: Effects of physical training and adiposity in glucose metabolism and I-insulin binding, *J Appl Physiol* 46:235, 1979.

46. Leon AS et al: Effects of a vigorous walking program on body composition and carbohydrate and lipid metabolism of obese young men, *Am J Clin Nutr* 32:1776, 1979.

47. Lewis SF, Haller RG: The pathophysiology of McArdle's disease: clues to regulation in exercise and fatigue, *J Appl Physiol* 61:391, 1986.

48. Lewis SF, Haller RG: Disorders of muscle glycogenolysis/glycolysis: the consequences of substrate-limited oxidative metabolism in humans, *Biochem Exerc* 21:211, 1989.

49. Lewis SF, Haller RG: Skeletal muscle disorders and associated factors that limit exercise performance, *Exerc Sport Sci Rev* 17:67, 1989.

50. Lewis SF et al: Metabolic control of cardiac output response to exercise in McArdle's disease, *J Appl Physiol* 57:1749, 1984.

51. Lewis SF et al: Availability of oxidative substrate and leg blood flow during exercise in McArdle's disease, *Fed Proc* 45:783, 1986.

52. Lewis SF et al: Disordered oxidative metabolism in muscle phosphofructokinase deficiency, *Neurology* 38(suppl 1):269, 1988.

53. Lithel HOL: Lipoprotein metabolism and physical training in normal men and diabetic and cardiac patients, *Biochem Exerc* 16:279, 1986.

54. McArdle B: Myopathy due to a defect in muscle glycogen breakdown, *Clin Sci* 10:13, 1951.

55. Minuk HL et al: Glucoregulatory and metabolic response in obese and non–insulin-dependent diabetes, *Am J Physiol* 240:E458, 1981.

56. Olefsky JM, Farquhar JW, Reaven GM: Reappraisal of the role of insulin in hypertriglyceridemia, *Am J Med* 57:551, 1974.

57. Oelfsky JM et al: Insulin resistance in non–insulin-dependent (type 2) and insulin-dependent (type 1) diabetes mellitus, *Adv Exp Med Biol* 189:176, 1985.

58. Paul P: Effects of long-lasting physical exercise and training on lipid metabolism. In Howald H, Poortmans JR, editors: *Metabolic adaptation to prolonged physical exercise,* Basel, 1975, Birkhauser Verlang.

59. Pavlou KN et al: Effects of dieting and exercise on lean body mass, oxygen uptake, and strength, *Med Sci Sports Exerc* 17:466, 1985.

60. Pearson CM, Rimer DG, Mommaerts WHFM: A metabolic myopathy due to absence of muscle phosphorylase, *Am J Med* 30:502, 1961.

61. Pernow BB, Havel RJ, Jennings DB: The second-wind phenomenon in McArdle's syndrome, *Acta Med Scand Suppl* 472:294, 1967.

62. Poussier P et al: Open loop intravenous insulin waveforms for postprandial exercise in type 1 diabetes, *Diabetes Care* 6:129, 1983.

63. Pruett EDR: Glucose and insulin during prolonged work stress in men living on different diets, *J Appl Physiol* 28:199, 1970.

64. Ravussin E, Burnand B, Schutz Y: Twenty-four hour energy expenditure and resting metabolic rate in obese, moderately obese, and control subjects, *Am J Clin Nutr* 35:566, 1982.

65. Reichman H: Disorders of lipid metabolism in muscle and their exercise implications, *Biochem Exerc* 21:243, 1989.

66. Reitman JS et al: Improvement of glucose homeostasis after exercise training in non–insulin-dependent diabetes, *Diabetes Care* 7:434, 1984.

67. Rowland LP, Araki S, Carmel P: Contracture in McArdle's disease, *Arch Neurol* 13:541, 1965.

68. Ruderman NB, Ganda OP, Johansen K: The effect of physical training on glucose tolerance and plasma lipids in maturity onset diabetes, *Diabetes* 28(suppl 1):89, 1979.

69. Russell DM et al: Skeletal muscle function during hypocaloric diets and fasting: a comparison with standard nutritional assessment parameters, *Am J Clin Nutr* 37:133, 1983.

70. Russell DM et al: Metabolic and structural changes in skeletal muscle during hypocaloric dieting, *Am J Clin Nutr* 39:503, 1984.

71. Saltin B et al: Physical training and glucose tolerance in middle-aged men with chemical diabetes, *Diabetes* 28(suppl 1):30, 1979.

72. Scarlato G et al: The syndrome of carnitine deficiency: morphological and metabolic correlations, *J Can Sci Neurol* 5:205, 1978.

73. Schneider SH et al: Studies on the mechanism of improved glucose control during regular exercise in type 2 (non–insulin-dependent) diabetes, *Diabetologia* 26:355, 1984.

74. Schutz Y et al: Spontaneous physical activity measured by radar in obese and control subjects studied in a respiratory chamber, *Int J Obes* 6:23, 1982.

75. Schutz Y et al: Decreased glucose-induced thermogenesis after weight loss in obese subjects: a predisposing factor for relapse of obesity, *Am J Clin Nutr* 39:380, 1984.

76. Segal KR, Gutin B, Albu J: Thermic effects of food and exercise in lean and obese men of similar lean body weight, *Am J Physiol* 252:E110, 1987.

77. Segal KR, Gutin B, Nyman AM: Thermic effect of food at rest, during exercise, and after exercise in lean and obese men of similar body weight, *J Clin Invest* 76:1107, 1985.

78. Segal KR, Pi-Sunyer FX: Exercise and obesity, *Med Clin North Am* 73:217, 1989.

79. Tarui S et al: Phosphofructokinase deficiency in skeletal muscle: a new type of glycogenosis, *Biochem Biophys Res Commun* 19:517, 1965.

80. Thompson JK, Jarvie GJ, Lahey BB: Exercise and obesity: etiology, physiology, and intervention, *Psych Bull* 91:55, 1982.

81. Tobin WE et al: Muscle phosphofructokinase deficiency, *Arch Neurol* 28:128, 1973.

82. Trovati M et al: Influence of physical training on blood glucose control, glucose tolerance, insulin secretion, and insulin action in non–insulin-dependent diabetic patients, *Diabetes Care* 7:416, 1984.

83. Turnbull DM et al: Short-chain acyl-CoA dehydrogenase deficiency associated with a lipid storage myopathy and secondary carnitine deficiency, *New Engl J Med* 311:1232, 1984.

84. Vranic M, Lickley HLA: Hormonal mechanisms that act to preserve glucose homeostasis during exercise: two controversial issues, *Biochem Exerc* 21:279, 1989.

85. Walberg JL et al: Exercise capacity and nitrogen loss during a high- or low-carbohydrate diet, *Med Sci Sports Exerc* 20:34, 1988.

86. Wallberg-Henriksson H et al: Increased peripheral insulin sensitivity and muscle mitochondrial enzymes but unchanged blood glucose control in type 1 diabetics after physical training, *Diabetes* 31:1044, 1982.

87. Wasserman DH, Vranic M: Interaction between insulin, glucagon, and catecholamines in the regulation of glucose production and uptake during exercise: physiology and diabetes, *Biochem Exerc* 16:167, 1986.

88. Welle S: Metabolic responses to a meal during rest and low-intensity exercise, *Am J Clin Nutr* 40:990, 1984.

89. Wiles CM, Jones DA, Edwards RHT: Fatigue in human metabolic myopathy. In Porter R, Whelan J, editors: *Human muscle fatigue: physiological mechanisms,* London, 1981, Pitman.

90. Zierz S, Engel A: Regulatory properties of a mutant carnitine palmitoyltransferase in human skeletal muscle, *Eur J Biochem* 149:207, 1985.

91. Zinman B: Diabetes mellitus and exercise, *Behav Med Update* 6:22, 1984.

92. Zinman B: Acute and long-term effects of exercise in type 1 diabetes, *Biochem Exerc* 16:241, 1986.

93. Zinman B et al: Glucoregulation during moderate exercise in insulin-treated diabetes, *J Clin Endocrinol Metab* 45:641, 1977.

94. Zinman B et al: The role of insulin in metabolic response to exercise in diabetic man, *Diabetes* 28(suppl 1):76, 1979.

STUDY QUESTIONS

■ Describe how muscle enzyme deficiencies affect lipid and glycogen metabolism and the resultant effect on the ability to exercise.

■ Describe the differences between type 1 and type 2 diabetes.

■ What are the benefits of diet and exercise training for persons with type 1 and type 2 diabetes?

■ Describe contraindications for exercise training in persons with diabetes.

■ What is the cause of obesity?

■ What are the benefits of diet and exercise training for patients with obesity?

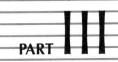

PART III

EXERCISE AND THE RESPIRATORY AND CARDIOVASCULAR SYSTEMS

■ *KEEP IN MIND WHILE YOU READ* . . . *Kathleen Westphal and Elizabeth Protas, in Chapters 4 and 6, respectively, describe normal pulmonary and cardiovascular anatomy and physiology. In Chapter 5 Donna Frownfelter compares normal ventilatory responses to responses in patients with restrictive and obstructive lung diseases. In Chapter 7 Lawrence Cahalin describes normal cardiovascular responses and responses for a variety of cardiac disorders. Once again, focus on indications and contraindications for exercise, and try to get a feel for how impairment in untrained patients limits their physical activity in comparison to that of persons in good health.* ■

NORMAL RESPIRATORY ANATOMY, PHYSIOLOGY, AND RESPONSES AT REST AND DURING EXERCISE

Kathleen Westphal

KEY TERMS

- Acid-base balance
- Alveolus
- Gas diffusion
- Hemoglobin
- Minute ventilation
- O_2 and CO_2 association and dissociation curves
- Partial pressures of O_2 and CO_2
- Ventilatory mechanics
- Ventilatory muscles

The respiratory system does not simply consist of the lungs functioning like isolated bellows or of "inflated balloons." The lungs are made up of airways that become progressively smaller, eventually terminating in minute sacs called *alveoli*. The volume and composition of the air within these airways and alveoli are influenced by the activity of the surrounding skeletal and muscular thorax, the information communicated along the controlling neural system, and the status of the circulating blood within the pulmonary vasculature. The respiratory "system" is, indeed, a coordinated network of structures that function in a dynamic fashion to attempt to meet the energy requirements of the body. The purposes of this chapter are to present the anatomy and physiology of the respiratory system, to discuss factors affecting respiration and ventilation, to explain how this system accommodates increases in metabolic demands, and to discuss how the system is controlled.

ANATOMY AND PHYSIOLOGY

The primary function of the respiratory system can be simply stated. This system is expected to oxygenate mixed venous blood and remove accumulated carbon dioxide (CO_2) to maintain homeostasis of the body's cellular environment. When both the lungs and the ventilatory pump are functioning optimally, the addition of oxygen (O_2) and the removal of CO_2 are easily accomplished, thereby maintaining a normal arterial blood composition. Depending on the demands of the body and pathologic structural alterations, however, the process may become less than perfect. For the process to occur as intended, the basic requirements are, first, that an adequate amount of air must reach the alveoli and must be distributed uniformly within these alveoli and, second, that this fresh air must then be able to diffuse from the alveoli to the blood within the pulmonary capillaries. These requirements imply that the barrier to diffusion be minimal and that there be adequate pulmonary blood flow. If the strength of the ventilatory pump is lessened, if the diffusion barrier is deleteriously affected, or if pulmonary blood flow is hindered, the composition of arterial blood may be affected, regardless of whether the alveoli are adequately ventilated. The third requirement for normal gas exchange is that the respiratory system must be energetically efficient. If the energy requirements of the respiratory system become excessive, other metabolically active cells of the body may be deprived, which would then place an even greater demand on the already overworked system. Once the requirements that allow the respiratory system to function optimally are recognized, it is important to understand how each requirement can be altered through anatomic and physiologic mechanisms.

As already stated, an important component of the respiratory system is the respiratory tree, or the airways. These, along with the alveoli, are the structures through which air travels on entering and leaving the system. The airways may be viewed as the sequential branching of the limbs of a tree, generally consisting of 23 branchings, or "generations," each successive generation of a smaller caliber (Fig. 4-1).[2] However, luminal diameter is not the only characteristic difference between the sequential airway generations. Based on general respiratory function, differences also exist in the amounts of smooth muscle, secretory cells, cilia, and macrophage activity. For general purposes the airways are identified either as part of the proximal *conducting zone* or as part of the distal *respiratory zone*, although the function of each zone must be considered of equal importance.

The conducting zone is the portion of the respiratory network that serves transport, purification, and humidification functions but does not participate in the exchange of gas between respiratory structures and the circulating blood. This zone begins at the nose, continues as the pharynx and the trachea (the first airway generation), and finally terminates at the level of the terminal bronchioles (generation 16). Within the conducting zone incoming air is warmed to 37° C and moisturized to a level of 100% saturation, so the air is fully conditioned before reaching the more distal airways. Just distal to the terminal bronchioles are the respiratory bronchioles (generation 17), which serve as the first generation of the respiratory zone, or the zone of actual gas exchange. At the level of the respiratory bronchioles the existence of occasional alveoli begins. The respiratory zone terminates at

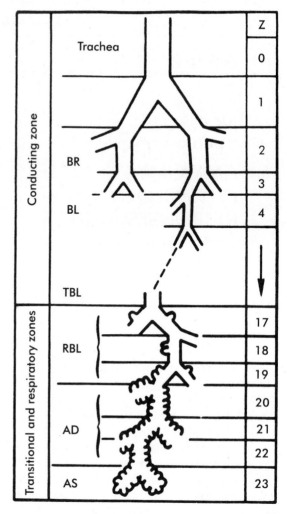

Fig. 4-1 Schema of the airway branches of the respiratory system. *AD,* Alveolar duct; *AS,* alveolar sac; *BL,* bronchiole; *BR,* bronchus; *RBL,* respiratory bronchiole; *TBL,* terminal bronchiole.

the most distally located respiratory structures, the alveoli.

On histologic examination the airways change as one moves through subsequent divisions, as would be expected because of the functional differences between zones. Ciliated, secretory, and goblet cells are seen within the epithelium of the bronchi, and deep to this epithelium exist the important bronchial submucosal glands.[6] The populations of these cells and glands decrease in the more distal airways, and the projecting cilia become shorter. The motile cilia, the mucous secretions provided by the goblet cells and submucosal glands, and the serous periciliary fluid layer all function together as a mucociliary escalator or mucociliary transport mechanism. The viscous and elastic mucus portion of the escalator is responsible for trapping foreign particles that have entered the airways. The cilia, which are bathed in the surrounding serous secretions, then complete the clearance of the particles by sweeping the mucus and particulate material cephaladad, where they may then be swallowed or expelled. The normally thin layer of mucus has two other important functions. First, its presence acts as a barrier against potential penetration by bacteria or other invading microorganisms. Second, this mucus acts as a defense against excessive water losses or gains at the level of the air passageways, since hydration of the incoming air is accomplished by the movement of water from the vascularized epithelium across the mucus. Then, as the fully hydrated air is expired, water moves in the opposite direction, back into the capillaries of the mucosal layer. Thus changes in the amount or consistency of the mucus, the presence or motility of the cilia, the temperature and humidity of the inspired air, or a combination of these factors may have profound effects on the clearance and hydration of the airways.

The debilitating symptoms of many respiratory diseases and disorders are the result of problems with the mucociliary transport mechanism. For example, the individual with chronic bronchitis has repeated respiratory infections and impairment of gas exchange because of excessive mucus production, which overpowers the sweeping ability of the existent cilia. Although individuals with bronchiectasis may have infections and gas exchange difficulties similar to those in persons with chronic bronchitis, the primary cause of poor bronchopulmonary hygiene in these individuals is a protein deficiency that interferes with the motility of the cilia. It is important to note, however, that for the function of the mucociliary escalator to be altered, the existence of a disease process is not necessary. Certain aerosols, including cigarette smoke, may have the effect of paralyzing cilia during the brief exposure to the noxious agent and may also result in altered mucus production with repeated exposures. Inspiration of excessively dry air, even in the absence of disease, results in the discomfort of a dehydrated airway and also increases the viscousness of the mucus. This explains the need for humidification in air-conditioning systems and in medical intervention devices such as respirators.[8] In the postsurgical patient or the patient with pulmonary disease this concern with removal of mucus is dealt with by means of positional techniques, cough encouragement, antibiotic intervention, and increased hydration in an attempt to decrease the viscousness of the secretions.

Although the mucociliary escalator is an excellent defense mechanism for the airways, the alveoli must also possess some avenue for removal of particulate matter, since the smallest inhaled particles often settle in these most distal respiratory structures. The defense against infection at the level of the alveoli is accomplished by alveolar macrophages, cells that originate as monocytes within the bone marrow. As is typical for any macrophage, these cells possess a strong phagocytic and lysosomal capability, which enables them to easily engulf and digest invasive organisms. The natural wandering characteristic of these alveolar macrophages allows them to travel between alveoli in search of foreign particles and then to enter the pulmonary interstitium or nearby capillaries for eventual removal. They may also be removed via the mucociliary escalator, as has been observed in sputum cultures. Although it may be relatively obvious that too few of these wandering macrophages could easily result in an eventual infection, it may not be as readily evident that serious pulmonary tissue damage may also result from an excess of these cells. However, any substance that stimulates an inflammatory reaction within the lungs also encourages an increase in macrophage numbers and activity. If the duration of exposure to this substance is excessive, the normally beneficial macrophages become involved instead in pulmonary tissue destruction, which is a simplistic explanation of the emphysematous result of long-term cigarette smoking.

Other histologic differences within the airways besides those involving the mucociliary transport mechanism have also been noted. If all the airways were composed solely of soft tissue, they would be easily collapsed by the excessive intrathoracic pressures especially evident during expiration. Such collapse would result in the trapping of gas within the lungs. However, the airways of the conducting zone are characterized by the presence of approximately 20 cartilaginous rings that do not completely encircle the airways but instead are bound to one another posteriorly by autonomically innervated smooth muscle. The cartilaginous rings are C or U shaped and function to maintain the patency of the airways. The presence of the smooth muscle between the ends of the rings along the posterior wall of the conducting airways allows the size of the lumen of the airways to be altered. Increasing or decreasing the relative level of stimulation to this layer of smooth muscle results either in bronchoconstriction or in bronchodilation, but because of the presence of the cartilaginous rings, these larger airways can never be completely occluded. The morphologic appearance of the cartilaginous rings changes as one moves distally in the respiratory tree. At the level of the smallest bronchioles in the conducting zone the rings eventually become irregular in appearance, acquiring a configuration often described as saddle shaped, and actually encircle the entire airway. At this level the smooth muscle remains but lies internal to the cartilaginous rings, so contraction of the muscle in these smaller airways may actually have a sphincteric effect, completely closing off the lumen. The cartilaginous rings are no longer evident at any point distal to the terminal bronchioles. Their absence suggests that airways in the respiratory zone may be collapsed if exposed to high extraluminal pressures. Should this occur, gas would become trapped in distal airways and expiratory volume and flow would decrease.

Most of the respiratory tree is centrally located within the chest. This portion of the chest is called the mediastinum and also includes such structures as the heart, various blood vessels and nerves, and portions of the gastrointestinal tract.[9] Extending peripherally from the mediastinum are the two lungs, which are protectively encased by the rib cage, sternum, thoracic vertebral column, and diaphragm. Additionally, each lung is surrounded by two serous membranes, the parietal and visceral pleurae, which are continuous with one another and differ only in location (Fig. 4-2). The parietal pleura is a thin membrane firmly adhered to the inner wall of the thorax. It reflects on itself at the hilum of the lung to become the visceral pleura, which is adhered to the outer wall of the lungs. During embryologic development these pleurae begin as two pleural sacs that are subsequently invaginated by the two developing lung buds. Since the two pleurae are actually one continuous anatomic structure, they display no major histologic differences, being made up primarily of a basement membrane, a mesothelial cell layer, and a connective tissue matrix. The mesothelial cells have the important responsibility of secreting the fluid that separates the two pleurae. The presence of this fluid is extremely important in permitting the two pleurae to smoothly glide past one another with each breath. Equally important is the composition of the fluid, which is controlled to some extent by the integrity of the basement membrane and the connective tissue matrix, since they jointly function to maintain the permeability of the pleurae. In some diseases or disorders, such as pleural inflammations, pleural tumors, or asbestosis, these structures may be singly affected or may all be damaged, resulting in an alteration in the oncotic state of the pleural fluid. This alteration in turn deleteriously affects the ease with which the lungs are able to inflate.

Although the two lungs function comparably, anatomic differences exist between them. The right lung consists of three lobes, whereas the left lung, which occupies a smaller area of the thorax because of the presence of the heart and associated vessels, has only two identified lobes (Fig. 4-3).[8] The lobes of the right lung are referred to simply as the upper, middle, and lower lobes. The left lung consists of an upper and a lower lobe. Each lobe is

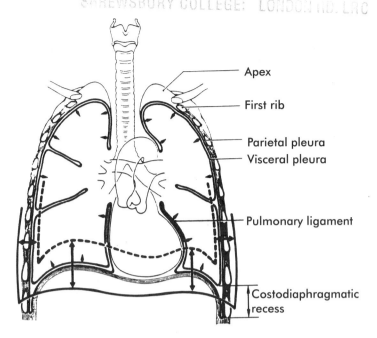

Fig. 4-2   Parietal and visceral pleurae of the thorax.

then further subdivided into bronchopulmonary segments, 8 on the left and 10 on the right, which are conveniently separated by interlobar connective tissue septa. This connective tissue is a continuation of the connective tissue matrix of the pleurae, which explains how forces are equitably distributed over the entirety of the lungs. The bronchopulmonary segments do not share bronchioles or blood vessels, allowing for the surgical removal of individual segments rather than entire lobes or lungs, if necessary.

FACTORS AFFECTING RESPIRATION AND VENTILATION

Whether because of individual differences, the natural process of aging, or various diseases or disorders, not all lungs expand to hold the same volume of air. For that matter, neither do all lungs contain the same amount of air after expiration. Norms have been established for the static lung volumes and capacities (capacities are defined as being more than one volume), but unless the values are interpreted along with the results

of other dynamic tests, they have little predictive value, since they are strictly anatomic measurements. These static lung volumes and capacities[4] include the following:

1. Tidal volume (TV): Amount of air inspired or expired during a quiet breath
2. Inspiratory reserve volume (IRV): Maximal volume that may be inspired beyond a tidal respiration
3. Expiratory reserve volume (ERV): Amount of air that can be maximally expired after a normal tidal expiration
4. Residual volume (RV): Volume of air remaining in the lungs after a forceful maximal expiration.
5. Inspiratory capacity (IC): Combination of TV and IRV
6. Functional residual capacity (FRC): Combination of ERV and RV; may also be described as the amount of air left in the lungs after a normal, quiet expiration
7. Vital capacity (VC): Combination of IRV, TV, and ERV

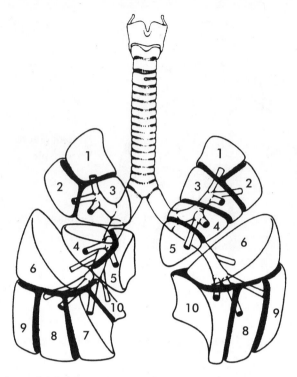

Fig. 4-3   The right and left lobes of the lungs. Segments of the lobes are, *1*, apical; *2*, posterior; *3*, anterior; *4*, lateral; *5*, medial; *6*, superior; *7*, anterior basal; *8*, lateral basal; *9*, posterior basal; and, *10*, medial basal.

8. Total lung capacity (TLC): Combination of TV, IRV, ERV, and RV

All these static lung volumes and capacities are approximately 20% to 25% lower in women than in men of equal age. Some decline in volumes is also seen with age, but the literature does not yet clearly suggest the effects of prolonged aerobic exercise in possibly preventing this change.

Most of the lung volumes and capacities may be determined by performing simple spirometry, with the exception of FRC, RV, and TLC. The measurement of FRC is accomplished by means of complicated tests that involve the inspiration of an insoluble gas such as helium (closed-circuit helium dilution technique), the inspiration of 100% O_2 (open-circuit nitrogen washout technique), or the use of a body plethysmograph.[2] The insoluble gas

technique is based on the principle that the helium used is not able to diffuse across the alveolar-capillary interface, so any changes in measured concentration must reflect changes in lung volume. In other words, if gas of a known concentration is inspired from a container of a known volume, the volume in the lungs may be computed from the measured differences in inspired and expired gas concentrations. The nitrogen washout technique allows the examiner to determine FRC by measuring expired gas volume and nitrogen concentration and comparing these to the known concentration of nitrogen in the inspired gas that was in the lung at the beginning of the test. The body plethysmograph method is based on Boyle's law, which states that at a constant temperature the volume of a perfect gas varies inversely as the pressure and the pressure varies inversely as the volume ($P_1V_1 = P_2V_2$). The individual to be tested is placed in a box comparable to a telephone booth and is instructed to breathe through a mouthpiece. The mouthpiece is then occluded, and the individual continues to attempt breaths against this occlusion. Changes in pressure measurements at the mouth and within the box allow calculation of FRC. Once the measure of FRC is established by any of these three direct methods, RV may be computed indirectly by subtracting ERV from the FRC. TLC may be determined by adding the measures for FRC and IC.

Important lung volume measurements other than those previously described assess "dead space ventilation."[5] Respiratory dead space, made up of areas of the respiratory system that do not participate in gas exchange, may be broken into two component parts, *anatomic dead space* and *physiologic dead space*. The conducting zone, which is responsible for delivering gas to the respiratory zone but does not participate in pulmonary gas exchange, constitutes the anatomic dead space. Thus the air that enters the conducting zone with each inspiration is simply wasted ventilation. It is approximately equal, in milliliters, to an individual's ideal predicted weight in pounds. Of more interest when assessing diseases and disorders is the physiologic dead space, which is made up of the anatomic dead space plus any additional areas of the respiratory zone that are not able to participate optimally in the exchange of gases between the alveoli and the pulmonary capillary blood. This deficiency could result from a number of causes, including a diffusion impairment between the alveoli and pulmonary capillaries or inadequate blood flow in the capillary network servicing the alveoli. Regardless of the cause, the energy expended in getting air to these alveoli is wasted, or dead space, ventilation.

Although changes in the various static lung volumes and capacities certainly provide some insight into pulmonary health, one must remember that ventilation is a dynamic process and must be assessed accordingly. Ignorance of a time factor disregards the

consideration that ventilation relies heavily on the rate of air flow, especially when maximal efficiency of function is a factor. For example, if the respiratory rate is too slow, the respiratory system may be inadequate in meeting the metabolic needs of the body, even in individuals who exhibit a relatively normal TV. On the other hand, the individual who demonstrates a normal respiratory rate may also have problems satisfying the metabolic needs of the body, if breathing is so shallow as to provide an inadequate TV. This is the reason for pulmonary function tests that measure flow, or the volume of air moved over a specified time.

The measure of the amount of gas that is moved during 1 minute is called the pulmonary minute volume ($\dot{V}_E$) and is a more important gauge than either TV or respiratory rate, considered individually. However, since the TV measure includes anatomic dead space ventilation, an even better assessment of how well the respiratory system is fulfilling the cellular needs of the body is a measure of exactly how much fresh air is entering those alveoli capable of participating fully in pulmonary gas exchange. This volume is called alveolar ventilation. When measured during the period of a minute, it is called the minute alveolar ventilation ($\dot{V}_A$). Minute alveolar ventilation should naturally increase as metabolic rate and CO_2 production increase, such as during exercise or in the patient with a fever or severe burn. Concurrent with this increase in $\dot{V}_A$ is an increased energy demand on the part of the ventilatory muscles responsible for lung and thorax movement.

Although $\dot{V}_E$ and $\dot{V}_A$ are extremely important measures, their assessment requires the collection of exhaled gases and arterial blood samples. If the instruments necessary to conduct these studies are unavailable, flow characteristics may also be approximated by means of simple spirometric studies that measure the volume of an individual's forced vital capacity (FVC), which is a measure of the amount of air moved during a timed period. For example, FEV_1 is a measure of the amount of air moved during the first second of the attempted measurement of FVC, and FEV_3 is the amount of air moved during the first 3 seconds.[9] Typically one should expire approximately 80% of the FVC within the first second of a forced expiratory maneuver. Although individual differences certainly exist, a markedly decreased FEV_1 may suggest some sort of obstructive disease or disorder. For example, luminal narrowing of the airways resulting from bronchoconstriction, increased mucus production, or excessive transmural pressure may prevent the rapid expiratory flow of air.

Examination of a normal lung and its multiple alveoli reveals the natural tendency for these structures to assume the smallest possible size. This tendency is partially the result of their inherent elasticity and the surface tension created by the fluid lining the alveoli. The elasticity exhibited by the alveoli is also exhibited by the thoracic cage. As the term ''elasticity'' implies, both the lungs and the thorax return to their original shapes after a deforming force is applied. This response, termed ''recoil,'' is an important principle in the processes of inspiration and expiration, since changes in recoil may alter the amount of air that is moved with a respiratory effort and the amount of energy required for that effort.[2] This recoil tendency is readily evident when the lung and thorax are observed in complete isolation from one another. In other words, if a lung is removed from the body, thereby negating the influence of any forces other than its own inherent elasticity, it recoils to a size at which it contains only its RV. Once the lungs are removed from the chest, the naturally balanced posture preferred by the thorax may be observed. The elasticity of the tissues of the chest wall makes the thorax assume a somewhat expanded position relative to that seen during normal, quiet respiration. In fact, the thorax prefers a position approximately 600 ml above the level of the resting expiratory volume.

The inherent elasticity in both the lungs and the thorax tends to cause each of these structures to recoil to a predetermined position when released from any other forces. A good practical example of the recoil force is to observe what happens when air is introduced into the intrapleural space, as in the case of a pneumothorax. After this introduction of air between the two pleurae the intrapleural pressure is no longer negative but is actually equal to atmospheric pressure. This means that the involved lung cannot be inflated on inspiratory effort because it is no longer influenced by the negative intrapleural pressure produced by the two juxtaposed pleurae. As a result the lung immediately recoils to its preferred size. Through the action of comparable elastic forces, the thorax also recoils. The principle of recoil is especially evident in various diseases and disorders and in the normal aging process. With aging the lung loses some of its elasticity and does not recoil to a size as small as that of the younger lung. This alteration can make expiration somewhat more difficult and may result in a larger FRC, or excess air in the lung. The loss of lung recoil ability can actually be seen on clinical examination. It is not unusual for the chests of some older individuals to take on a more barrel-like appearance, which results when the thorax recoils to its preferred position and an equal recoil force is not exerted on it by the older, less elastic lungs.

As already mentioned, the tendency for the lungs to recoil to a smaller size results not only from the intrinsic elasticity of the tissue but also from the existence of surface tension within the alveoli. This surface tension is due to the strong attraction between the waterlike molecules that make up the fluid layer inside each alveolus.[8] As these molecules are attracted to one another, they tend to pull the alveolus closed, so a pressure greater than the surface tension of water must be produced to prevent atelectasis. This inherent surface tension is decreased by the presence of surfactant in the normal alveolus. Surfactant, with its detergent-like characteristics, decreases the desire water molecules have for one another, and thereby the tendency for atelectasis. Surfactant is produced by organelles in the type 2 alveolar cells and may be detrimentally affected by substances such as cigarette smoke or by the process of aging. The lack of surfactant is the cause of the major respiratory disturbances seen in preterm infants with respiratory distress syndrome. Surfactant production does not begin until approximately the twenty-third week of gestation, and sufficient quantities are not available to allow the lung to maintain inflation until approximately the twenty-eighth week of fetal life.[6] Without adequate surfactant the respiratory muscles of the infant require extraordinary amounts of energy to inflate the geometrically small alveoli, which causes respiration to become a fatiguing activity. Medical intervention for these infants is directed toward assisting with each respiratory effort by mechanical means and by artificial stimulation of surfactant production.

The variation in the pressure necessary to inflate alveoli of differing sizes and surface tensions is explained by Laplace's law. This law states that the pressure necessary to inflate a bubble is directly proportional to the tension in the walls of the sphere and indirectly proportional to the radius of the sphere ($P = 4T/r$). In other words, if the tension in the walls of the alveolus is reduced by the presence of surfactant, the pressure required to maintain the alveolar volume is less than the pressure required to maintain the same volume in an alveolus of the same size without surfactant. The size of the alveolus is also a factor. In the absence of surfactant, less energy is required to maintain a large lung volume than to maintain a small lung volume. Thus without surfactant the pressure required to maintain the volume of a geometrically small alveolus may be greater than can be generated, which would result in eventual atelectasis. To minimize the pressure required to keep an alveolus open, the surface tension must be decreased or the radius must be increased. However, increasing the radii of multiple alveoli would have the deleterious effect of decreasing the total surface area of the lung available for diffusion, so the reduction of surface tension by surfactant is the better alternative.

The characteristics of recoil and surface tension obviously have an effect on ventilation, that is, the ability to move air in and out of the lungs. Changes in these properties can make ventilation easier or more difficult by altering the existent pressure gradients required for the movement of air. Since the pathway that the air travels is between the mouth and the distant alveoli, a pressure gradient must exist between these structures during inspiration and expiration, when air is moving. This gradient is the difference between the atmospheric pressure seen at the mouth and the pressure measured within the alveoli, or the alveolar pressure (P_A). Since atmospheric pressure does not change from breath to breath, the value that changes must be the P_A. At rest, that is, during the brief period between the phases of inspiration and expiration, $P_A = 0$, the same as mouth or atmospheric pressure. Alveolar pressure increases with inspiration, when air mass enters the alveoli, and then decreases as air exits the alveoli during expiration.

Although flow of air occurs once a pressure gradient is established between the mouth and alveoli, the establishment of the pressure gradient is the result of the changes in size of the thorax and lungs. The competing recoil characteristics of the thorax and lungs create a subatmospheric, or negative, pressure between the two attached pleurae, which is referred to as the intrapleural pressure (P_{IP}). This pressure is evident even during the short rest period between inspiration and expiration, since the intrapleural pressure is responsible for maintaining the partial inflation of the lungs and the retention of the RV. As the diaphragm descends and the thorax expands during inspiration, this pressure becomes increasingly negative, since the lung is being forcefully pulled farther and farther from its preferred recoil shape.

Fig. 4-4 demonstrates how the lung pressures and volumes interrelate during normal, quiet inspiration and expiration. During normal inspiration the diaphragm descends after receiving a message to do so from the phrenic nerve. Although the diaphragm is the primary muscle of inspiration, further enlargement of the thorax is generally accomplished through the action of other skeletal muscles such as the intercostals and scalenes.[1] When this enlargement of the thorax is occurring, the parietal pleura attached to the diaphragm and the chest wall is simultaneously pulled outward and downward. This movement of the parietal pleura increases the negativity of the pressure that exists between it and the visceral pleura. As the diaphragm descends and the intrapleural pressure becomes more negative, the lungs and their corresponding alveoli are pulled open. Once these empty alveoli are expanded, the gas within them exhibits a negative pressure relative to the atmospheric pressure that is present at

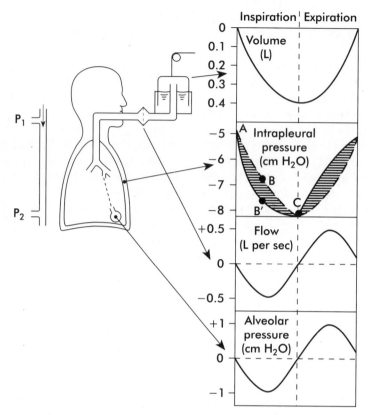

Fig. 4-4 Pressures during the breathing cycle. *A,* Intrapleural pressure before inspiration begins; *B,* intrapleural pressure during inspiration; *B′,* the difference between *B* and *B′* is the alveolar pressure at any instance; *C,* intrapleural pressure as inspiration ends; *P₁*, atmospheric pressure; *P₂*, alveolar pressure.

the mouth. This difference in pressure between the mouth and the alveoli serves as the pressure gradient necessary for air to enter the lungs from the environment. The entrance of gas into the alveoli increases the pressure within these lung units until the pressure within the alveoli once again equals mouth pressure. At the same time, contraction of the inspiratory muscles ceases and their consequent relaxation results in a decrease in thorax and lung volumes, with a concomitant increase in alveolar pressure and decrease in the negativity of the P_{IP}. The positive pressure at the level of the alveoli is then greater than the atmospheric pressure at the mouth, and the difference between the

two serves as the necessary pressure gradient for expiration. Air is exhaled until a pressure gradient no longer exists between the alveoli and the environment, at which time the process initiated by diaphragm descent and inspiratory muscle contraction begins again.

The description of the static lung pressures and volumes necessary for normal respiration is, indeed, convenient to an understanding of some of the forces that influence the flow of air into and out of the lungs. However, such a simple explanation must be considered in concert with certain other factors that may mediate this flow of air. Even if the existent alveolar and mouth pressures favor inspiration or expiration,

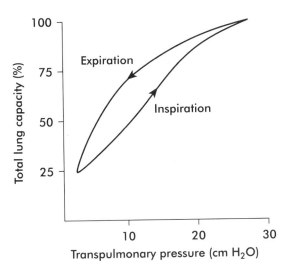

Fig. 4-5 Pressure and volume (capacity) curves during inspiration and expiration.

this movement of air is also positively or negatively affected by certain resistive factors.

Opposition to airflow is considered elastic or nonelastic. Elastic resistance is determined by calculating the separate measures for the compliance, or stiffness, of the lungs and chest wall. Changes in the ease with which either of these structures moves may have a profound influence on the ability to inflate the lungs. Compliance is defined as a change in volume relative to a given change in pressure (V/P) (Fig. 4-5). As shown in Fig. 4-5, as the slope of the graphed line increases, so does the compliance, or distensibility, of the measured system. Concomitantly stiffness decreases.

Nonelastic resistance consists of both the usual minimal resistance afforded by movement of overlying lung tissues and the typically greater resistance offered by the tubular anatomy of the airways. The effect of the change in the luminal diameters of these airway tubes is described by Poiseuille's law. This law states that the volume flow in a tube (1) is directly proportional to the pressure drop along the length of the tube and to the fourth power of the radius of the tube and (2) is inversely proportional to the length of the tube and to the viscosity of the fluid (F = (P_1 − P_2)r4/η1).[2] Although a direct relationship exists between the driving pressure gradient (P_1 − P_2) and the resultant flow (F), the effect of a change in radius (r) on flow is even greater. In fact, for every one-unit change in luminal radius, flow changes by a factor of 4. Therefore anything that alters the size of the airways also alters the amount of air entering or exiting the system. Airway diameter may be altered by several influences, which are usually mediated by a neural system response to a chemical, a foreign body, or an emotion. Of particular importance to the exercising individual is the decrease in airway resistance that occurs simply as a result of switching from nose to mouth breathing. Indeed, if the nasal turbinates could be bypassed, the opposition to airflow by the airways would be lessened but the conditioning of the air would also be seriously affected.[10]

Consideration of all the previously described characteristics is important to a study of the work of breathing. In other words, what has to be overcome, to get air in and out of the lungs? Of course, the natural recoil forces must be overcome. If the lungs become less compliant or less elastic, more work is required to inflate them. If the lungs become excessively compliant, or floppy, it may not be difficult to fill them with air but more work is required to empty them because the lungs do not recoil to the same small shape as when compliance was normal. Quiet expiration becomes an energy-consuming process, although it is normally a passive activity.

EFFECT OF METABOLIC DEMAND ON THE RESPIRATORY SYSTEM

Usually the work of breathing is minimal. For example, the active respiratory structures typically use only about 1% to 2% of the O_2 consumed by the body at rest (approximately 2 ml/kg per min).[7] This statistic implies that the O_2 demands of the respiratory structures in a healthy individual do not limit maximal exercise capabilities. Although this is generally true, the potential for a limitation exists at high exercise intensities, since the ventilatory muscle's minute oxygen consumption may increase to as much as 15% or 20% of the body's volume of oxygen consumption (Vo_2).[7]

Under less than healthy conditions ventilatory energy demands may increase precipitously as a result of such problems as narrowed airways or noncompliant lungs. In other words, a large portion of the respiratory reserve is already being used, even during rest, and the ventilatory structures are functioning at approximately 40% of their maximal capacity, whereas in the healthy individual they function at 5% of maximal capacity. As energy substrate consumption is increased by the respiratory structures, the active skeletal muscles are prematurely relegated to function in an anaerobic state, unlike in the individual with a healthy respiratory system. The resultant production of fatigue may limit not only exercise activities but also functional activities of daily living, depending on the extent of the disease or disorder.[3]

The energy required to overcome the disease involved determines the respiratory pattern the individual exhibits. Every attempt will be made by the system to minimize energy expenditure. The primary alternative available for the respiratory system to meet an increase in metabolic demands is to increase the depth of breathing or to increase the respiratory rate, or both. (Recall that $\dot{V}_E = \dot{V}_T \times f$ [f = Respiratory frequency]). For lung disorders that deleteriously alter the compliance, or distensibility, of the lung-thorax complex, an increase in f is generally the preferred option, since increasing TV simply increases the elastic energy demands of tissues already exhibiting abnormal volume and pressure characteristics. At the opposite end of the spectrum of diseases and disorders are problems with airway luminal diameter, whether caused by airway hyperreactivity, excessive mucus production, or tissue destruction. In these disorders there is a tendency to respond to a greater metabolic demand by preferentially increasing respiratory depth rather than respiratory frequency, since an increase in rate would increase the work required to generate the force necessary to move air through airways of inadequate size. As would be expected, most disorders lie someplace along the continuum between these two extremes.

What is the basic function of the ventilatory activity? As a result of lung ventilation the cells of the body are normally supplied with O_2 and excess CO_2 is removed. These results are accomplished by means of pressure gradients that are established for the movement of these gases across the alveolar membrane. The partial pressure of O_2 in the alveoli (PA_{O_2}) is approximately 100 mm Hg, whereas the partial pressure of O_2 in the returning venous blood (PV_{O_2}) is approximately 38 mm Hg. This difference provides a large pressure gradient for O_2 to enter the venous blood as it passes through the capillaries lining the alveoli. This same venous blood has a CO_2 partial pressure (PV_{CO_2}) of approximately 45 mm Hg, whereas the partial pressure of CO_2 in the alveoli (PA_{CO_2}) is about 40 mm Hg, thus establishing a driving force for CO_2 to enter the alveoli. If these pressure gradients are not maintained to favor the diffusion of O_2 and CO_2 in the appropriate directions, cellular equilibrium is eventually affected.

The diffusion of gases across a membrane may be best explained with the assistance of Fick's law of diffusion. This law states that the rate of diffusion is directly proportional to the surface area involved in the diffusion process, the concentration gradient between the two compartments, and the solubility of the gas.[9] An inverse relationship exists between both the rate of diffusion and the thickness of the barrier that is traversed and the molecular weight of the gas. A variable that is not considered in Fick's law is the rate of blood flow. In other words, even in the healthiest lungs and under ideal conditions is adequate time available for dynamic equilibration to occur between alveolar air and the circulating pulmonary capillary blood? The answer appears to be affirmative, even during periods of intense exercise, when the rate of blood flow is considerably accelerated.

When the principles of Fick's law of diffusion are applied to the lung, one sees that the healthy lung is ideally suited for its function of allowing the movement of gases across the alveolar and pulmonary capillary membranes. Because of the presence of approximately 300 million alveoli within the two adult lungs and their associated capillary network, a tremendous alveolar-capillary surface area is available for gas exchange in healthy lungs.

This area is estimated to be between 50 and 100 m^2. One may also use Fick's law to explain many of the difficulties encountered in various pulmonary diseases and disorders. A clear example of the existence of this direct relationship between surface area and diffusion rate is observed when alveoli are destroyed, such as in patients with emphysema. The destruction of multiple small alveoli in these patients results in a loss of alveolar-capillary surface area, thereby causing a diffusion impairment.

Less obvious examples of relative loss of alveolar-capillary surface area are seen when ventilation or perfusion is diminished, that is, when a "ventilation-perfusion mismatch" occurs. For the metabolic needs of the body to be adequately met by the respiratory system, pulmonary capillary perfusion and alveolar ventilation must be closely matched. The match or mismatch between these two variables is assessed by determining the ratio of alveolar ventilation to pulmonary capillary blood flow, $\dot{V}_A/\dot{Q}$. If the average normal resting $\dot{V}_A$ is estimated to be 4 L per minute and the average normal resting right ventricular output is 5 L per minute, the ratio that depicts the ideal match between ventilation and perfusion is 0.8 (5.0/4.0).[8] Both acute and chronic respiratory disorders may result in mismatches of ventilation and perfusion, since they typically result in some degree of mucus plugging in the airways, which precludes adequate ventilation of alveoli distal to the plug. The surface area of these nonventilated atelectatic alveoli must be subtracted from the alveolar surface area that is normally available in the healthy, well-ventilated lung. Although blood flow to the alveolus may be adequate, a ventilation-perfusion mismatch results because the alveolus is insufficiently ventilated. The $\dot{V}_A/\dot{Q}$ ratio would be less than the ideal of 0.8.

At the other end of the ventilation-perfusion spectrum is an alveolus that is insufficiently perfused. Although this alveolus may be ventilated and thus fully capable of exchanging O_2 and CO_2, the volume of gas in this alveolus would be considered physiologic dead space if the gas were unable to communicate with the mixed venous blood in the pulmonary capillary. Like the previously described alveolus, this alveolus, too, has a ventilation-perfusion mismatch, since it has a $\dot{V}_A/\dot{Q}$ greater than 0.8. This type of mismatch occurs when there is a decrease in blood flow distal to the site of obstruction during a pulmonary embolus or in the case of a weak right ventricle that is incapable of providing the pressure necessary to force its stroke volume through the pulmonary vasculature.

The uniformity or nonuniformity of blood flow in the pulmonary vasculature can best be described in terms of Poiseuille's law, as previously presented. Flow is directly proportional to the driving pressure and the radius of the vessel and is inversely proportional to the viscosity of the blood and the length of the vessel segment. For the purposes of this chapter the variables of driving pressure and radius are most important. The pressure that drives blood through the pulmonary vessels is considerably less than the pressure responsible for pushing blood through the peripheral systemic vessels. The driving pressure is the difference between the pressure produced at the level of the right ventricle (normally approximately 15 mm Hg) and the filling pressure at the level of the left atrium (normally 5 mm Hg). Thus the possibility exists for problems with either the right or the left ventricle to potentiate problems with the flow of blood within the vessels of the lung. For example, pulmonary hypertension may be caused either by an increase in left ventricular filling pressure such as may occur with stenosis of the mitral valve or by right ventricular hypertrophy.

Blood flow depends on the caliber of the vessel through which it is traveling, as well as on the driving pressure. However, several factors influence the patency of the pulmonary vessels located within the different regions of the lungs. Some level of smooth muscle control exists, but the vessels of the pulmonary system have much less smooth muscle than do the vessels of the systemic peripheral system.

Although equity of ventilation and perfusion is the ideal circumstance, this balance is never achieved throughout the lung, even in a normal, healthy individual. Since the lungs comprise more than 300 million alveoli of different sizes and their corresponding pulmonary capillaries, it is impossible for all the alveoli and capillaries to be equally ventilated and perfused at the same time. When the diaphragm descends during inspiration, the alveoli at the basilar portions of the lungs are more fully expanded and therefore better ventilated than are those at the apices. Blood flow is also greater at the base than at the apex. Since the relative difference in blood flow is greater than the difference in ventilation between these two regions of the lung, the ventilation-perfusion ratio exhibited at the base of the lung is generally less than 1. The ratio at the apex, however, is greater than 1, since pulmonary blood flow has decreased more than ventilation has.

Assigning a number, or a ratio, to the balance that exists between ventilation and perfusion mistakenly implies that this balance is a fixed or static phenomenon. As with all other processes associated with respiration, however, the inequality between alveolar ventilation and capillary blood flow is easily changed. For example, the normal individual achieves an increase in alveolar-capillary surface area with the increased ventilatory demands of exercise. This increase in surface area is accomplished by an accentuation of the distracting forces on the airways, improved ventilation of alveoli, and an increase in pulmonary blood pressure, which promote an improved balance between ventilation and perfusion throughout all regions of the lung. A change in posture or body position also has an effect on both ventilation and perfusion. The ratios previously described are typically observed in individuals in the standing posture. When the individual moves to a supine posture, however, the forces exerted on the airways and blood vessels are altered in such a way that the anterior portion of the lung is better ventilated than perfused ($\dot{V}_A/\dot{Q} > 0.8$) and the posterior portion is better perfused than ventilated ($\dot{V}_A/\dot{Q} < 0.8$).

As Fick's law of diffusion suggests, diffusion impairments are not only caused by surface area deficits but also may be associated with an increase in the thickness of the diffusion barrier. Although gases must traverse numerous structural obstacles to move from alveolus to red blood cell or from red blood cell to alveolus, this distance is minimal and

easily accommodated in the normal lung. A molecule of gas must diffuse through the gases within the alveolus and then pass through the surfactant, alveolar epithelium and basement membrane, pulmonary interstitium, capillary basement membrane and endothelium, plasma, and finally the membrane of the red blood cell before binding with a hemoglobin molecule. If the diffusion barrier is thickened because of an increase in the size of any of these obstacles, the rate of diffusion may be deleteriously affected. An altered diffusion rate may become evident on clinical assessment by the presence of abnormal blood gas values or by simple observation of skin coloration, both of which provide some measure of gas exchange equilibrium. The patient with emphysema provides an excellent example of this principle. Individuals with emphysema have an increase in diameter of their remaining alveoli, so a molecule of gas has a greater distance across which it must diffuse before being able to enter the pulmonary capillary. Often this increase in travel time decreases the chance for adequate equilibration of the involved gases. Similar diffusion impairments are observed in patients with pulmonary edema or interstitial fibrosis. Both conditions exhibit an abnormal thickening in the alveolar capillary pathway.

The physical properties of the diffusing gases as well as the thickness of the diffusion barrier, affect equilibration. Although O_2 and CO_2 exhibit dissimilarities in solubility and molecular weight, the differences in the normally existent pressure gradients between alveolar air and pulmonary arterial blood for these two gases provide the forces necessary for adequate diffusion. Since the rate of diffusion is indirectly proportional to the square root of the molecular weight of the gas, a large difference in density would be necessary for a substantial diffusion effect to occur. Oxygen has a molecular weight of 32 and CO_2 has a molecular weight of 44, so density characteristics obviously do not play a major role in diffusion differences. However, CO_2 is approximately 20 times more soluble than is O_2, which explains its ability to achieve equilibrium at a much lower pressure gradient than for O_2 at the level of the alveolus. When the returning deoxygenated pulmonary arterial blood possesses a Pao$_2$ of 60 mm Hg and the alveolus has a PAo$_2$ of 100 mm Hg, the gradient driving the movement of O$_2$ approximates 40 mm Hg. The gradient for CO$_2$ ranges between 5 and 6 mm Hg, since Paco$_2$ and PAco$_2$ are 40 mm Hg and 45 mm Hg, respectively.

Distinct differences exist in the way O$_2$ and CO$_2$ are transported in the plasma and the red blood cell. Oxygen may be carried either dissolved in solution or in combination with hemoglobin. The amount of O$_2$ that is carried dissolved in plasma is directly proportional to the alveolar pressure. However, despite the driving pressure of approximately 100 mm Hg, only a small portion of O$_2$ is transported in this fashion (about 0.3 ml per 100 ml blood). In fact, if dissolved plasma O$_2$ were the only source of circulating oxygen available to active tissues, the resting cardiac output would need to be increased approximately 60 to 70 times.

Since a maximal cardiac output during intense exercise activity approximates 25 to 30 L per min, another method of transporting and delivering O$_2$ to the metabolically active tissues must obviously be available. Hemoglobin, a protein within the red blood cell, is actually the primary means of O$_2$ transport within the body. Each hemoglobin molecule basically functions like a minivan that has enough seats to carry four O$_2$ passengers. Although the total amount of hemoglobin in the blood varies from individual to individual, 15 g per 100 ml of blood is a normal estimated total amount. These 15 g of hemoglobin allow for the carriage of a total of 20.1 ml of O$_2$, since each gram of hemoglobin binds with 1.34 ml of O$_2$. The importance of hemoglobin in the carriage of O$_2$ is obvious, since any process that results in diminished levels of hemoglobin decreases in turn the oxygen-carrying capacity of the affected blood. Without adequate levels of O$_2$ the tissues have difficulty functioning aerobically, which pushes the body toward early fatigue.

Just as the amount of O$_2$ transported in plasma in the dissolved state depends on Po$_2$, so does the amount of O$_2$ transported chemically bound to hemoglobin. However, a significant difference exists: a linear relationship does not exist between Po$_2$ and O$_2$ associated with hemoglobin, whereas a proportional relationship exists between Po$_2$ and dissolved O$_2$. The O$_2$ association-dissociation curve depicts the lack of proportionality between Po$_2$ and the O$_2$ associated with hemoglobin (Fig. 4-6). The sigmoid shape of the curve characterizes the advantageous relationships that have been established to ensure the optimal carriage and release of O$_2$ to meet physiologic needs. The flat plateau portion to the right of the curve is the "association" part of the curve. In other words, even if Po$_2$ should drop to as low as 60 to 65 mm Hg, hemoglobin remains saturated at 97% to 98%, that is, highly "associated" with oxygen. Thus the use of the hemoglobin saturation value as a measure of a patient's pulmonary health can be extremely misleading. A patient with a definite mismatch between ventilation and perfusion could easily have near-normal saturation values, yet an examination of arterial blood gas levels might reveal a Pao$_2$ low enough to merit modification of the patient's activity level. The steep portion of the curve to the left of the plateau corresponds to a decrease in affinity between hemoglobin and O$_2$ and is the "dissociation" part of the curve. The advantage of this dissociation is that O$_2$ is more easily provided to oxygen-starved tissues that possess a Po$_2$ of approximately 40 mm Hg.

The position of the O$_2$ association-dissociation curve may be changed by an altered physiologic environment. For example, the change in cellular environment that occurs with exercise clearly depicts this change in position. With an increase in activity an individual generally has an increase in temperature, an increase in Pco$_2$ with a resultant decrease in pH, and an increase in 2,3-diphosphoglycerate. These changes cause a shift of the O$_2$ dissociation curve to the right, which is called the Bohr effect. The Bohr effect assists in the unloading of the O$_2$ at the level of the tissues. This decrease in hemoglobin's affinity for O$_2$ is fortuitous, since the tissues are generally in dire need of O$_2$ during exercise.

Just as the curve may be shifted to the right, it may also be shifted to the left. This alternate

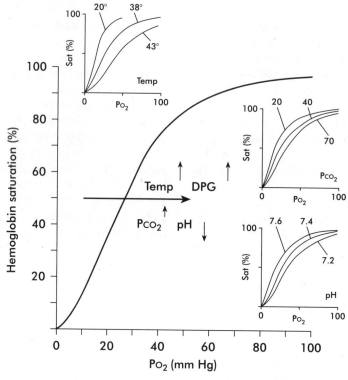

Fig. 4-6 Oxygen association-dissociation curve. *DPG,* 2, 3 Diphosphoglycerate; *Temp,* Celsius scale.

change in position can be observed when comparing the O_2 dissociation curves of maternal and fetal blood. Because of differences in hemoglobin, the curve for the fetus is to the left of that of the mother. This difference in curves appears to represent a "safety valve" that ensures adequate availability of O_2 to the developing fetus, even during occasional times when the arriving maternal blood has a lower Pao_2, regardless of the cause.

Although CO_2, like O_2, is carried in the plasma and red blood cell, differences in the characteristics of the two gases result in differences in their means of transport. Carbon dioxide is much more readily soluble than O_2, which means that CO_2 can attain equilibration with a lower driving pressure than that required for equilibration of O_2. Also, a much larger portion of CO_2 than O_2 can be transported in solution in the plasma. In fact, approximately 10% of transportable CO_2 is dissolved in

the plasma, as compared with only 0.03% of O_2. However, CO_2 is not transported as CO_2 but instead travels in one of two other forms. The CO_2 may bind with the plasma proteins to form carbamino compounds or may react with plasma water to form carbonic acid ($CO_2 + H_2O \rightleftharpoons H_2CO_3$). This H_2CO_3 then dissociates to bicarbonate (HCO_3^-) and a hydrogen ion (H^+). This bicarbonate (or CO_2) is released across the alveolar-capillary membrane at the level of the lungs and exists with the expired air. At the same time, O_2 is being transported in the reverse direction onto the red blood cell "minivan." This loss of CO_2 plays a vital role in the maintenance of the body's acid-base equilibrium.

Since only 10% of the CO_2 produced from metabolism is dissolved within the plasma, an alternate, preferred method of transport must also be available. Indeed, most of the CO_2 actually enters

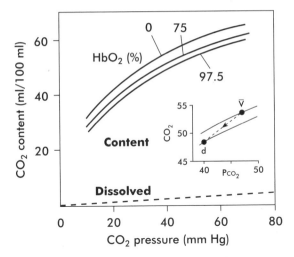

Fig. 4-7 Carbon dioxide association-dissociation curve.

the erythrocyte, where it may once again be transported in combination with a protein or as HCO_3^-. The protein with which it binds within the red blood cell is hemoglobin, and the resultant carbamino compounds account for approximately 45% of CO_2 transport. However, most of the CO_2 that enters the blood ultimately enters the red blood cell and participates in the chemical processes that allow for the production of bicarbonate. This movement of CO_2 is assisted by the presence of a positive pressure gradient and the ready solubility of CO_2, both of which aid its entrance into the plasma. The portion of CO_2 that is not carried in the plasma enters the red blood cell. Once within the erythrocyte, the CO_2 may bind with water, just as it may within the plasma. The red blood cell, however, unlike the plasma, possesses a catalytic enzyme called "carbonic anhydrase," which serves to markedly accelerate the formation of H_2CO_3. The negatively charged HCO_3^- that dissociates from this H_2CO_3 then exits the cell and is transported in the plasma. To maintain the electrical neutrality of the red blood cell, a chloride ion enters the cell from the plasma in a process called "the chloride shift."

Just as there is an O_2 dissociation curve, there is a CO_2 dissociation curve (Fig. 4-7).[9] Clear com-

parisons and distinctions may be made between the two. Although the carriage of each gas depends on the existent driving pressure, the relationships between the amount of gas that is being transported and the driving pressure are characteristically different. The difference is most evident in the differences in the shapes of the two curves. The CO_2 dissociation curve lacks the sigmoid shape of the O_2 dissociation curve. Instead, the CO_2 dissociation curve demonstrates a relatively linear relationship between CO_2 content and Pco_2.

The amount of CO_2 carried in the blood not only depends on Pco_2 but also is affected by the degree of O_2 saturation in hemoglobin. The dependence between these two variables is referred to as the Haldane effect, which reflects the ability of hemoglobin to serve a dual carriage function. As soon as the hemoglobin gives up O_2 at the level of the needy tissues, the loading of CO_2 on the hemoglobin molecule for return to the lungs is facilitated. The loss of CO_2 at the alveolus facilitates loading of O_2. Thus three different curvilinear lines appear on the CO_2 dissociation curve. The curve to the right depicts hemoglobin that is almost fully saturated with O_2 and coincidentally has the lowest CO_2 content. The curves to the left reflect hemoglobins that are less saturated with O_2 and therefore have a greater CO_2 content.

To explain the transport and release of CO_2, a discussion of acid-base homeostasis is necessary. Obviously, since the lungs are prime controllers of the movement of acidic CO_2, they may function to maintain or disrupt the normal pH of the body's cellular environment. For example, an individual may be in a hyperventilatory state as a result of exercise, hyperthermia, or general anxiety. Regardless of the cause, if too much CO_2 is expired, or "blown off" by these excessive respirations without the initiation of immediate compensatory mechanisms, the internal chemical environment of the body could become less acidic. This condition is referred to as respiratory alkalosis, or an alkalotic state caused by the respiratory system. The body initiates certain metabolic activities to correct this problem and attempts to return the pH closer to 7.4. These activities generally involve ridding the body of a base such as HCO_3^- at the level of the kidneys. Thus the respiratory alkalosis is compensated for by metabolic mechanisms.

When a state of respiratory acidosis occurs, for example, when ventilatory status is depressed by certain drugs, the body must compensate by retaining excessive levels of base so that the pH remains at least near the normal level. In other words, much work is done to maintain a pH of near 7.4, but other, highly abnormal laboratory measures may persist. In the previously described alkalotic state the pH may return to a near-normal level, but HCO_3^- levels are lower than the normal level of 21 to 23 mEq/L. During respiratory acidosis HCO_3^- levels are higher than normal. An acid-base disequilibrium is not considered "corrected" until all blood gas values return to normal along with the pH.

CONTROL OF RESPIRATION

The control of respiration is an interesting, controversial subject. Although respiration is often thought of as a completely automatic process, common sense dictates that this is not the case. It is true that most of the time, the rate and depth of breathing are involuntarily determined, but the individual also possesses the ability to voluntarily change these values. Normally, however, when the individual alters activity from sleeping to high levels of exercise, the individual does not consciously think of how to change the respiratory pattern to ensure effective alveolar ventilation. Instead, the metabolic needs of the body are met because a need has been sensed by receptors sensitive to changes in Pao_2, Pco_2, or pH.

How are the changes in chemical status detected by the body? As with any other organism that must maintain homeostasis, the human body has sensors that function to provide information about changes in chemical equilibrium. The information detected by these sensors is communicated to a comparator. This comparator compares the afferent information with an established set point before a decision is made as to whether some efferent response is indicated. In the case of the respiratory system the comparator is at the level of the medulla within the brain stem. Afferent information about chemical status is sent to cells within the medulla from peripheral and central chemoreceptors. The peripheral chemoreceptors are located close to the carotid and aortic baroreceptors. The carotid peripheral chemoreceptors are the more responsive of the two and are located at the bifurcation of the carotid artery. The much less reactive aortic chemoreceptors reside in the arch of the aorta. Afferent information from the carotid and aortic receptors is transmitted via the glossopharyngeal and vagus nerves, respectively, to the respiratory "center" of the medulla. By necessity, of course, the peripheral chemoreceptors are highly vascularized, since they are detecting changes in the chemical constituents of the blood. They are primarily responsive only to changes in the Po_2 and generally are not highly reactive until Po_2 falls below 60 to 65 mm Hg, which coincidentally is the partial pressure that demarcates the beginning of the dissociation section of the O_2 dissociation curve. On the other hand, the central chemoreceptors located within the medulla near the site of the exit of the vagus nerves are highly reactive to changes in Pco_2 and hydrogen ion concentration. Should a chemical imbalance relative to the established set point at the medulla be noted by either the peripheral or the central chemoreceptors, efferent information may be sent to any of a number of sites to attempt correction so that alveolar ventilation remains adequate to meet the metabolic needs of the body.

The transmission of chemical information to the medulla should not imply that this brain stem structure functions independently in regulating respiratory rate and rhythm. Although it has been recognized for years that cells within two separate nuclei on the dorsal and ventral surfaces of the medulla function as the primary controllers of respiratory rhythm, the cells are strongly influenced by much afferent input from other sources.[2,4,6] The two nuclei are the nucleus tractus solitarius and the nucleus retroambiguous, both of which contain cells that are active during inspiration and others that discharge during expiration. The inspiratory cluster of cells rhythmically and tonically discharge and must be inhibited in some way so that inspiration can cease. This inhibition is provided by afferent information from a variety of sources, including higher respiratory areas in the cortex or pons, the hypothalamus, and input from autonomic afferents responsible for sensing changes directly within respiratory tissues and structures.

Respiration is normally established by integrating all the afferent input, but scientific studies have clearly shown that as long as the medulla remains intact, removal of this incoming information is not a requirement for continued inspiratory initiation. In other words, respiration ceases with loss of medullary output to respiratory structures. The medulla has been established as the controller of respiratory rhythm on the basis of studies in which the respiratory communication networks have been altered by chemical or surgical means during automatic, or involuntary, breathing. First, when cortical and cerebellar input to the brain stem is removed, respiratory rhythm remains unaffected. This response is not surprising, since the cortex functions primarily in the control of voluntary breathing. Second, when the proximal third of the pons, or the pneumotaxic center, is removed, the observed respiratory pattern varies depending on whether vagal input is present. With vagal input, respiration continues but a prolonged inspiratory phase is evident. This sustained inspiration, or apneusis, is not evident in the presence of vagal input. Instead, little change in rate and rhythm is noted other than some slight slowing and, perhaps, an increase in TV, if the vagi are intact. Removal of the lower portion of the pons, or the apneustic center, results in continued respiration, although the pattern of breathing is somewhat irregular and gasping, with or without vagal input. Third, removal of the medulla results in the cessation of breathing, or apnea.

Because input from the vagi is capable of altering respiratory rhythm, the importance of information being sensed in peripheral structures is evident. For example, the impulses transmitted from stretch receptors in the alveoli convey information about the distention of the alveolar units. This afferent arm of a stretch reflex is intended to protect the alveoli from becoming overinflated and permits the prevention of apneusis, even after the pneumotaxic center has been removed. Other important information is conveyed to the respiratory centers via the vagus nerve from irritant receptors in the trachea, bronchi, bronchioles, and cough receptors in the larynx. Most but not all of this information travels to the central nervous system in the vagus nerves, although other respiratory-related information may travel in the trigeminal and glossopharyngeal nerves. Efferent information reaches the respiratory structures either parasympathetically in the vagus nerve or by sympathetic impulses transmitted through the cervical or upper thoracic sympathetic ganglion. The cholinergic responses that occur with parasympathetic stimulation are bronchoconstriction and glandular secretion, whereas the adrenergic responses are bronchodilation and an inhibition of secretions. These differences in response explain why many of the pharmacologic agents used in the treatment of pulmonary disorders are designed either to mimic the effect of sympathetic receptor stimulation or to inhibit the parasympathetic respiratory effect.

REFERENCES

1. Celli BR: Respiratory muscle function, *Clin Chest Med* 7(4):567, 1986.
2. Comroe JH: *Physiology of respiration,* St Louis, 1977, Mosby.
3. DeTroyer A, Estenne M: Functional anatomy of the respiratory muscles, *Clin Chest Med* 9(2):175, 1988.
4. Forster RE et al: *The lung: physiologic basis of pulmonary function tests,* ed 3 Chicago, 1986, New York Medical.
5. Martin DE, Youtsey JW: *Respiratory anatomy and physiology,* St Louis, 1988, Mosby.
6. Netter FN: *The CIBA collection of medical illustrations: respiratory system,* New Jersey, 1980, CIBA-Geigy.
7. Pardy RL, Hussain SNA, Macklem PT: The ventilatory pump in exercise, *Clin Chest Med* 9(2):35, 1984.
8. Scanlan CL et al: *Egan's fundamentals of respiratory care,* ed 5, St Louis, 1993, Mosby.
9. West JB: *Respiratory physiology: the essentials,* ed 3, Baltimore, 1985, Williams & Wilkins.
10. Whipp BJ, Wasserman K: *Exercise: pulmonary physiology and pathophysiology,* New York, 1991, Marcel Dekker.

STUDY QUESTIONS

- Describe the anatomy of the lungs.
- Define minute ventilation, and discuss the variations on minute ventilation from rest to exercise. What are the differences in trained and untrained individuals?
- Describe the role of hemoglobin in O_2 and CO_2 transport and acid-base balance.
- Describe the relationship between P_{O_2} and hemoglobin saturation.
- Describe the changes that occur in the O_2 association-dissociation curve with exercise.

CHAPTER 5

EXERCISE TOLERANCE AND TRAINING FOR PATIENTS WITH RESTRICTIVE AND OBSTRUCTIVE LUNG DISEASE

Donna Frownfelter

EFFECT OF EXERCISE TRAINING ON VENTILATION AND Po_2

In normal individuals exercise is limited by hemodynamic factors, particularly the level to which the cardiac output can be elevated efficiently. No limitations are imposed by ventilatory capability, pulmonary gas exchange, or elevation of the pulmonary capillary wedge pressure. In normal individuals low-intensity exercise results in an increase in cardiac output (that is, stroke volume and heart rate), a widening of the arterial-venous oxygen difference ($Pa - Vo_2$) and an increase in oxygen consumption (Vo_2) and carbon dioxide production (Vco_2). The minute ventilation (tidal volume multiplied by respiratory rate) increases sufficiently to maintain the alveolar ventilation at a level high enough to remove all the CO_2 produced; therefore the arterial carbon dioxide pressure ($Paco_2$) remains within normal limits. Increased levels of exercise cause the alveolar-arterial oxygen pressure difference $P(A - a)o_2$ to decrease as a result of an improved ventilation-perfusion ratio (V/Q). During exercise pulmonary blood flow increases, and the pulmonary perfusion becomes more evenly distributed than during a period of rest. When exercise levels are increased, there comes a time when the blood flow available to the exercising muscles is inadequate to provide the needed oxygen. At that point, termed the *anaerobic threshold,* anaerobic metabolism occurs. Lactic acid enters the venous circulation and blood pH falls. In response to metabolic acidosis, minute alveolar ventilation rises disproportionately to the Vo_2, providing another indicator that the anaerobic threshold has been reached. When the Pco_2 falls, the extent of metabolic acidosis is moderated. If exercise is continued, however, a more severe acidosis follows; the Pao_2 is not significantly affected. In normal individuals cardiac output and the resultant increase in blood flow to the muscles are the limiting factors in exercise.[15]

The normal sequence of relationships among the previously described pulmonary function values during exercise changes when an individual has pulmonary dysfunction. Patients with either restrictive or obstructive lung disease are limited not by hemodynamic capabilities but by ventilatory limitations or pulmonary gas-exchange compromise, or by a combination of the two factors. Disturbances in the ventilation-perfusion relationship (such as increased dead space ventilation in patients with emphysema) must be taken into account. The work of breathing, defined as the perception of difficulty in breathing, may be thought of as the percentage of the vital capacity that the tidal volume occupies. For example, if a patient's vital capacity is 2000 cc and the tidal volume is 500 cc, 25% of the vital capacity is used during each breath. If the vital capacity drops to 1000 cc and the tidal volume is 500 cc, 50% of the vital capacity is used for the work of breathing. Such a patient has little reserve and probably has a sense of fatigue and difficulty breathing during exercise.

To understand the problems that individuals with pulmonary dysfunction exhibit during exercise, the classification of pulmonary diseases must be identified. Before pulmonary function testing was widely available, there was no easy, noninvasive way to document and monitor trends in the physiologic effects of pulmonary disease on the lungs. Pulmonary function tests help determine the following:

1. The volume of gas the lungs can move in and out
2. How fast the gas can be moved
3. How stiff the lungs and chest wall may be
4. The diffusion capabilities of the alveolar capillary membrane
5. How efficiently the O_2 is used and the CO_2 is removed

A complete pulmonary function test, including determination of arterial blood gas levels, permits an assessment of lung function.

Determination of normal pulmonary function values is based on variables that affect lung function. The variables are body size (height and weight), age, and sex. Height has the greatest impact. For the patient who is wheelchair bound, arm span may be used to correlate to height. Weight has less effect than height, although weight can be a significant factor when weight gain results from increased musculature (which might increase lung volumes) or when the patient has morbid obesity (in which case a restrictive component might be expected). Age is a factor in lung function because an individual's vital capacity may increase during the twenties and then decrease with continuing aging. A 20-year-old man may have a predicted vital capacity of slightly more than 5000 cc, whereas by 70 years of age the same person's predicted vital capacity will have fallen to approximately 25%. In addition to height, weight, and age variations, when men and women are matched for size, the lungs are larger in men. Other, poorly defined predictors mentioned in the literature are race and environmental factors, including altitude.

Many of the pulmonary function tests require the patient to give maximal effort. Consequently the practitioner must consider this aspect of patient performance when evaluating the pulmonary function results. Abnormal pulmonary function test results can be categorized into obstructive or restrictive lung defects. This grouping is based on the two basic components, air flow and volume, measured in the routine spirogram, the centerpiece of pulmonary function tests. An easy-to-understand distinction is that when flow is impeded, the defect is obstructive and when volume is reduced, a restrictive defect is responsible.[11,31,35]

An obstructive lung defect is usually one of several abnormalities associated with chronic obstructive pulmonary disease (COPD), asthma, chronic bronchitis, and emphysema. Obstruction can occur in the upper airways (larynx, trachea, or right or left main-stem bronchi), large airways (diameter greater than 2 mm), or the small airways (diameter less than 2 mm). The anatomic site of obstruction to flow may be suggested by the part of the spirogram that is abnormally affected.

When restrictive lung disease processes are present, results of the routine spirogram or the other studies of volume (such as body plethysmography) demonstrate reduced values. This category of disease includes chest wall dysfunction, neurologic disease such as muscular dystrophy or spinal cord injury, dysfunction of the diaphragm, and scarring of the lung as a result of interstitial lung disease or radiation therapy to the chest.

Some disease processes, such as sarcoidosis and emphysema, demonstrate a combined obstructive-restrictive component. For example, in patients with emphysema the residual volume in the lung slowly increases and eventually forces a restriction of the volume of air that can be inspired. The result is both obstructive and restrictive. Untreated bronchospasm can also cause a decrease in inspired volume.

Pulmonary function tests often are repeated after administration of a bronchodilator, if airway obstruction is identified. Measures of forced vital capacity (FVC), forced expiratory volume in 1 second (FEV_1), and forced expiratory flow (FEF) during the middle range of the expiratory curve (FEF of 25% to 75%) are used as indicators of the effect of the bronchodilator. Forced vital capacity should increase by 10%; FEV_1, by 15%; and FEF of 25% to 75%, by 20%. Bronchodilators are often prescribed when no significant increase in test values is evident, to determine whether an effect will occur over time.

A determination of arterial blood gas levels is usually obtained during a pulmonary function test, to detect the oxygenation, ventilation, and O_2 saturation deficits. In the evaluation of pulmonary function test results it is important to consider that the range of results can be wide, depending on the site of the test and the equipment used. Wanger and Irvin[34] compared test results for five trained, healthy individuals studied in 13 Denver-area pulmonary function test laboratories. The researchers performed an analysis of variance on the commonly used test values. They found no significant difference in measures of FVC, FEV_1, FEF of 25% to 75%, and functional residual capacity (FRC) obtained by helium dilution technique. There was a significant difference in diffusing capacity for carbon monoxide and total lung capacity (TLC). In the 13 hospitals studied six different brands of pulmonary function test instruments were used. There were differences in the sequence of the test items, the number of trials performed, and the calculation of the diffusing capacity for carbon monoxide and breath-hold time. The researchers concluded that hospitals in a given area should consider standardizing test techniques and adopt common reference equations for calculations, to minimize variability of results.

Exercise Testing

Exercise testing is an important part of patient assessment, since it provides information that is not available when patients are at rest. The decision to perform an exercise test is based on a need for additional information about a patient. Gallagher[13] cited the following reasons to perform an exercise test on a patient with COPD:

1. Assessment of exercise capacity
2. Aid in diagnosing cause of exercise limitation and symptoms
3. Assessment of factors contributing to exercise limitation
4. Prescription of exercise training program
5. Assessment of need for specific therapy that may improve exercise performance
6. Assessment of response to therapy

Exercise testing is generally used in patients with pulmonary disease to evaluate the anaerobic threshold, the point at which the body is stressed when oxygen need exceeds the oxygen availability. In addition, when patients begin to demonstrate a low oxygen pressure (Po_2) (that is, 55 to 60 torr), the patient might be expected to demonstrate oxyhemoglobin desaturation during exercise. The desaturation level would be easily observed during monitoring with an oxygen saturation meter.

Pulse oximetry. Pulse oximetry is a noninvasive method used to measure the oxygen carried by hemoglobin in pulsating blood vessels. A sensor or probe is attached to a number of body sites such as the ear, finger, nose, toe, or heel. The probes alternately shine red and infrared light supplied by means of light-emitting diodes through a pulsating vascular bed.

The accuracy of pulse oximetry is plus or minus 3%. However, Chapman et al.[5] reported that accuracy is greater with arterial oxygen saturation (SaO_2) levels above 75%. Falsely elevated readings were found when SaO_2 levels dropped below 75%. The researchers found that the lower the level of SaO_2, the greater the level of error in readings. This rate of error presents a problem in patients with severe COPD, in whom desaturation occurs more dramatically than normal. These patients may have profound desaturation, whereas the practitioner may have a false sense of security during the testing.[29] The following situations[23] limit the effectiveness of oximetry:

1. Dyshemoglobinemias (that is, CO hemoglobin, methemoglobin, and fetal hemoglobin)
2. Dyes and pigments (methylene blue, indocyanine green, and bilirubin)
3. Low perfusion
4. Anemia
5. Increased venous pulsations

It is important to compare the SaO_2 levels obtained by oximetry to actual arterial blood gas measurements for accuracy. Even when differences occur, trends can be monitored by means of oximetry. In severe hypoxemia the practitioner can be aware of the potential differences that may occur in SaO_2 values.

Shortness of breath on exertion is one of the most common complaints that lead patients to seek medical advice. Since dyspnea is subjective, further evaluation is required. An exercise test often is indicated. Mild COPD may be asymptomatic for many years. In patients who have a sedentary life-style 60% of lung function may be lost before shortness of breath occurs during daily activity. Spirometry may detect mild to moderate air flow obstruction in asymptomatic patients.[19]

Exercise Training

Normally exercise training methods are geared toward increasing strength, power, speed, and endurance. As described in Chapter 1, principles of training for healthy individuals and patients usually revolve around intensity, duration, frequency, and specificity of training, which are reviewed briefly here.

Intensity is important for any body system: to improve, it must be stressed to work harder than normal. Intensity, an "overload" phenomenon, refers to the extent of overload. The amount of the overload greatly influences the rate at which physiologic improvement occurs. Usually the greater the intensity, the greater the effect. Duration refers to the intensity repeated over time to provide sufficient overload to produce optimal physiologic function.

Frequency refers to periods of rest and exercise. Rest is needed to help in rebuilding the overloaded system to a new, higher level of function. Frequency also refers to how often exercise must be performed to attain a training level. Currently a frequency of three to four times per week is suggested.

The general concept of specificity of training is that training should be directed toward specific muscular groups used in an activity. To achieve specific training, the specific activity should be simulated. For example, if a patient chooses to increase his or her ability to walk, a treadmill would be a better instrument to use than a bicycle.

The choice of equipment gives the practitioner many options. Indoor treadmills are available and can be a good choice in winter or during inclement weather. However, to increase strength and avoid boredom, alternative exercise is helpful. Stationary cycles are excellent at home, since resistance can be applied. The seat must be at a comfortable level, with a 10% to 15% flexion at the knees. Toe clips are helpful and are recommended so that the cycler can pull up the pedals, as well as push them down. Patients often complain that the seat is uncomfortable; placing a towel, a cushion, or lambswool on the seat often helps. Semirecumbent cycles are available for patients who have poor trunk support or poor balance, or both. These cycles can facilitate the work load by increasing comfort and providing needed support for patients with severe disease.[14]

The practitioner functions much as a coach functions in setting goals for an athlete. We often have the following goals in mind during rehabilitation for patients with lung disease: (1) to improve the patients' physiologic function, (2) to improve the patients' skill and coordination, and (3) to motivate patients to achieve and maintain optimal levels of function.

Endurance is one of the most important components of training. Endurance is defined as the sustained ability of the heart, lungs, and circulatory system to take oxygen from the air and deliver it throughout the body. The body undergoes an adaptive response to the demands of repeated aerobic exercise. The heart pumps faster, and the arteries become dilated so that more blood can be carried to the muscles. The increased blood volume induces capillary formation so that the muscles are better supplied with blood. The muscles become more efficient at absorbing oxygen from the blood and converting stored carbohydrates and fats into energy. These effects are referred to as training effects.

The components of a physical therapy program for pulmonary rehabilitation of patients with obstructive lung disease are generally evaluation, patient education, airway clearance techniques, breathing retraining, relaxation techniques, exercise conditioning, and endurance training to increase activities of daily living.[12]

In an effective patient evaluation a determination is made regarding the limiting factors in the patient's functional status. If the patient has copious secretions, it makes sense that airway clearance techniques such as postural drainage, percussion and vibration, controlled cough, and hydration are started first. The patient is taught the techniques and usually is able to take the responsibility for self-treatment after the first few therapy sessions. Ross and Dean[28] have documented the beneficial role of positioning and mobilization as therapeutic interventions that can enhance oxygen transport in patients with cardiopulmonary dysfunction.

Before conditioning exercise is initiated, breathing retraining is initiated to help the patient gain control of breathing and understand how the perception of shortness of breath can be cognitively adjusted. Most patients can learn to use a controlled breathing technique when they begin to feel breathless; the technique allows them to continue to exercise and progress in endurance. Initially a simple pursed-lip breathing technique can help them pace their breathing.

The patient's breathing pattern should be assessed at rest and during activity and exercise. It is helpful to observe the patient when he or she is unaware of being observed. Is the patient using accessory muscles at rest? During activities? During exercise? Is posture normal? Does the chest wall move symmetrically during inspiration? Does the patient appear comfortable or stressed? What postures are chosen? Is he or she able to follow directions to alter the breathing pattern?

In a normal breathing sequence the diaphragm contracts, causing the central portion to descend and displace the abdominal viscera, which causes an anterior displacement of the abdomen. When the central tendon stabilizes on the viscera, the lateral fibers of the diaphragm cause the ''bucket handle'' effect and lift and elevate the lower ribs. Finally, the middle and upper regions of the chest expand. The practitioner must become aware of the components of the normal breathing pattern, to increase skill in identifying abnormal components in the patient's breathing pattern. A practical approach to changing abnormal breathing patterns in patients with pulmonary disease is to do the easiest thing first. For example, if a patient has a high respiratory rate and is using accessory muscles of respiration, simple relaxation techniques alone may be needed.

Relaxation techniques are helpful in gaining control. Visualization and contraction-relaxation exercises (Jacobsen's relaxation exercise) have been found helpful by many patients and have been reported to enhance the training benefit.[12] If relaxation techniques do not succeed in returning the patient's breathing pattern to normal, specific intervention must be initiated in the form of breathing retraining.

Diaphragmatic breathing must be taught in a developmental sequence. Generally the patient's progression is from the supine, or sidelying, position to sitting, standing, walking, and climbing stairs. Since exercise is task specific, it is important to remember to reinforce the use of diaphragmatic breathing in various postures and during a variety of activities of daily living (see the boxes on pp. 90 to 95). In the author's experience patients learn the breathing pattern more effectively when they can ''feel'' the movement of the diaphragm than when the practitioner tells them what

---

RELAXATION TECHNIQUE No. 1
Relaxation of arms (duration: 4 to 5 min)

First Settle back as comfortably as you can, and allow yourself to relax to the best of your ability. Clench your right fist, tighter and tighter, and study the tension as you tighten. Keep it clenched and feel the tension in your fist, hand, and forearm. Relax. Let the fingers become loose. Observe the contrast in your feelings. Let yourself go, and try to become more relaxed all over.

Second Clench your right fist tightly again. Hold it and notice the tension. Relax. Your fingers straightened out, and you notice the difference once again.

Third Repeat the procedure with your left fist. Clench the fist while the rest of your body relaxes. Clench the fist tighter and feel the tension. Relax, then repeat the procedure, enjoying the contrast. After clenching, relax for a minute or two.

Fourth Clench both fists, tighter and tighter. Both fists and forearms should be tense. Study the sensations. Relax. Straighten your fingers and feel the relaxation. Continue relaxing your hands and forearms more and more.

Fifth Bend your elbows and tense your biceps. Tense them harder and study the feelings. Straighten your arms, then let them relax. Feel the difference. Let the relaxation develop. Once more, tense your biceps. Hold the tension and observe it carefully. Straighten your arms and relax. *Pay close attention to your feelings each time you tense and relax.*

Sixth Straighten your arms until you feel most tension in the triceps muscles along the back of your arms. Stretch your arms and feel the tension, then relax. Get your arms back into a comfortable position. Allow the relaxation to proceed on its own. The arms should feel comfortably heavy as you allow them to relax. Straighten the arms once more so that you feel the tension in the triceps muscles. Feel the tension. Then relax.

Seventh Concentrate on pure relaxation in the arms without any tension. Get your arms into a comfortable position, then let them relax. Continue to relax them even more. Even when your arms seem fully relaxed, try to go that extra bit further; try to achieve deeper and deeper levels of relaxation.

From Frownfelter DL: *Chest physical therapy and pulmonary rehabilitation: an interdisciplinary approach,* ed 2, St Louis, 1987, Mosby.

to do. The practitioner places his or her hand on the patient's upper abdomen below the xiphoid. During the end of exhalation the practitioner provides a slow, gentle stretch upward into the diaphragm and gives the command ''Now, breathe into my hand'' to guide the patient's inspiratory effort. Later the pattern can be brought to the patient's cognition by the following statement: ''Notice that when you breathe in, your abdomen rises and when you exhale, it goes down.'' The practitioner should remind the patient to use the proper

pattern and to be aware of his or her breathing when performing various activities during the day. The preceding is not ''breathing exercise'' but the instruction in normal sequence of breathing.

The practitioner must be aware that the patient with severe COPD may have a flat diaphragm. This condition is generally diagnosed by means of radiograph and is noted on the interpretation. If the patient has a flat diaphragm, teaching diaphragmatic breathing is pointless, since in such patients diaphragmatic breathing causes a negative, down-

---

RELAXATION TECHNIQUE No. 2
Relaxation of facial area, neck, shoulders, and upper back (duration: 4 to 5 min)

First   Let all your muscles go loose and heave. Settle back quietly and comfortably. Wrinkle your forehead; wrinkle it tighter. Stop, relax, and smooth it out. Picture the entire forehead and scalp becoming smoother as the relaxation increases.

Second   Frown and crease your brows and study the tension. Release the tension. Smooth out the forehead once more. Close your eyes tighter and tighter. Feel the tension. Relax your eyes. Keep your eyes closed (good luck reading this with your eyes closed). They should be closed gently, comfortably. Notice the relaxation.

Third   Clench your jaws, studying the tension throughout your jaws. Relax. Let your lips part slightly. Appreciate the relaxation.

Fourth   Press your tongue hard against the roof of your mouth. Feel the tension. Let your tongue return to a comfortable and relaxed position.

Fifth   Purse your lips, pressing them tighter and tighter together. Relax. Notice the contrast between tension and relaxation. Feel the relaxation all over your face, forehead, scalp, eyes, jaws, lips, tongue, and throat. The relaxation progresses further and further.

Sixth   For the neck: Press your head back as far as it can go, and feel the tension in the neck. Roll your head to the right and feel the tension shift; now roll it to the left. Straighten your head and bring it forward. Press your chin against your chest. Let your head return to a comfortable position and study the relaxation. Let the relaxation develop.

From Frownfelter DL: *Chest physical therapy and pulmonary rehabilitation: an interdisciplinary approach,* ed 2, St Louis, 1987, Mosby.

ward pull on the chest that does not improve breathing. For patients with flat diaphragms it is more appropriate to teach energy conservation and pacing techniques that increase the ability to cope with shortness of breath.

Inspiratory Muscle Fatigue

Muscle weakness or muscle fatigue can lead to hypoventilation. Muscle weakness is a failure in the generation of an expected force or the chronic reduction in a contractile force, whereas muscle fatigue is a failure to maintain an expected force during repeated or sustained contractions. Inspiratory muscle fatigue occurs when the inspiratory effort exceeds the capacity of the inspiratory muscles to sustain that effort.[30]

Assessment of inspiratory muscle fatigue is basically a clinical evaluation of physical signs such as tachypnea, decreased tidal volume, discoordinated breathing pattern or paradoxic breathing, increased P_{CO_2}, bradypnea, and decreased pulmonary minute volume (V_E). In a research setting electromyography and force-frequency curves could be used in the evaluation.

Inspiratory Muscle Training

Inspiratory muscle training, like skeletal muscle training, attempts to condition and train the inspiratory muscles for strength and endurance. Training involves subjecting a muscle to stress greater than its usual load (overload). The training should be directed toward the development of strength or endurance and must be maintained or regression occurs.

The clinical technique most generally used is inspiratory muscle resistance training. In this technique either a commercially available narrow tube with a variable orifice size or a tube with a specific inspiratory load is used. The size of the orifice determines the load. Patients may begin training by

---

RELAXATION TECHNIQUE No. 3
Relaxation of chest, stomach, and lower back (duration: 4 to 5 min)

First   Relax your entire body to the best of your ability. Feel the comfortable heaviness that accompanies relaxation. Breathe easily and freely in and out. Notice how the relaxation increases as you exhale. Feel that relaxation as you breathe out.

Second   Breathe in and fill your lungs; inhale deeply and hold your breath. Study the tension. Now exhale; let the walls of your chest grow loose and push the air out automatically. Continue relaxing, and breathe freely and gently. Feel and enjoy the relaxation.

Third   With the rest of your body as relaxed as possible, fill your lungs again. Hold your breath. Breathe out and appreciate the relief. Just breathe normally. Continue relaxing your chest and let the relaxation spread to your back, shoulders, neck, and arms. Let go and enjoy the relaxation.

Fourth   Now pay attention to your abdominal muscles. Tighten your muscles to make your abdomen hard. Notice the tension, then relax. Let the muscles loosen and notice the contrast. Once more, press and tighten your stomach muscles. Hold the tension and study it. Relax. Notice the general well-being that comes with relaxing your stomach.

Fifth   Draw your stomach in. Pull the muscles right in and feel the tension this way. Now relax and let your stomach out. Continue breathing normally and easily, and feel the gently massaging action all over your chest and stomach. Pull your stomach in again and hold the tension. Now push out and tense. Hold the tension. Once more, pull in and feel the tension.

Sixth   Relax your stomach fully. Let the tension dissolve as the relaxation grows deeper. Each time you breathe out, notice the rhythmic relaxation both in your lungs and in your stomach. Notice how your chest and stomach relax more and more. Try to let go of all contractions anywhere in your body.

From Frownfelter DL: *Chest physical therapy and pulmonary rehabilitation: an interdisciplinary approach,* ed 2, St Louis, 1987, Mosby.

---

working up to breathing into and out of the tube for 15 to 30 minutes, three times per day. Nose clips are provided, but compliance is a problem. The patient must be taught to swallow with the tube in the mouth and lips closed before the procedure can be performed for 15 minutes.

The previously described treatment has been reported to prevent acute deterioration of respiratory status, improve ventilatory function and decrease work of breathing, increase exercise tolerance, and facilitate weaning from mechanical ventilation.[1,2,9,17,24-26]

Exercise Programs

During exercise programs for patients with lung disease patients often complain about dyspnea with upper-extremity exercise, yet few therapists prescribe upper-extremity exercise. Generally, breathing exercise and some form of walking or bicycle program for endurance are used. Ries et al.[27] studied upper-extremity exercise training in patients with COPD. They grouped patients into the following categories: (1) those who performed gravity-resisted exercise, (2) those who received modified proprioceptive neuromuscular upper-extremity training, and (3) those who received no upper-extremity training (control group). Groups 1 and 2 demonstrated improved performance over the control group for the tasks specific to the training performed. Ratings of perceived breathlessness decreased in the trained groups. The researchers concluded that

---

RELAXATION TECHNIQUE No. 4
Relaxation of shoulders and upper and lower back

First Using your imagination, think of yourself on a soft, fluffy white cloud. Your whole body is floating. Let yourself go. Let your muscles go loose and heavy. Feel that comfortable "all is well" feeling as you totally relax. Notice how the relaxation increases as you exhale.

Second Feel tension in your shoulder muscles as you shrug your shoulders. Pretend you are a turtle pulling its head into its shell. Hold the tension. Now relax and let go. Move your shoulders about until you sense the feeling of relaxation. Try to remember the feeling of tightness and tension as you shrug your shoulders again. Bring your shoulders up and forward. Hold the tension, being aware of the feeling. Now let go. Feel the muscles across your shoulders and the back of your neck grow limp. As you shrug your shoulders this time, bring them up and back. Tense those muscles, hold, then let go. Be aware of the change in feeling.

Third As you tense your shoulder muscles this time, tighten your neck, throat, jaws, and facial muscles. Bring your shoulders up and forward now, as you squeeze muscles in your neck, throat, jaws, and face. Hold it. Relax and notice the difference in feeling. Feel the relaxation spread deeply into your shoulders, right into the back of your neck, throat, and face. Let go. Let the feeling go deeper and deeper.

Fourth Now direct your attention to your lower back. Arch your back, making it hollow, and feel the tension along the spine. Recognize that feeling, and settle down again, relaxing the lower muscles. Keep the rest of the muscles throughout your body as relaxed as possible as you do that again. Arch your back, tighten the muscles, recognize the feelings as you localize the areas of tension. Now let go, settle down, feel the ease, warmth, and comfort. Notice the changed feeling and how restful it is.

Fifth With your attention focused on the lower back, bend sideways to the right, and feel the tension of the muscles on the left of your lower spine. Straighten your back and notice the relaxed feeling. Bend sideways to your left; bend a little more. Think of the muscles in your lower back. Now straighten and relax.

Sixth This time, try to flatten your lower back so that your spine is as straight as possible. Lying on the floor, flatten your back so that you can't put a finger between it and the floor. Feel the tension, then release. Study the difference between the tensed and relaxed states.

Seventh Relax your entire body as well as you can. Move your shoulders and upper back until they are comfortably positioned. Now do the same with your lower back, moving from side to side as necessary to find the most comfortable position. Mentally check your back muscles for looseness. Mentally talk to these muscles, telling them to let go.

From Frownfelter DL: *Chest physical therapy and pulmonary rehabilitation: an interdisciplinary approach,* ed 2, St Louis, 1987, Mosby.

upper-extremity exercise appeared to be beneficial and warranted more study.

During exercise in patients with low Po_2 it is helpful to have an oximeter available for evaluation of desaturation during exercise. In any patient with a Po_2 of 65 torr or less, desaturation should be suspected. Oximeters have been demonstrated to be helpful in monitoring saturation levels. Escourrou et al.[8] found by measuring direct arterial blood gas levels that the oximeter readings were not always exact, but oximetry was useful for tracking increases or decreases in saturation and looking at trends.

RELAXATION TECHNIQUE No. 5
Relaxation of hips and calves and complete body relaxation

First
Let go of all tensions, and relax. Now flex your buttocks and thighs. Flex your thighs by pressing down your heels as hard as you can. Relax and notice the difference. Straighten your knees and flex your thigh muscles again. Hold the tension. Relax your hips and thighs. Allow the relaxation to proceed on its own.

Second
Press your feet and toes downward, away from your face, so your calf muscles become tense. Study the tension. Relax your feet and calves.

Third
This time, bend your feet toward your face so that you feel tension along your shins. Bring your toes right up. Relax again. Keep relaxing for a while. Let yourself relax further, all over. Relax your feet, ankles, calves, shins, knees, thighs, buttocks, and hips. Feel how heavy and relaxed you have become.

Fourth
Now spread the relaxation to your stomach, waist, and lower back. Let go more and more. Feel that relaxation all over. Let it proceed to your upper back, chest, shoulders and arms, and right to the tips of your fingers. Keep relaxing more and more deeply. Make sure that no tension has crept into your throat. Relax your neck and jaws and all your facial muscles. Keep relaxing your whole body like that for a while.

Fifth
Now you can become twice as relaxed as you are, merely by taking in a really deep breath and slowly exhaling. With your eyes closed to avoid distractions and to keep surface tensions from developing, breathe in deeply and feel yourself becoming heavier. Take in a long, deep breath and let it out very slowly. Feel how heavy and relaxed you have become.

Sixth
In a state of perfect relaxation, you should feel unwilling to move a single muscle in your body. Think about the effort that would be required to raise your right arm. Now you decide not to lift the arm but to continue relaxing. Observe the relief and the disappearance of tension.

Seventh
Continue relaxing like that. When you wish to get up, count backwards from 4 to 1. You should then feel refreshed, wide awake, and calm.

From Frownfelter DL: *Chest physical therapy and pulmonary rehabilitation: an interdisciplinary approach*, ed 2, St Louis, 1987, Mosby.

Use of Supplemental Oxygen During Exercise

Light et al.[18] demonstrated a relationship between improvement in exercise performance when supplemental oxygen was used and hypoxic ventilatory drive in patients with chronic air flow obstruction. A concern exists that increasing inspired oxygen in patients who retain CO_2 results in an oxygen-induced hypercarbia. This result has been documented by Dunn et al.[7] in patients receiving oxygen. The author's experience, however, is that when supplemental oxygen is used during exercise, a titration is made of a proper dose to prevent desaturation during exercise. For example, if desaturation occurs after the administration of 1 L per minute of oxygen by nasal cannula, 2 L of oxygen is administered. If 2 L of oxygen prevents desaturation, only 2 L of oxygen is used. When exercise is ended, the amount of supplemental oxygen is reduced to the level prescribed for the patient at rest. Since increased oxygen is used during exercise, if the oxygen is brought back down within a short time

---

RELAXATION TECHNIQUE No. 6
Total body relaxation

First   Position yourself as comfortably as possible, with a pillow under your head and another one under your knees. Bring the pillow under your head close to your shoulders. Allow your knees to fall apart, supported by the pillow under them.

Second   Beginning with your scalp and ending with your toes, you are going to tense and relax groups of muscles. Be conscious of the feeling of tension and the opposite feeling of release. You may sense feelings of hostility, aggravation, frustration, fear, and similar emotions as you tense your muscles. You may feel peaceful, loving, restful, accepted, forgiven, and similar comfortable feelings as you relax.

Third   Tense your scalp—relax. Wrinkle your forehead, hard—relax. Frown, crease your brows tightly—relax. Study the tension and relaxation feelings. Close your eyes, squeeze hard—relax. Press your tongue hard against the roof of your mouth—relax, allowing your tongue to go flat and limp. Clench your jaws, bite your teeth together—relax. Purse your lips and press them together hard—relax. Press your head back, study the neck muscles—relax. Press your head forward onto your chest—relax. Roll your head to the left and press—relax. Roll your head to the right—relax.

Fourth   Clench both fists—relax. Stretch your fingers—relax. Flex your biceps with clenched fists—relax. Straighten your arms, bending the backs of your hands upward—relax.

Fifth   Take in a deep breath and hold it—relax as you exhale. Tighten your abdominal muscles, pinch, and squeeze—relax. Push out and tense the muscles that way—relax.

Sixth   Shrug your shoulders up and forward—relax. Shrug your shoulders up and backward—relax. Arch your back—relax. Push back with the small of your back—relax.

Seventh   Flex your buttocks and thighs—relax. Press your feet and toes away from you; feel the pull on the leg calf muscles—relax. Press your feet and toes toward your face so that you feel tension along the shins—relax. Curl your toes, squeezing hard—relax. Now bend your toes out and relax.

Eighth   Take in a long, deep breath, and feel how heavy you are. Let your muscles go limp, sort of flow. Listen to your heart beat and notice the slow inhalation and exhalation of your breathing. Mentally check out each area of your body and let it go—head and face, arms, chest and abdomen, back, hips, legs, and feet. You are totally relaxed.

From Frownfelter DL: *Chest physical therapy and pulmonary rehabilitation: an interdisciplinary approach,* ed 2, St Louis, 1987, Mosby.

(that is, recovery time of 5 minutes), after the patient's heart rate and blood pressure have returned to baseline values, the oxygen is reduced. When the previously described method is used, the patient does not have increasing hypercarbia.

Long-term oxygen therapy is the only therapy that has been shown to improve survival in patients with COPD.[32] New techniques such as transtracheal oxygen therapy have been found to actually increase the patient's room air blood gas Pao_2 (ambient air) measure. In a study by O'Donohue[21] in 20% of the patients the Po_2 level improved to more than 55 mm Hg, which made them ineligible for home oxygen supplementation at rest. However, desaturation still occurred in these patients during walking. The study concluded that it was inappropriate to terminate the oxygen therapy because of the beneficial effects and the potential for patient deterioration if oxygen were removed.

When maximal exercise response is the goal, patients should be monitored during exercise for cardiac arrhythmias. Most patients with primary pulmonary disease who are asymptomatic at rest do not have arrhythmias during exercise. Cheong et al.[6] studied cardiac arrhythmias during exercise in patients with COPD and found that 87% of patients who were asymptomatic at rest did not have arrhythmias during exercise. However, cardiac monitoring revealed unsuspected problems in other patients. The researchers strongly suggested that cardiac monitoring be routinely performed during exercise testing in patients with COPD.

Normal fitness indicators are a lower heart rate at rest than during exercise, which shows that the heart is processing the same amount of blood with less effort at rest; decreased blood pressure at rest; and an adapted, lower blood pressure during exercise. The maximal volume of oxygen that the body is capable of taking in and using for one minute during intense exercise is the Vo_2max. A high Vo_2max is a sign of fitness. The Vo_2max of a runner in long-distance races can be twice that of a sedentary individual.

Exercise has been linked to "feeling better." Significant changes in attitude and mood seem to occur shortly after the initiation of exercise and may continue for the length of the workout and beyond. Explanations of these changes have ranged from "release of endorphins" and "psychologically" to "I work out, therefore I am in control of my life."[33]

Painter and Blackburn[22] have concluded that most patients with chronic disease can benefit from rehabilitation to optimize their functioning within the limitations placed on them by their disease or treatment. In addition, rehabilitation increases their level of personal responsibility and helps them cope with the disease more effectively. The researchers thought that a supervised exercise setting was best, since it increases exercise compliance and provides the primary physician with a

feedback mechanism. The support of the primary physician was found to dramatically enhance the rehabilitation efforts.

SPECIFIC EXERCISE TRAINING

There have been questions in pulmonary rehabilitation programs addressing whether there is a physiologic basis for increased exercise tolerance. Cassaburi et al.[4] attempted to answer the question by evaluation of reduction in blood lactate levels and ventilation, or pulmonary minute volume, (V_E) at given levels of exercise. They also attempted to determine whether training work rate would determine the size of the training effect. The researchers divided 19 patients with moderately severe COPD into two groups; each group performed exercise tests at either a low or a high work rate on a cycle ergometer for 15 minutes or to tolerance. Arterial blood samples were drawn so that blood gas levels and blood lactate measurements could be determined. The researchers concluded that although the work load was the same in both groups, training at a high work rate was more effective than training at a low work rate. They also found that the patients who trained at a high work rate had a smaller decrease in V_E for a given decrease in blood lactate level than did normal individuals. The premise of the researchers was that patients with COPD do not hyperventilate in response to lactic acidosis. Based on these findings, the authors thought that a physiologic rationale exists for the use of exercise training for COPD patients.

Foster et al.[10] studied patients with COPD who had elevated Pco_2 and severe impairment and might benefit from pulmonary rehabilitation. No data existed to indicate that hypercapnic COPD patients would benefit from intensive rehabilitation. There was a concern that in these severely sick patients a detrimental effect might result from exercise insofar as the respiratory muscles might be overtaxed. From 1983 to 1986, 317 patients in an inpatient pulmonary rehabilitation program were studied. Ambulation distance during a 6-minute walking test was used as an objective measurement of functional status. Patients were grouped according to P_{CO_2} levels. Eucapnic patients (normal P_{CO_2}; N = 197 patients) significantly increased ambulation distance from 409 to 816 feet, (p [significant value] less than 0.001). Hypercapnic patients improved as well. Patients grouped as moderately hypercapnic (P_{CO_2} of 45 to 54 torr; N = 86 patients) increased their ambulation distance from 330 to 663 feet (p less than 0.001). Patients with severe hypercapnia (P_{CO_2} greater than 54 torr; N = 34 patients) increased their ambulation distance from 336 to 597 feet (p less than 0.001). The researchers concluded that patients with COPD, despite severe ventilatory impairment and weak respiratory muscles, tolerate exercise well and benefit significantly from intensive pulmonary rehabilitation.

Pulmonary function test results rarely have been shown to change after a pulmonary rehabilitation program. However, data support the hypothesis that a short-term inpatient program of general exercise conditioning can improve work output, gas exchange, and mechanical efficiency (capacity) without significantly affecting spirometric indices. Carter et al.[3] observed that the positive changes may translate into improved performance of activities of daily living and give patients a general sense of well-being.

Results similar to those previously described have been observed in outpatient pulmonary rehabilitation programs. Zu Wallack et al.[37] reported on 50 ambulatory outpatients who completed a 6-week pulmonary rehabilitation program. The 12-minute walking distance (12 MD) was used as an indicator of improvement. An overall increase in the distance walked in 12 minutes in all patients resulted, and other interesting data emerged. Patients with lower peak levels of oxygen consumption ($V_{O_2}max$) showed a greater percentage of improvement in the 12 MD. The increase in 12 MD was inversely related to the percentage of its improvement. The combination of a smaller initial 12 MD and a larger forced expiratory volume in 1 second (FEV_1) was a significant predictor of success. The researchers concluded that patients with poor performance either on the 12 MD or on the maximal exercise test are not necessarily poor candidates for a pulmonary rehabilitation program.

Neiderman et al.[20] evaluated the improvement in 33 patients who completed an outpatient pulmonary rehabilitation program. The authors attempted to determine what types of improvement were seen and whether improvement was related to the degree of pulmonary dysfunction. They found that endurance measurements based on sustained submaximal performance on a cycle ergometer and the 12 MD increased significantly. Maximal exercise performance during a graded cycle test improved very little. A correlation existed between the sustained submaximal exercise performance and the FEV_1 (r = 0.5, p less than 0.01) but only when FEV was expressed in an absolute number (liters) and not as a percentage predicted. Pulmonary function did not correlate with the magnitude of change in both physiologic and psychologic values. These researchers, too, like others previously mentioned, concluded that the benefits of rehabilitation can extend to all patients with COPD, regardless of severity of pulmonary function impairment.

One of the training effects observed in individuals in good health is the improved sense of well-being. Kersten[16] attempted to describe the changes in self-concept that occurred during and after a formal pulmonary rehabilitation program. Thirty-seven patients with COPD were given a 20-item semantic-meaning differential scale. They were asked to evaluate their past, present, and future selves on admission to the program, on discharge from the program, and at intervals of 2 and 6 months after the program. The mean total self-concept score for the present self significantly increased from the time of program admission to the time of discharge to home 3 weeks later. No significant decline in score was noted at 2 months and 6 months after the program. Men showed a greater increase in total self-concept score than did women during the 3-week program; however, the decrease in the men's score was greater after home discharge. The authors suggested that this decrease might indicate a greater need for more intensive follow-up in men.

CASE STUDY

Mrs. H., a 69-year-old widow, was referred to physical therapy after a hospitalization for an acute exacerbation of asthma secondary to pneumonia of the right lower lobe, which was complicated by congestive heart failure. Pulmonary function test results demonstrated a decreased FEV_1 (60% of predicted) and increased total lung capacity (110%). Arterial blood gas levels were pH, 7.37; Pco_2, 45 torr; Po_2, 59 torr; and Sao_2, 93% on room air. An oximetry study revealed desaturation within 2 minutes when patient was walking on a treadmill at a rate of 1.2 mph at 0% grade. Blood pressure increased to 176/90, heart rate to 140 beats per min. Patient was discharged on a regimen of Alupent and Vanceril metered-dose inhalers (MDIs) three times per day and prednisone, 10 mg daily.

Patient assessment revealed the following: breath sounds decreased, right lung greater than left, rales bilaterally at bases, wheezing on inspiration and expiration. Cough was productive of moderate amount of thick greenish yellow mucus. Exercise tolerance was poor; patient was unable to perform activities of daily living. Supplemental oxygen was prescribed during exercise at 3 L per minute. Patient was given a peak-flow meter to monitor her progress but did not understand how to use it or her MDIs properly. Instruction was given at first therapy session.

PT plan of treatment

1. Review proper use of MDIs and peak-flow meter, encourage exercise and activities of daily living after use of bronchodilators for maximal lung function.
2. Airway clearance techniques: Postural drainage, percussion and vibration, proper cough techniques, encourage hydration.
3. Breathing exercises, relaxation, controlled, paced breathing with activities.
4. Graded exercise program with supplemental oxygen at 3 L per minute.
5. Increase walking program and use of stairs (patient lives on second floor of a condominium).

Results

After 6 weeks of therapy twice a week with patient follow-through for home exercise program, results included the following:

1. Breath sounds clear, decreased at bases, no wheezing.
2. Cough minimally productive, good hydration.
3. Increased activity tolerance, able to perform activities of daily living independently, with rest periods in between.
4. Patient stopped using supplemental oxygen with exercise at home. Physician notified; patient was retested and desaturation did not occur during exercise. Oxygen supplementation discontinued, acute pneumonia considered resolved, patient more stable.
5. Dosage of prednisone decreased to 2.5 mg.
6. Inspiratory resistance exercise initiated; patient was not compliant.
7. Patient ambulating for a distance of 2 blocks, climbing three flights of stairs.
8. Patient expressed an increased feeling of security in being alone and increased well-being; compliant with home exercise program and independent chest physical therapy when necessary. Daughter instructed in chest physical therapy techniques in case patient becomes ill and unable to perform chest physical therapy.

SUMMARY

We can feel confident as physical therapists that exercise has an important role to play in the rehabilitation of patients with COPD. Pulmonary rehabilitation is effective, regardless of the severity of pulmonary dysfunction. Both physical and psychologic improvements are evident. However, the literature contains little information about restrictive pulmonary disease.

REFERENCES

1. Aldridge T, Kaysel J: Inspiratory muscle resistive training in respiratory failure, *Chest* 86(2):302, 1984.
2. Belman MJ, Sieck GC: The ventilatory muscles: fatigue, endurance and training, *Chest* 82(6):761, 1982.
3. Carter R et al: Exercise conditioning in the rehabilitation of patients with chronic obstructive pulmonary disease, *Arch Phys Med Rehabil* 69(2):118, 1988.
4. Cassaburi R et al: Reductions in exercise lactic acidosis and ventilation as a result of exercise training in patients with obstructive lung disease, *Am Rev Respir Dis* 143(1):9, 1991.
5. Chapman KR et al: Range of accuracy of two wavelength oximetry, *Chest* 89:540, 1986.
6. Cheong TH et al: Cardiac arrhythmias during exercise in severe chronic obstructive pulmonary disease, *Chest* 97(4j):793, 1990.
7. Dunn WF et al: Oxygen-induced hypercarbia in obstructive pulmonary disease. I, *Am Rev Respir Dis* 144 (3):526, 1991.
8. Escourrou PJ et al: Reliability of pulse oximetry during exercise in pulmonary patients, *Chest* 97(3):635, 1990.
9. Flynn MG et al: Threshold pressure training breathing pattern and exercise performance in chronic airflow obstruction, *Chest* 95(3):535, 1989.
10. Foster S et al: Pulmonary rehabilitation in COPD patients with elevated Pco_2, *Am Rev Respir Dis* 138(6):1519, 1988.
11. Frownfelter DL: Review of respiratory physiology. In Frownfelter DL: *Chest physical therapy and pulmonary rehabilitation, ed 2*, St Louis, 1987, Mosby.
12. Frownfelter DL: Relaxation techniques. In Frownfelter DL: *Chest physical therapy and pulmonary rehabilitation, ed 2*, St Louis, 1987, Mosby.
13. Gallagher C: Exercise testing in patients with COPD, *Respiratory Management* 21(6):140, 1991.
14. Goldman B, Katz R: *The ''E'' factor: the secrets of new-tech training and fitness for the winning edge,* New York, 1988, William Morrow.
15. Irwin S, Tecklin J: Abnormal exercise physiology. In Irwin S, Tecklin J: *Cardiopulmonary physical therapy,* St Louis, 1990, Mosby.
16. Kersten L: Changes in self-concept during pulmonary rehabilitation. I. *Heart Lung* 19(5):456, 1990.
17. Kigin CM: Breathing exercises for the medical patient: the art and science, *Phys Ther* 70(11):700, 1990.
18. Light RW et al: Relationship between improvement in exercise performance with supplemental oxygen and hypoxic ventilatory drive in patients with chronic airflow obstruction, *Chest* 95(4):751, 1989.
19. Make B: COPD: management and rehabilitation, *Am Fam Physician* 43(4):1315, 1991.
20. Neiderman MS et al: Benefits of a multidisciplinary pulmonary rehabilitation program: improvements are independent of lung function, *Chest* 99(4):798, 1991.
21. O'Donohue WJ Jr: Effect of oxygen therapy on increasing arterial oxygen tension in hypoxemic patients with stable chronic obstructive pulmonary disease while breathing ambient air, *Chest* 100(4):968, 1991.
22. Painter P, Blackburn G: Exercise for patients with chronic disease, *Post Grad Med* 83(1):185, 190, 1988.
23. Ralston AC et al: Potential errors in pulse oximetry: effects of interference, dyes, hemoglobins and other pigments: *Anaesthesia* 46:291, 1991.
24. Reid WD, Loveridge BM: Ventilatory muscle training in patients with chronic obstructive airways disease, *Physiother Can* 35(4):197, 1983.
25. Reid WD, Warren CPW: Ventilatory muscle strength and endurance training in elderly subjects and patients with chronic airflow limitation: a pilot study, *Physiother Can* 36(6):305, 1984.
26. Richardson J et al: Inspiratory resistive endurance training in patients with chronic obstructive pulmonary disease: a pilot study, *Physiother Can* 41(2):85, 1990.
27. Ries AL et al: Upper-extremity exercise training in chronic obstructive pulmonary disease, *Chest* 93(4):688, 1988.
28. Ross J, Dean E: Integrating physiological principles into the comprehensive management of cardiopulmonary dysfunction, *Phys Ther* 69(4):255, 1989.
29. Severinghaus JW, Naifeth KH: Accuracy of response to six pulse oximeters to profound hypoxia, *Anesthesiology* 67:551, 1987.
30. Shekleton M: Respiratory muscle fatigue. In Frownfelter DL: *Chest physical therapy and pulmonary rehabilitation, ed 2*, St Louis, 1987, Mosby.
31. Singleton M, Branch E: Interpreting arterial blood gas measurements in the patient with pulmonary disease. In *Physical therapy and the pulmonary patient: aspects of evaluation and treatment,* New York, 1986-1987, Haworth.
32. Swarski, K et al: Predictors of survival in patients with chronic obstructive pulmonary disease treated with long-term oxygen therapy, *Chest* 100(6):1522, 1991.
33. Time-Life Books: *Building endurance.*
34. Wanger J, Irvin C: Comparability of pulmonary function results from 13 laboratories in a metropolitan area, *Respir Care* 36:1375, 1991.

35. Wilkins R, Sheldon R, Krider SJ: *Clinical assessment in respiratory care,* ed 2, St Louis, 1990, Mosby.
36. Reference deleted in proofs.
37. Zu Wallack RL et al: Predictors of improvement in the 12-minute walking distance following a six-week outpatient pulmonary rehabilitation program, *Chest* 99(4):805, 1991.

SUGGESTED READINGS

Bjure J et al: Respiratory impairment and airway closure in patients with untreated idiopathic scoliosis, *Thorax* 25:451, 1970.

Carter R et al: Demand oxygen delivery for patients with restrictive lung disease, *Chest* 986(6):1307, 1989.

Demling RH et al: Restrictive pulmonary dysfunction caused by the grafted chest and abdominal burns, *Crit Care Med* 16(8):743, 1988.

Goldstein RS et al: Intermittent positive pressure ventilation via a nasal mask in patients with restrictive ventilatory failure, *Chest* 97(suppl 3):805, 1990.

Hickey SA et al: Tracheostomy closure in restrictive respiratory insufficiency, *J Laryngol Otol* 104(11):883, 1990.

Kafer ER: Respiratory and cardiovascular functions in scoliosis and the principles of anesthetic management, *Anesthesiology* 52:339, 1980.

Robb-Nicholson LC et al: Effects of aerobic conditioning in lupus fatigue: a pilot study, *Br J Rheumatol* 28(6):500, 1989.

Schwartz DA: Determinants of restrictive lung function in asbestos-induced pleural fibrosis, *J Appl Physiol* 68(5):1932, 1990.

STUDY QUESTIONS

- Describe common physical therapy techniques for improving airway clearance and breathing retraining.

- Describe the differences between obstructive and restrictive pulmonary disease.

- Describe the responses during exercise and after an exercise training program for patients with COPD.

- What is the role of supplemental oxygen for patients with pulmonary disorders?

NORMAL CARDIOVASCULAR ANATOMY, PHYSIOLOGY, AND RESPONSES AT REST AND DURING EXERCISE

Elizabeth J. Protas

Chapter 6 focuses on normal cardiovascular anatomy and physiology. The material in this chapter is considered essential to an understanding of normal exercise responses and the consequences of disease or disability. After reading this chapter, the reader will be able to discuss normal myocardial structure, the components of the cardiovascular system, myocardial activation and contraction, hemodynamics, and circulatory control. Knowing both the structure and the function of the cardiovascular system greatly enhances the practitioner's ability to apply this knowledge to clinical exercise situations.

MYOCARDIAL STRUCTURE: BASIS FOR PUMPING BLOOD
General Structure of the Heart

The heart is composed of specialized muscle known as cardiac muscle or myocardium, which is organized in a multichambered system for the purpose of pumping blood either to the lungs or to the rest of the body. The heart is effectively two pumping systems, the right side and left side of heart. These systems are controlled by specialized nerve cells within the myocardium that can be modulated by the central nervous system. Coordination between the mechanical and electrical events of the heart and system reserves allows the heart to function well at rest and respond to the demands of heavy exercise.

Myocardial muscle. Cardiac muscle has a number of features in common with skeletal muscle. The muscle fibers are striped or striated. The muscle has small myofibril units containing actin and myosin filaments that interdigitate and slide along one another during contraction.

Unlike skeletal muscle fibers, however, cardiac muscle fibers are highly interconnected and have a latticework appearance. Fibers are separated by cell membranes known as intercalated disks, which serve to drastically reduce the resistance to an electrical current when it flows from one fiber to

Sincere thanks to Kay Sarver for creating illustrations for this chapter.

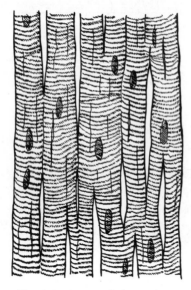

Fig. 6-1 Myocardial synctium.

another.[23] This interconnection enables the individual cells of the myocardium to act as a functional whole with other cells, since the activation of one cell is rapidly spread to all the others.[15] This structure is known as a syncytium, or the fusion of multinucleated cells into a unit (Fig. 6-1).

There are atrial and ventricular syncytiums in the heart, which are separated by a fibrous band between the atria and the ventricles. These two systems permit an action potential to spread and depolarize either the atrium or ventricles as a unit.[34] The specialized conduction system carries the depolarization from the atrium through the fibrous band to the ventricles.

The syncytial arrangement of the cardiac muscle permits the stimulation of any atrial cell to result in the stimulation of the entire atrium. The same is also true for the stimulation of any ventricular cell. In this way cardiac muscle works on the "all-or-none" principle. Unlike the application of the "all-or-none" principle to nerve cells, in which a single cell is fired, the entire atrium or ventricle depolarizes.

Four chambers of the heart. The heart is divided into right and left sides; each side has an atrium and a ventricle (Fig. 6-2). The right side of the heart receives and pumps blood to the lungs, whereas the left side pumps blood to the trunk, head, and extremities. The bulk of the work of the heart is done by the main pumps, the ventricles. The atria act as auxiliary pumps that contract to inject blood into the ventricles just before the ventricles contract.[25]

A considerable difference exists in the demands made on the right and left ventricles. The right side of the heart has to move the blood a relatively short distance to the lung. The left side of the heart, however, has to ensure that oxygenated blood is delivered to the farthest periphery of the toes. The difference in the work produces a much thicker left ventricular wall.[18]

The ventricular muscle contains three layers (Fig. 6-3). Two layers are arranged in spiral S fashion from the superior portion of the heart near the aorta and pulmonary artery to the inferior apex of the heart. Contraction of these layers produces a wringing-type motion of the ventricle. The other layer is arranged more circumferentially and constricts the ventricular diameter when contracted. This action has been compared to the motion of a bellows.[34]

Valves. Four valves operate to move blood in a unidirectional fashion into and out of the ventricles (Fig. 6-4). Two valves between the atria and ventricles, the atrioventricular (AV) valves, allow blood to pass into the ventricles during ventricular filling and prevent blood from flowing back into the atria during ventricular contraction. The valve between the right atrium and ventricle has three leaflets and is called the tricuspid valve. The left AV valve has two leaflets and is referred to as the bicuspid valve. Because the bicuspid valve looks like a bishop's hat, a miter, it is also called the mitral valve. Another set of valves, the semilunar valves, is positioned between the ventricles and the aorta and pulmonary arteries. These are called the aortic and pulmonic valves, respectively. When the ventricles contract, a rise in pressure in the ventricles passively opens the aortic and pulmonic valves and extrudes blood into the great arteries. The pressure drops again after enough blood exits and the valves close.[25]

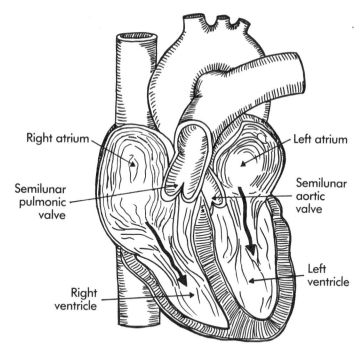

Fig. 6-2   The four chambers of the myocardium. The wall of the left ventricle is thicker than that of the right ventricle, and both atria have relatively thin muscular walls. The mitral and tricuspid valves are shown open (*large arrows*) during diastole.

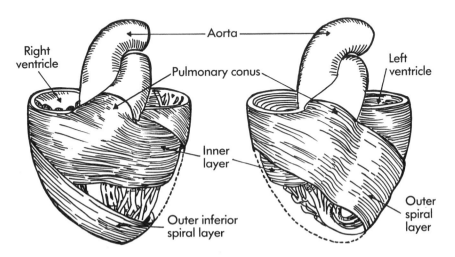

Fig. 6-3   The outer spiral layers and the inner circumferential layers of the ventricular muscle.

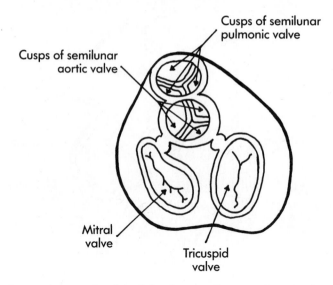

Cusps of semilunar pulmonic valve

Cusps of semilunar aortic valve

Mitral valve

Tricuspid valve

Fig. 6-4 The heart valves consist of the following: semilunar aortic and pulmonic valves and the atrioventricular tricuspid and mitral valves.

The AV valves open and close during the opposite time of the cardiac cycle from the aortic and pulmonic valves. The AV valves allow ventricular filling, and the semilunar valves allow ventricular emptying. The AV valves are relatively delicate tissues that, when closed, have to withstand the large pressures developed in the ventricles. If the valves were not supported in some way, leaking from the ventricle back into the atria would occur during ventricular contraction. Support for the AV valves is provided by the papillary muscles in the ventricular walls, which are attached to the ventricular surface of the valves by the chordae tendineae. The papillary muscles contract with the ventricle and literally hold the AV valves closed against the tremendous ventricular pressures.[25] Any damage to these fine structures, such as may occur with a myocardial infarction, results in a leaky or incompetent valve. Scarring of valve leaflets, which does not allow enough blood to flow from one chamber to another, can also occur. This condition is known as valvular stenosis.

Pacemaker and specialized conduction system. The heart's internal pacemaker and its associated conduction system ensures that the heart beats at a regular rate and that timing of the firing is carefully orchestrated (Fig. 6-5). The sinoatrial (SA) node located in the right atrium is the pacemaker and has an intrinsic firing rate of 70 beats per minute at rest. A depolarization emanating from the SA node depolarizes both atria and moves into the AV node. The AV node is also known as the junctional node, since it is at the junction between the right atrium and ventricle. The conduction velocity of an electrical impulse through the AV node is slow, which allows for a delay between atrial contraction and ventricular depolarization. The action potential then proceeds down the specialized conduction system consisting of the bundle of His, the right and left bundle branches, and the Purkinje fibers. The conduction system enables rapid deployment of an action potential through the right and left ventricles.[8]

In addition to the SA node, other parts of the specialized conduction system can pace the heart. The SA node usually is the pacemaker because it has the highest intrinsic rate and suppresses the other components. The rate in the AV node of 50 to 60 beats per minute at rest is slightly lower than that in the SA node.[19] A failure of both the SA and

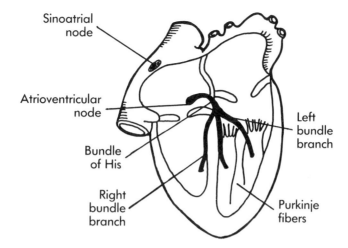

Fig. 6-5 Electrical pacemaking and conduction system of the heart. The sinoatrial node is the principle pacemaker of the heart.

the AV nodes, such as with a complete heart block, can result in the exceedingly slow rate of 30 to 40 beats per minute produced by the bundle of His and the Purkinje fibers.

Autonomic control. Both sympathetic and parasympathetic nerves innervate the SA and AV nodes. This neural influence can increase or decrease the firing rate of the heart. The parasympathetic nerves in the vagus nerve release acetylcholine, which hyperpolarizes the membrane and increases the permeability of the membrane to potassium. These actions slow the rate of the SA node. In contrast, the release of norepinephrine from sympathetic nerves increases the rate of firing.[21] The autonomic controls provide a means for the heart to rapidly respond to the demands of exercise and to slow the heart rate after exercise ceases.

Heart transplantation removes the nervous connections to the heart, thus leaving a denervated heart without autonomic control. The result is that the resting heart rate is usually higher, the heart rate responds slowly to an exercise stimulus via circulating catecholamines, and the heart rate recovery period is prolonged.[10]

Coronary circulation. The left main and right coronary arteries branch from the aorta to supply blood to the heart (Fig. 6-6). The left main coronary artery branches into the circumflex coronary artery, which supplies much of the posterior myocardium and the left anterior descending coronary artery.[22]

The coronary arteries are often compromised as a result of arteriosclerotic processes that reduce the size of the artery or block the blood flow entirely. Arteriograms (Fig. 6-7) are obtained after a radiopaque dye is introduced into the coronary circulation to examine the patency of the arteries. In Fig. 6-7, *A*, a normal coronary arterial tree is evident; Fig. 6-7, *B*, demonstrates vessel blockage. When blockages are present, coronary artery bypass surgery is often required, or the blockages can cause a myocardial infarction.

Pericardium. The heart is surrounded by a thin, membranous sac known as the pericardium. The pericardial sac holds a small amount of fluid that lubricates the heart as it moves in the chest cavity.[30] An inflammation of the pericardium, called pericarditis, can produce severe chest pain similar to the pain created by coronary artery disease.

SYSTEMIC AND PULMONARY CIRCULATION
Components

The circulatory system is a closed system connected by blood vessels of various sizes. Each category of blood vessels performs a different function. The system is divided into arterial and venous sides.

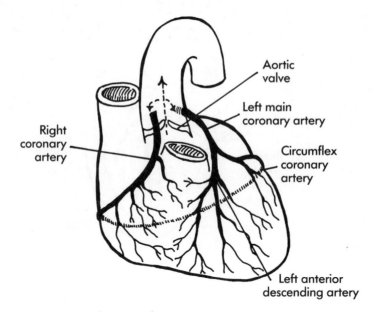

Fig. 6-6 The main coronary arteries.

The arteries carry blood away from the heart to the rest of the body. Arteries must be able to withstand the considerable pressure of a large bolus of blood coursing through their channels, therefore the arteries have thick, muscular walls to contain the pressure and move the blood.[38]

The arterioles are the most distal vessels of the arterial system. These act to regulate the flow of blood in an area. The arterioles, like the arteries, have thick walls consisting of vascular smooth muscle. The smooth muscle is responsive to several factors that can produce contraction or relaxation, including nervous impulses, local metabolites, vasoactive hormones in the circulation, and drugs. The arterioles are implicated in hypertension, since an increase in the contractile state of the vessels can increase the pressure in the large arteries.[11]

The capillaries function to exchange oxygen and carbon dioxide, fluid, nutrients, and other substances between the blood and the interstitial spaces or air sacs of the lung. To allow the passive exchange of these substances, the capillaries must have thin walls. The capillary membrane contains pores that make the membrane permeable to water and other substances.[32]

The movement of fluid across the capillary membranes is controlled by two different types of pressure gradients. A hydrostatic pressure gradient between the inside of the capillary and surrounding tissue spaces in the periphery facilitates the movement of fluids from an area of high pressure to an area of lower pressure. An osmotic pressure created by the large plasma proteins in the blood within the capillaries encourages fluid to move in the opposite direction, from an area of low osmotic pressure to an area of high osmotic pressure. These two pressures tend to be in equilibrium and minimize the flow of fluids through the capillary membranes. Other substances such as carbon dioxide and sodium tend to diffuse through the membranes following a concentration gradient by moving from areas of high concentration to areas of low concentration.[32]

Compared to the pressure in the systemic capillaries, the pressure in the pulmonary capillaries is relatively low. The low pressure keeps the hydrostatic force to move fluids from the capillaries into the alveolar space rather small. A high osmotic pressure within the pulmonary capillaries tends to attract fluids into the capillaries and out of the in-

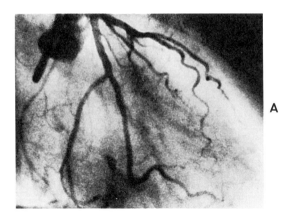

A

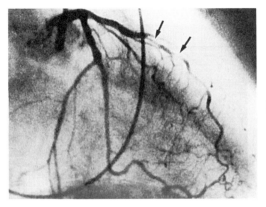

B

Fig. 6-7 Arteriograms. Arrows indicate, **A,** normal coronary arteries and, **B,** restricted coronary arteries.

terstitial space in the lung. The pressures in the pulmonary system act to keep fluid out of the alveolar and interstitial spaces. Under normal circumstances fluids cannot interfere with the gas exchange function of the pulmonary capillaries.[38]

The venules act like a low-pressure collecting system in gathering the blood from the capillaries. The walls of the venules are thinner than those of the arteries or arterioles and contain smooth muscle innervated by the automomic nervous system. Contraction and relaxation in the venules can affect the pressure in the capillaries.[28]

The veins are thin-walled and more distensible than the arteries. In addition to taking blood back to the heart, the veins can act as a reservoir for the blood. The veins generally contain about 60% of the body's blood volume. Small changes

in venous pressure can produce major changes in blood volume.[28]

Systemic or peripheral circulation. The function of the peripheral circulation is to deliver oxygenated blood to the tissues and return the blood to the heart. High pressure on the arterial side ensures that blood is distributed throughout the large network of arteries and arterioles to the capillaries, whereas lower pressures in the venules and veins assist in returning the blood to the heart.[11]

A large pressure gradient exists between the aorta and the vena cava (Fig. 6-8). The pressure in the aorta reflects the pressure in the left ventricle. During systole, when blood is ejected into the aorta, the pressure is about 120 mm Hg in an individual at rest. During diastole the aortic pressure drops to 80 mm Hg. The mean arterial pressure in the aorta at rest is 100 mm Hg.

The drop in pressure in the peripheral circulation is directly related to increasing vascular resistance. In large vessels such as the aorta the resistance is practically nonexistent. The increasingly smaller diameters of the arterioles and capillaries serve to increase the resistance to blood flow and decrease the pressure. The pressure drops to about 30 mm Hg while the blood is entering the capillaries and drops to about 10 mm Hg at the venous end of the capillaries. The pressure continues to drop in the venules and veins until minimal pressure is reached in the right atrium.[14]

The resistance in the venous system is mostly external pressure applied to the vessels. For example, the pressure on veins that occurs as a result of muscle contractions can collapse veins in the area of the contraction. The large veins of the abdomen and thorax are subjected to intraabdominal or intrathoracic pressures that often lead to partial collapse of these vessels. Vessel collapse increases the pressure and resists blood flow. These factors keep the pressure in the venous system 4 to 9 mm Hg higher than in the right atrium, ensuring that the blood continues to flow back to the right side of the heart.[14]

Pressure in the right atrium is determined by the amount of blood returning from the periphery and the ability of the heart to pump blood out of the atrium. Since the blood returned by the veins to the

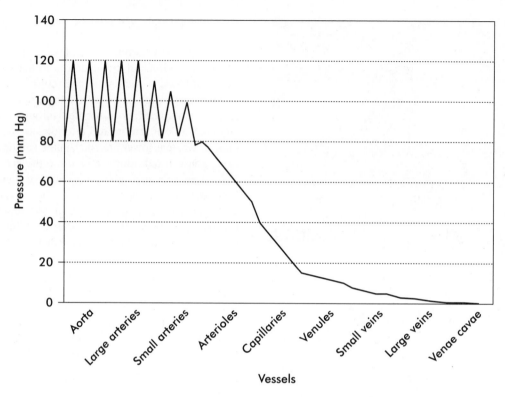

Fig. 6-8   Blood pressures in the vessels of the circulatory system.

heart converges at the right atrium, the pressure in the right atrium is often referred to as the central venous pressure.

Central venous pressure is an important indicator of blood volume and the heart's pumping action. An indirect assessment of the status of the central venous pressure is always included in a physical examination by observation of the jugular veins in the neck. These veins are normally not distended when a person is sitting; however, an increase in central venous pressure can distend these veins. Increased central venous pressure and right atrial pressure can result from an increase in blood volume or a failing right side of the heart, or both. Central venous pressure can also be measured directly by inserting a catheter with a pressure recorder into the vena cava or the right atrium. This procedure is often performed after heart surgery to monitor the pumping ability of the heart.[16]

Pulmonary circulation. The pulmonary circulation is essentially a low-pressure system. Fig. 6-9 compares the pressure-pulse curves for the right ventricle, the pulmonary artery, and the aorta. The systolic pressure for the right ventricle and pulmonary artery peak at about 22 mm Hg, and the diastolic pressure is 0 to 1 mm Hg for the right ventricle. The diastolic pressure for the pulmonary artery, however, is approximately 8 mm Hg. In contrast, the pressure in the vessels returning blood from the lungs to the heart, the pulmonary veins, and the left atrium is even lower and averages around 2 mm Hg.[17]

The purpose of the pulmonary circulation is to oxygenate the blood when it passes through the lungs. The distribution of the blood volume is not necessarily even and is influenced by the oxygen pressure in areas of the lung. Areas with low alveolar oxygen pressure cause blood vessel con-

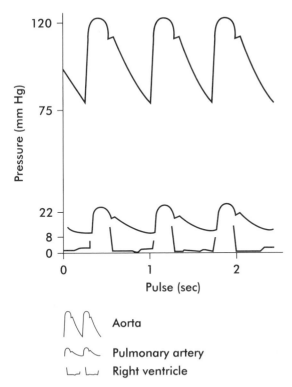

Fig. 6-9 Pressure-pulse curves in the aorta, the pulmonary artery, and the right ventricle.

striction, which in turn causes an increase in vascular resistance. The net effect of higher vascular resistance is to reduce blood flow through areas with low oxygen concentrations. This effect ensures that the pulmonary blood flow is shunted to areas with higher oxygen concentrations. The phenomenon is known as ventilation-perfusion matching in the lung.[37] This reaction in the pulmonary circulation is opposite to what occurs in the systemic circulation. Systemic blood vessels dilate rather than constrict in response to low levels of tissue oxygenation.

Posture plays an important role in blood flow distribution in the lung. To match the ventilation with the perfusion, a fine balance must exist between the low pressures in the alveoli and the pulmonary capillaries, where the gas exchange occurs. During erect stance these pressures are altered slightly as a result of hydrostatic pressure

(Fig. 6-10). In the uppermost region of the lung, the apex, the capillary pressure drops below the alveolar pressure, forcing the collapse of the capillaries. In the middle region of the lung at the level of the heart, the difference between alveolar and capillary pressures is lessened, allowing intermittent blood flow. In the base of the lung, the hydrostatic pressures within the capillaries keep the capillary pressure higher than the alveolar pressure, which enhances the blood flowing through these open capillaries. Postural hydrostatic pressures increase the blood flow in the most dependent portion of the lung and decrease blood flow in the uppermost areas.[7]

The lungs also have a large capacity for increasing the gaseous exchange during exercise. The demand for oxygen can be 7 to 20 times greater during maximal exercise than at rest, depending on the fitness of the individual.[39] The lung supplies more oxygen during exercise by increasing the number of open capillaries and by accommodating a greater cardiac output. Greater perfusion allows more blood to be exposed to alveolar oxygen.[31]

Many clinical conditions can upset the delicate balance of the gas exchange function of the lung. For example, an individual who is having heart failure in the left side of the heart begins to have increased left atrial pressure. This causes an increase in pressure in the pulmonary capillaries and veins. In turn, this increased pressure causes fluid to leak out of the capillaries into the interstitial spaces and alveoli. A condition known as pulmonary edema results.[33] Excessive fluid in the lung interferes with blood oxygenation by increasing the thickness of the tissues through which oxygen must diffuse to reach the capillaries. Another clinical condition is atelectasis, the collapse of a portion of the lung. The collapse could be due to several causes, such as surgery in which the thorax is open or a mucus plug that blocks a bronchus. The poor ventilation in regions of the lungs often constricts blood vessels so that little gas exchange occurs. If atelectasis affects a large enough area of the lung, the partial pressure of systemic arterial oxygen can be reduced.[38]

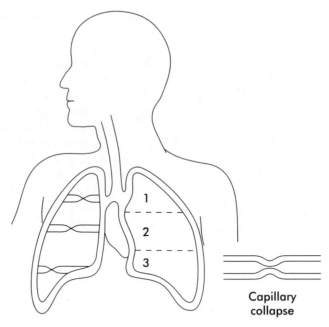

Fig. 6-10 Influence of posture on blood flow in the lung. In the apex, *1,* high alveolar pressures collapse the capillaries. At the level of the heart, *2,* the pressures in the alveoli and the capillaries are nearly equal, causing only intermittent problems in capillary blood flow. In the base of the lung, *3,* the hydrostatic pressures keep capillary pressure higher than alveolar pressure.

MYOCARDIAL ACTIVATION AND CONTRACTION
Electrical Activity

Rhythmic depolarization of the cardiac pacemaker initiates the electrical events that lead to myocardial depolarization and contraction. Membrane depolarization, the coordination between the excitation and contraction, and how these events are related to the electrocardiogram (ECG) are discussed in this section.

The resting membrane potential of a cardiac cell generally ranges from -60 to -90 mV. That is, the charge in the intracellular region is negative compared to that in the extracellular region. The negative intracellular charge is maintained by a chemical concentration gradient between the inside and outside of the cell, by differences in electrical forces across the membrane, and by the membrane itself. An excess of potassium ions is present within the cell, and an excess of sodium and calcium ions exists externally. All these ions would tend to move from areas of high concentration to areas of low concentration, if other factors were not influencing them. A negative intracellular charge tends to hold the positively charged potassium within the cell and to attract the positively charged sodium ions into the cell. The cell membrane, however, maintains the level of intracellular potassium by being selectively permeable to potassium over sodium or calcium and by actively pumping sodium out of the cell. The intracellular potassium is primarily responsible for maintaining the resting membrane potential of cardiac cells.[12]

An action potential is generated when there is a quick change in the membrane permeability to sodium. The sodium moves down its concentration gradient into the cell. The intracellular area becomes less negative with the higher sodium con-

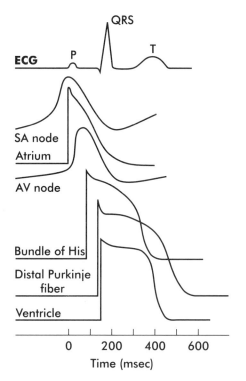

Fig. 6-11 Diagram of an ECG and the action potentials of the myocardial conduction system.

centration until a critical threshold is reached. At this threshold there is rapid depolarization of the cell membrane, producing an action potential. The cell membrane potential reaches about +10 mV, then slowly declines over several hundred milliseconds until the negative resting membrane potential is again reached (Fig. 6-11). The slow plateau that delays repolarization results from a slow inward migration of calcium that occurs while the sodium is being pumped outward. The increase in intracellular calcium ensures that calcium is available for the contraction process.[36] The action potential labeled *ventricular* in Fig. 6-11 is typical of the fast-response action potentials seen in atrial and ventricular muscles and the Purkinje fibers. These action potentials have a fast upstroke and a rapid conduction velocity.

Slow-response action potentials are characteristic of the SA and AV nodes (Fig. 6-11). The slower

initial upward responses of these action potentials seem to be due to a slow inward movement of calcium, which differs from the rapid influx of sodium seen in fast-response cells. The initial portion of the slow-response action potential is more like the calcium movements of the fast-response cells later in the action potential than the early response. Slow-response cells, as the name implies, also have a slowed initial response and a slow conduction velocity.[38]

The understanding of the slow-response characteristics of the pacemaker cells and their relationship to calcium movement has led to the use of medications known as calcium antagonists. These drugs, such as verapamil and nifedipine, partially block the slow calcium response and decrease the firing of the pacemaker cells. Therefore calcium antagonists can be used to control rapid-firing arrhythmias.[35]

Once the cell has depolarized, there is a period when the cell cannot be depolarized again. This period is known as the absolute refractory period (Fig. 6-12). The absolute refractory period is about as long as the contraction duration, which means that the myocardial cells cannot have serial contractions or tetany. As the cell continues to repolarize, a relative refractory period occurs in which a stronger-than-normal stimulus can cause another action potential. The refractory periods control the rate of depolarizations in myocardial cells and protect against retrograde depolarization in the AV node and Purkinje cells. A supernormal phase of increased excitability follows the refractory periods.[24]

The action potential initiates a chain of events that results in contraction of the myocardial fiber, which is called excitation-contraction coupling. As suggested earlier, the increased intracellular calcium during the plateau of the action potential activates the release of bound, stored calcium in the sarcoplasmic reticulum and fibril cisternae. Calcium also combines with the myocardial proteins in the troponin complex to trigger the linkages of actin with myosin. The actin and myosin form cross-bridges that shorten the myofibrils to produce a contraction. When the cell membrane repolarizes, calcium again becomes bound to the

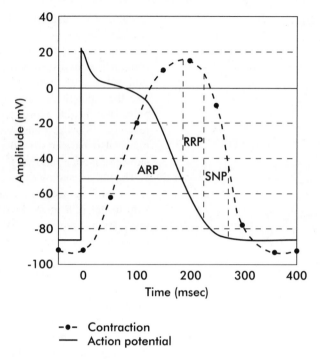

Fig. 6-12 Relationship between the action potential of ventricular muscle and the muscle contraction. The graph shows the absolute refractory period (ARP), the relative refractory period (RRP), and the supernormal period (SNP).

sarcoplasmic reticulum or is removed from the cell. Without the extra intracellular calcium, the myofibril relaxes. The amount of calcium available influences the magnitude of the contraction. The greater the concentration of calcium, the greater the number of cross-bridges formed and the higher the magnitude of the contraction. In contrast, the contractility of skeletal muscle is not responsive to external calcium.[29]

Digitalis is a medication used in the treatment of heart failure to increase the force of myocardial contraction. The contraction force is increased because of increased movement of calcium into the cell during an action potential. The force can be enhanced by as much as 50% or 60% to assist a failing heart.[35]

The ECG is a recording of all the electrical changes in the myocardium (Fig. 6-13). The depolarization is initiated in the SA node in the right atrium and quickly spreads through the atria. The

wave of atrial depolarization is reflected as the first positive upstroke on the ECG, the P wave. The P wave is followed by atrial contraction. The ECG then returns to the baseline, when there is a slowing of the depolarization as it passes through the AV node. A large depolarization wave, the QRS complex, reflects the depolarization of the ventricles and precedes the contraction of the ventricles. Again the electrical activity returns to the baseline, followed by a positive upstroke, the T wave, which represents the repolarization of the ventricles. The myocardium is electrically silent, as indicated by the ECG returning to baseline until another wave of depolarization is initiated by the SA node.[9]

Mechanical Activity

The mechanical events that make up the cardiac cycle are divided into systole and diastole (Fig. 6-13). Systole begins with the increase in ventricular pressure during the ventricular contraction and

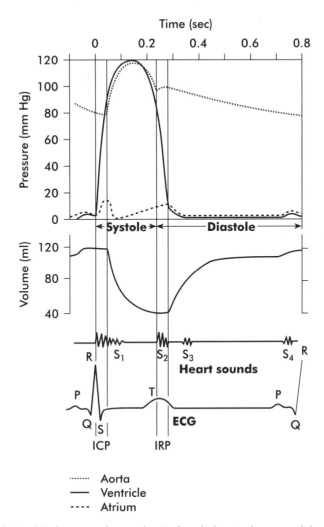

Fig. 6-13 Relationship between the mechanical and electrical events of the cardiac cycle. During the isovolumetric contraction period (ICP) and the isovolumetric relaxation period (IRP) the ventricular volume remains the same because the valves are closed. When the aortic valve opens and the blood is ejected into the aorta, the ventricular volume rapidly decreases.

continues until the closure of the aorta or pulmonic valve, when blood is no longer pumped into the arterial circulation. During diastole the ventricles relax and are filled with blood in preparation for the next cycle.

Fig. 6-13 shows the relationship between the mechanical and the electrical events of the heart.[15] The pressure curves show that at the beginning of ventricular systole the ventricular contraction causes a rapid rise in ventricular pressure. This

pressure rise occurs because the ventricles are a closed system. The myocardium is contracting on the blood within its walls. This period is known as the isovolumetric period, since the ventricles are isometrically contracting with the same volume of blood. When the ventricular pressure rises to the same level as the pressure in the aorta, generally about 80 mm Hg, the aorta opens. The pressure in the ventricle continues to rise during the ventricular contraction until the pressure reaches about 120 mm Hg at rest. Ventricular pressure begins to fall rapidly during the reduction of blood volume in the ventricle. When that pressure drops below the level of pressure in the aorta, the aortic valve closes, marking the end of ventricular systole. The ventricular pressure continues to fall because of the low ventricular blood volume until the ventricular pressure drops below the level of pressure in the atrium. The semilunar valves then open and allow blood to flow from the atria into the ventricle. This is a passive activity, since blood flows from an area of high pressure to one of lower pressure. The passive activity continues until the end of diastole, when the atria contract to move an additional volume of blood into the ventricle just before ventricular contraction and the beginning of a new systolic cycle.

The atrial pressure is significantly lower than the ventricular pressure, which facilitates the return of blood from the low-pressure venous system. A slight rise in pressure at the end of diastole reflects the atrial contraction. The relationship is evident between the P wave on the ECG and the atrial pressure curve just before the increase in atrial pressure. As soon as the ventricular pressure begins to build rapidly, the ventricular pressure becomes greater than the atrial pressure and the atrioventricular valve closes. The atrial pressure continues to rise at this time because of the bulging of the valve into the atrium and the effect of the ventricular contraction on the atrial muscle. After a slight pressure drop the atrial pressure begins to rise slowly as blood begins to fill the atria, and the mitral valve remains closed.

The volume curve represents ventricular volume change during the cardiac cycle.[15] The volume of the ventricles at the end of diastole, the end-diastolic volume, is about 120 ml, whereas the end-systolic volume is about 40 ml. The difference in the two is the average stroke volume of about 80 ml at rest. The percentage of the end-diastolic volume that is ejected as the stroke volume is the ejection fraction, or about 67%. A drop in the ejection fraction can indicate disease such as a failing ventricle.

The heart sounds are created by turbulence of the blood that occurs when the valves close and by the movement of the valves themselves.[20] The first heart sound (S_1) is due to the closing of the atrioventricular valves, the mitral and tricuspid valves. The second heart sound (S_2) is due to the closing of the aortic and pulmonic valves. Third heart sounds (S_3) can occur during the passive filling of the ventricles in children and young adults, but when the sound is present in adults beyond the age of 40 years, it is generally caused by disease such as heart failure or fever. The fourth heart sound (S_4) is not audible and can be detected only by means of phonocardiography. This sound is associated with the active filling of the ventricles that results from atrial contraction.

The waves of the ECG have to be closely linked to the mechanical events. The pause between atrial and ventricular depolarization, the PR interval, allows the atria to contract and contribute more blood volume to the ventricle before the ventricle contracts.[15] As stated earlier, this pause is caused by a slowing of conduction through the AV node. Disease such as ischemia or scarring around the AV node can increase this pause by increasing the conduction time and may change the timing between atrial and ventricular contraction.

The long pause between ventricular depolarization and repolarization, the ST segment, is the period when the ventricular contraction occurs. When ventricular ischemia exists, this segment may be depressed below the baseline or elevated above the baseline.[26]

CONTROL OF VENTRICULAR PERFORMANCE
Cardiac Output

The cardiac output is the amount of blood ejected by the right or left ventricle per minute. In the adult at rest, the stroke volume is about 80 ml and the resting heart rate is about 70 beats per minute. Thus the resting cardiac output is approximately 5.6 L per minute.[1] The cardiac output is the same for both the right and the left sides of the heart.

Determinants of Ventricular Function

The major determinants of ventricular function in humans are the preload, or the length of the myocardium before contraction; the afterload, or the systemic systolic blood pressure; the myocardial contractility, or inotropic state; and the heart rate.[38]

The ventricular end-diastolic volume or the end-diastolic pressure can be used to indicate preload on the myocardium. The volume or pressure directly affects the resting length of myocardial cells. As end-diastolic volume increases, such as during increased venous return, stroke volume increases because of the increased resting length of the cells. This response is known as the Frank-Starling mechanism.[38]

The determinant of afterload is the force against which the myocardium works to pump blood. This force is the systolic blood pressure. The higher the systolic pressure, the lower the stroke volume and ejection velocity.[27]

Myocardial contractility can be either increased, which is a positive inotropic effect, or decreased, which is a negative inotropic influence. Ordinarily myocardial contractility occurs through reflex autonomic control. For example, the sympathetic nervous system stimulates myocardial contractility, whereas stimulation of the vagus nerve (parasympathetic) decreases contractility. Many medications also affect inotropic state. Digitalis has a positive inotropic influence by increasing contractile strength. Barbiturates and β-blocking drugs have a negative influence.[35]

Besides stroke volume, heart rate is an important determinant of cardiac output. Heart rate is linearly related to cardiac output, since an increased heart rate is associated with an increased cardiac output.

Control of Heart Rate

The specialized conduction system of the heart displays spontaneous depolarization of the cells. The heart rate is normally generated by the spontaneous rate of the fastest pacemaker, the SA node. The resting rate of the SA node, which is not innervated by the autonomic nervous system, is around 100 beats per minute. This rate is evident in patients who have had heart transplantation, whose hearts are denervated.[10] Normally the autonomic nervous system inhibits the intrinsic rate of the SA

node by 30 or more beats per minute. Thus the resting heart rate is 70 beats per minute. This heart rate is mostly attributable to constant stimulation by parasympathetic fibers on the SA node.

CIRCULATORY RESPONSES DURING EXERCISE

Exercise places demands on the cardiovascular system to increase the blood supply to the exercising muscles, to meet the increased metabolic demands, and to cool the body. The cardiac output can increase from a resting value of 5.6 L per minute to 35 or 40 L per min, a 7- or 8-fold increase, during strenuous exercise in a young man.[1,3] Although there are various types of exercise, this discussion focuses on cardiovascular responses to dynamic, aerobic exercise rather than the responses to isometric or strenuous isotonic work.

Heart Rate

A rapid increase in the heart rate occurs in response to exercise. This rapid increase results from a decrease of vagal or parasympathetic stimulation. The removal of this inhibition allows the heart rate to increase. The response may be controlled by the central nervous system or mechanoreceptors in the exercising muscles. As the exercise continues for a minute or 2, increases in heart rate result from decreases in vagal inhibition, increases in sympathetic tone, and increases in circulating catecholamines. The heart rate can increase from 70 beats per minute at rest to a maximum of 200 beats per minute during high-intensity exercise in the young adult.[3] The maximal heart rate, and thus the circulatory response to exercise, decreases with age.[2]

An interesting situation arises in individuals who have had heart transplantation. Hearts in these individuals are denervated and are no longer under nervous system control (Fig. 6-14). Because of the lack of vagal inhibition, the individual's heart rate after transplantation is higher than it was before transplantation.[10] The heart rate also responds more sluggishly to a single level of moderate exercise, since increasing heart rate now depends on stimulation from circulating catecholamines. For

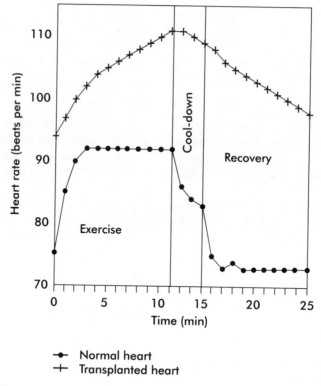

Fig. 6-14 Difference in heart rate between a patient with a denervated, transplanted heart and a healthy person during low-intensity exercise. The transplantation patient has a higher heart rate at rest, and heart rate increases more slowly than normal during exercise. During cool-down and recovery after exercise the heart rate response of the transplantation patient is more gradual than normal. (Modified from Fick AW, Holloway V. In Payton O et al, editors: *Manual of physical therapy*, New York, 1989, Churchill-Livingstone.)

the same reason the recovery rate is slower after the exercise is stopped.

The heart rate increases linearly with increasing exercise intensities (Fig. 6-15). The range of heart rate responses to different exercise intensities is broad. A number of factors influence the heart rate responses, such as age, level of fitness, gender, body size, and the existence of cardiac disease.[3] An adult who exercises regularly has a more gradual increase than normal in heart rate in response to increasing levels of exercise, whereas an individual with heart disease has higher-than-normal heart rate responses to low-intensity exercise and often has a lower-than-normal maximal heart rate.

Stroke Volume

The stroke volume generally increases early in an exercise session but tends to level off as the exercise intensity continues to increase (Fig. 6-16). Much of this early increase is the result of increasing venous return that occurs when the muscles begin to exercise, which increases end-diastolic volume and thus the stroke volume. A slight drop in central venous pressure during exercise also encourages venous return.[4] A positive

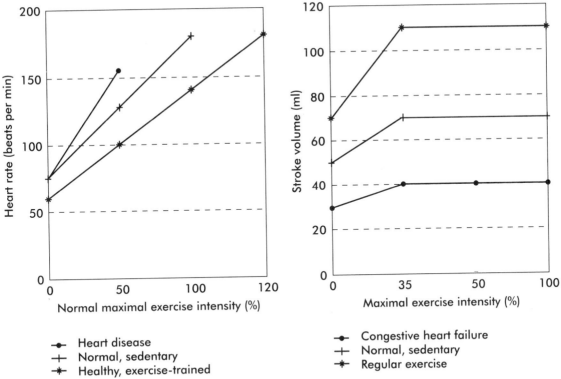

Fig. 6-15   Comparison of the increase in heart rate during increasing exercise intensity for the individual with heart disease; the normal, sedentary individual; and the healthy, exercise-trained individual.

Fig. 6-16   Comparison of the changes in stroke volume during increasing exercise intensity for the individual with congestive heart failure; the normal, sedentary individual; and the individual who regularly exercises.

inotropic effect of sympathetic nervous stimulation increases myocardial contractility during exercise, thereby increasing stroke volume.

Cardiac Output

Since the cardiac output is directly related to heart rate and stroke volume, it is easy to recognize that cardiac output increases in response to increasing exercise demands (Fig. 6-17). In healthy individuals the range of the cardiac output responses provides a reserve for increasing exercise demands.[13]

A significant shift in the distribution of the cardiac output occurs during exercise (Fig. 6-18). By the time maximal exercise intensity is reached, most of the increased cardiac output is flowing to the exercising muscles.[5] The increased blood flow to the skeletal muscles is stimulated by the buildup of local vasodilator metabolites within the muscles. The increased volume is the result of a shift in distribution caused by vasoconstriction in the splanchnic and renal blood vessels. A slight increase in blood flow to the myocardium also provides for the increased work being done by the heart during exercise.

Arteriovenous Oxygen Difference

The rate of extraction of oxygen in the tissues of an individual at rest is about 4 to 5 ml oxygen per 100 ml blood. This rate increases to between 13

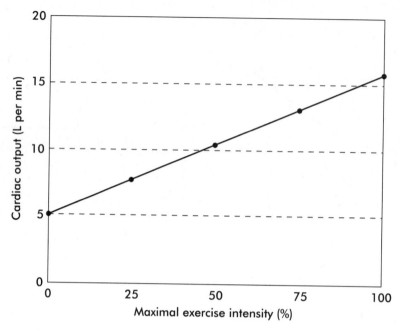

Fig. 6-17 Relationship between cardiac output and increasing exercise intensity.

and 16 ml per 100 ml blood during exercise of maximal intensity. The increase in oxygen consumption during exercise is directly related to the increased peripheral oxygen extraction and increased cardiac output.[3]

Hemodynamic Responses

The amount of increase in the heart rate, stroke volume, cardiac output, and rate of oxygen extraction depends on the intensity of the exercise and the amount of active muscle mass.[6] During strenuous exercise the work of the left ventricle may increase fourfold. The vasodilation in the active skeletal muscles reduces total peripheral resistance, but the mean arterial oxygen pressure increases. An increased resistance resulting from vasoconstriction in the gut also occurs and contributes to an increased afterload for the left ventricle. Using small muscle masses, for example, using the arms rather than the legs, can also increase blood pressure and heart rate responses during submaximal exercise.

REFERENCES

1. Asmussen E, Nielsen M: The cardiac output at rest and work determined simultaneously by the acetylene and the dye solution methods, *Acta Physiol Scand* 27:217, 1952.
2. Astrand PO: Human physical fitness with special reference to age and sex, *Physiol Rev* 36:307, 1956.
3. Astrand PO, Rodahl K: *Textbook of work physiology,* New York, 1987, McGraw Hill.
4. Bevegard BS et al: Circulatory studies in well-trained athletes at rest and during heavy exercise, with special reference to stroke volume and the influence of body position, *Acta Physiol Scand* 57:26, 1963.
5. Bevegard BS, Shepherd JT: Regulation of the circulation during exercise in man, *Physiol Rev* 47:178, 1967.
6. Blomqvist CG et al: Similarity of the hemodynamic responses to static and dynamic exercise of small muscle groups, *Circ Res* 48:187, 1981.
7. Cumming G: The pulmonary circulation. In Guyton AC, Jones CE, editors: *Cardiovascular physiology: MTP international review of science,* Baltimore, 1974, University Park.
8. Davies MF, Anderson RH, Becker AE: *The conduction system of the heart,* London, 1983, Butterworths. 102.
9. Dubin D: *Rapid interpretation of EKGs,* Tampa, Fla, 1975, Cover.

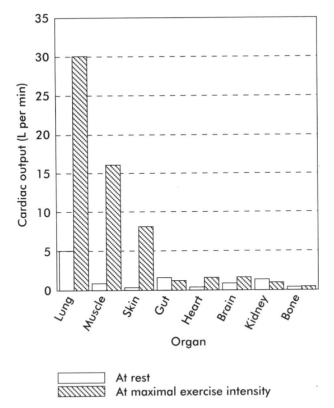

Fig. 6-18 Relative distribution of cardiac output during rest and at maximal exercise intensity. The lung distribution represents the entire cardiac output of the right ventricle; the cardiac output of the left ventricle is being distributed primarily to the working muscles and skin during maximal exercise intensity.

10. Fick AW, Holloway V: Rehabilitation of the postsurgical cardiac patient. In Payton O et al, editors: *Manual of physical therapy,* New York, 1988, Churchill-Livingstone.
11. Folkow B, Neil E: *Circulation,* London, 1971, Oxford University.
12. Fozzard HA: Heart: excitation-contraction coupling, *Ann Rev Physiol* 39:201, 1977.
13. Grimby G et al: Cardiac output during submaximal and maximal exercise in active middle-aged athletes, *J Appl Physiol* 21:1150, 1966.
14. Guyton AC: Pressure-volume curves of the entire arterial and venous systems in the living animal, *Am J Physiol* 184:253, 1956.
15. Guyton AC: *Human physiology and mechanisms of disease,* ed 5, Philadelphia, 1992, WB Saunders.
16. Guyton AC, Jones CE: Central venous pressure: physiological significance and clinical implications, *Am Heart J* 86:431, 1973.

17. Hughes JMB: Pulmonary circulatory and fluid balance, *Int Rev Physiol* 14:135, 1977.
18. Hurst JW, editor: *The heart, arteries and veins,* ed 7, New York, 1990, McGraw-Hill.
19. James TN, Sherf L: Specialized tissues and preferential conduction in the atria of the heart, *Am J Cardiol* 28:414, 1971.
20. Leon DF, Shaver JA, editors: *Physiologic principles of heart sounds and murmurs,* Monograph no. 46, Dallas, 1974, American Heart Association.
21. Levy MN, Mil NG, Zieske H: Functional distribution of the peripheral cardiac sympathetic pathways, *Circ Res* 19:650, 1966.
22. McAlpine, WA: *Heart and coronary arteries,* New York, 1975, Springer-Verlag.
23. McNutt NS, Weinstein RS: Membrane ultrastructure of mammalian intercellular functions, *Prog Biophys Mol Biol* 2:45, 1973.

24. Milnor WR: Properties of cardiac tissue. In Montcastle VB, editor: *Medical physiology,* ed 14, St Louis, 1980, Mosby.

25. Moore KL: *Clinically oriented anatomy,* ed 3 Baltimore, 1992, Williams & Wilkins.

26. Protas EJ: Cardiac rehabilitation during the acute phase of recovery. In Payton OD et al, editors: *Manual of physical therapy,* New York, 1989, Churchill-Livingstone.

27. Ross J et al: Contractile state of heart characterized by force-velocity relations in variably afterloaded and isovolumic beats, *Circ Res* 18:149, 1966.

28. Rothe CF: The venous system: the physiology of the capacitance vessels. In Abboud FM, Shepherd JT, editors: *Handbook of physiology. II. The cardiovascular system,* vol 3, Bethesda, Md, 1982, American Physiological Society.

29. Rushmer R: *Structure and function in the cardiovascular system,* Philadelphia, 1978, WB Saunders.

30. Shabetai R: *The pericardium,* New York, 1981, Grune & Stratton.

31. Shephard RJ: Oxygen costs of breathing during vigorous exercise, *J Exp Physiol* 51:336, 1966.

32. Smith JJ, Kampine JP: *Circulatory physiology,* Baltimore, 1984, Williams & Wilkins.

33. Staub NC: Pulmonary edema, *Physiol Rev* 54:678, 1974.

34. Streeter DD: Gross morphology and fiber geometry of the heart. In Berne RM et al, editors: *Handbook of physiology,* vol 1, Washington, DC, 1979, American Physiological Society.

35. Van Camp SP: Pharmacologic factors in exercise and exercise testing. In Blair SN et al, editors: Resource *manual for guidelines for exercise testing and prescription,* Philadelphia, 1988, Lea & Febiger.

36. Vassalle M: Cardiac automaticity and its control, *Am J Physiol* 233:H625, 1977.

37. West JB: Blood flow in the lung and gas exchange, *Anesthesiology* 41:124, 1974.

38. West JB: *Best and Taylor's physiological basis of medical practice,* ed 11, Baltimore, 1985, Williams & Wilkins.

39. Whipp BJ, Mahler M: Dynamics of pulmonary gas exchange during exercise. In West JB, editor: *Pulmonary gas exchange,* vol 2, New York, 1980, Academic.

STUDY QUESTIONS

■ Describe the changes that occur in the cardiac cycle in relationship to electrical and mechanical events.

■ Define cardiac output, and describe the changes that occur from rest to exercise.

■ Describe the importance of the ventilatory and muscle pump systems for venous return and cardiac output.

■ Describe the changes in blood flow distribution from rest to exercise.

■ Describe the relationship of cardiac output and peripheral vascular resistance to blood pressure.

CHAPTER 7

EXERCISE TOLERANCE AND TRAINING FOR HEALTHY PERSONS AND PATIENTS WITH CARDIOVASCULAR DISEASE

Lawrence P. Cahalin

The legend of the run of Pheidippides from the battlefield of Marathon to Athens (a distance of approximately 24 miles) is an extreme example of cardiovascular performance and is the basis for the present-day marathon. In the legend, Pheidippides, a trained runner, runs the 24 miles to report of a victory over the Persians.[67] On his arrival in Athens, however, he gasps out the victorious news and falls dead of exertion. Although this classic event apparently occurred in 490 B.C., it has great implications for today's exercise enthusiasts because it demonstrates that extremes of exercise can be not only harmful but also fatal. Such a consideration is of utmost importance when prescribing exercise for individuals with cardiovascular, or any, disease.

The assessment of cardiovascular response to exercise can provide important prognostic and therapeutic information (such as effects of training or of specific medications and dosages on hypertension, angina, and the like) for individuals with and without coronary artery disease. Cardiovascular performance can be thoroughly assessed via interpretation of physiologic response to exercise

and exercise testing.[36] Consistent, reproducible evaluation of symptoms, heart rate, blood pressure, electrocardiogram (ECG), respiratory rate, and oxygen saturation level during progressive exercise training or testing can objectively determine the status of the cardiovascular and musculoskeletal systems. Additional assessment of cardiovascular performance by echocardiography, radionuclide study (cardiac catheterization and thallium or adenosine testing), respiratory gas analysis, or other methods (see the box on p. 122) can provide useful information regarding cardiovascular function.[49] For example, Douglas, O'Toole, and Woolard[29] recently observed echocardiographic changes in myocardial performance that are suggestive of myocardial fatigue during the Hawaii Ironman Triathlon.

The purpose of this chapter is to review the responses during exercise and the effects of exercise training on cardiovascular performance in both the absence and the presence of cardiovascular disease. This review is followed by a discussion of the effects of medications, cardiac arrhythmias, myocardial infarction, peripheral vascular disease,

---

METHODS USED TO ASSESS CARDIAC PERFORMANCE

Echocardiography
Impedance cardiography
Radionuclide ventriculography
Thallium and technetium imaging
Cardiac catheterization
Multigated acquisition study or multiple gated
    acquisition (MUGA) scan (radionuclide imaging
    of the ventricle)
Transesophageal echocardiography
Computerized tomography (CT) or CT scan
Magnetic resonance imaging (MRI) or MRI scan
Indirect assessments of cardiac performance
    (heart rate, blood pressure, rate-pressure product,
    and tension-time index)

---

renal failure, and cardiovascular procedures (coronary artery bypass graft surgery, valvular replacement, and percutaneous transluminal coronary angioplasty) on cardiovascular performance. The clinical implications of each factor for exercise training is also discussed. Several fundamental concepts of exercise testing and training are presented, including the *clinical* use of the target heart rate, metabolic equivalents of oxygen consumption (METS), steady-state exercise, and the Borg ratings of perceived exertion.

EXERCISE TOLERANCE AND CARDIAC PERFORMANCE IN THE ABSENCE OF CARDIOVASCULAR DISEASE
Peripheral Adaptations

The physiologic responses to exercise depend greatly on the status of the circulation,[5] which is schematized in Fig. 7-1. The upper scale demonstrates that a large percentage of blood (80% to 85% of cardiac output) is diverted to exercising muscles, and at rest (as shown in the lower scale) the blood is relatively evenly distributed.[5]

The distribution of blood to active muscles depends primarily on the level of metabolism in the muscle cells and appears to be regulated locally.[5] The peripheral adaptations during exercise therefore contribute significantly to the observed physiologic responses to specific types of exercise or work. Submaximal levels of exercise and work redistribute less of the total blood supply to active muscles, since the level of work is adequately maintained by fewer muscle fibers. Fewer muscle fibers utilize less oxygen and aerobically maintain adenosine triphosphate (ATP) supplies as food nutrients are broken down via oxidative phosphorylation (see Chapters 1 to 3).[5] Therefore submaximal exercise produces lower heart rates, blood pressures, respiratory rates, levels of oxygen consumption, and Borg ratings of perceived exertion.

As greater levels of work are performed, more muscle fibers are recruited, which increases the need for oxygen to supply the active muscle fibers with needed energy from the breakdown (again, via oxidative phosphorylation) of food nutrients. However, the greater the level of work, the less likely it is that adequate supplies of oxygen will be delivered for the breakdown of food and nutrients. The efficiency of the cardiovascular system dictates not only the maximal amount of oxygen that can be consumed (Vo_2 max) but also the ability to perform physical exercise.

When the oxygen demand outweighs the supply available, anaerobic glycolysis becomes the predominant metabolic process to provide the needed energy.[5] The specific point, or threshold, of greater dependence on glycolysis than on oxidative phosphorylation is a controversial topic and has been ascribed several descriptive terms, including the *anaerobic threshold, ventilatory threshold,* and *lactate threshold.*[7,95] Whatever term is used and whatever method is used to analyze this inflection (or deflection) point, it appears to be a useful tool in evaluating cardiovascular fitness and in prescribing exercise.

Various methods are used to identify the previously described point; respiratory gas analysis and blood sampling are the most common. Another method used to determine the anaerobic threshold is evaluation of the heart rate response to gradual increases in exercise work loads (every 30 to 45 seconds).[62] Continuous heart rate measurement during *bicycle* exercise testing has allowed for the

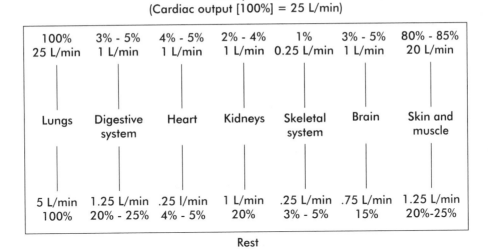

Fig. 7-1 Schema depicting blood flow (cardiac output) relationship to organ systems, *lower scale,* at rest and, *upper scale,* during heavy exercise.

identification of a "downward deflection" in the linear increase in heart rate.[62] However, the application of this method to identify the anaerobic threshold is questionable for *other* modes of exercise and may not always coincide with the anaerobic threshold under steady-state conditions.[62] Despite these shortcomings, the assessment of heart rate alone can provide important information regarding peripheral vascular function and central (cardiac) performance.

Central Adaptations

Perhaps the most useful noninvasive method for assessing cardiac performance is the rate-pressure product, which evaluates the heart rate and systolic blood pressure relationship. The product of heart rate and systolic blood pressure (double product) is a good indicator of coronary blood flow and of myocardial oxygen consumption. In 1972 Kitamura et al.[61] observed in young, healthy men a high correlation (r = 0.88 to 0.90) between coronary blood flow and myocardial oxygen consumption by using the rate-pressure product. In addition, the use of the rate-pressure product during maximal work on a bicycle ergometer has provided a *specific* assessment of cardiac performance.[42] This indirect measurement of cardiac performance has been termed the *myocardial efficiency index* (MEI), and it appears to correlate maximal work load (during bicycle exercise) with myocardial oxygen uptake (represented by the rate-pressure product) and body surface area. To derive the MEI, Garber et al.[42] used the following equation:

$$\frac{kg - m \text{ per min}}{(\text{heart rate} \times \text{systolic blood pressure})10^{-2}}/m^2$$

The researchers observed that the MEI correlated well with patients who had flat or depressed exercise ejection fractions (the percentage of blood ejected from the left ventricle, with an average value of 0.67 ± 0.08 in healthy subjects). Lower MEIs were observed in such patients and in patients with three-vessel coronary artery disease. The MEI therefore may be useful. Its use may provide a more complete assessment of patient response to exercise than rate-pressure product alone. Although only bicycle ergometry was studied, it seems likely that other modes of exercise could be used to determine the MEI.

Obtaining the MEI involves dividing the maximal rate-pressure product into the maximal work load on a bicycle ergometer (in kg − m/min) and finally dividing this quotient by the body surface area (m^2). Use of the rate-pressure product and MEI may provide important information regarding progression or deterioration in patient response to therapeutic exercise or medical treatment.

One additional method of assessing cardiac performance that is worthy of discussion is the tension-time index (TTI), which utilizes the duration of systole, obtained by evaluating the QT interval, and the mean systolic blood pressure.[86] The product of these two variables estimates the efficiency of left ventricular work (or *total tension* developed by the myocardium[86]) per beat; mm Hg is used as the scale of measure. The TTI per minute is the product of the two values (duration of systole × mean systolic blood pressure) and heart rate.[86] Tension-time index and myocardial oxygen consumption have a strong correlation; therefore TTI may be another useful clinical measure in documenting patient response to therapy.

An important component of the rate-pressure product, MEI, and TTI is the systolic blood pressure, which is the product of the total peripheral resistance (TPR) and cardiac output (CO) (systolic blood pressure = TPR × CO).[81] The previous discussion regarding the redistribution of the circulation during exercise should enhance one's understanding of the acute response to exercise in general and, specifically, the differences between upper-extremity and lower-extremity exercise.

When exercise begins, blood is distributed to active muscles, which readily accept the increased blood volume via arterial and capillary vasodilation.[5] The inactive muscles receive less blood via sympathetic arteriole vasoconstriction, thereby increasing TPR.[5] The mechanism of vasodilation in active muscles and vasoconstriction in inactive muscles can be profound and may be one reason why upper-extremity exercise appears to produce a more significant cardiovascular response than does lower-extremity exercise at comparable work loads. During upper-extremity exercise, vasodilation in the arms and vasoconstriction in the legs

(the larger muscle mass) produce a greater TPR than during lower-extremity exercise, when vasoconstriction occurs in the smaller muscles of the arms. Therefore heart rate, blood pressure, respiratory rate, and oxygen consumption are generally greater during upper-extremity exercise and lower during lower-extremity exercise at comparable work loads.[5]

Likewise, different types of muscle contraction produce different cardiopulmonary responses. Static and dynamic types of exercise have previously been compared, and the heart rate and blood pressure responses are typically greater during static exercise than during dynamic exercise. The effects of isokinetic exercise on cardiopulmonary function have also been evaluated and compared, and substantial increases in heart rate and blood pressure have been observed.[45] In fact, the cardiopulmonary responses are at times comparable to those obtained during maximal exercise stress testing.[70]

The heart rate, blood pressure responses, and other values (the exercise duration, rate-pressure product, and TTI) have been documented in experimental and clinical trials during a variety of exercise tests. These documented values provide clinical data that can be used to thoroughly analyze cardiopulmonary responses to exercise.[5,95] Such "normative data" enable practitioners to make patient comparisons and improve their understanding of the cardiovascular system. During dynamic exercise such as treadmill walking, heart rate and systolic blood pressure increase progressively in a linear manner as work load is increased. The expected increase in heart rate, systolic blood pressure, and oxygen consumption is in the range of 20 to 40 beats per min, 10 to 20 mm Hg, and 4 to 8 ml/kg per min each exercise stage, respectively.[36] However, the work load during each exercise stage varies considerably from one protocol to another.

The diastolic blood pressure, on the other hand, has been observed to decrease during dynamic treadmill exercise. This decrease is in the range of 2 to 4 mm Hg per exercise stage but in many patients may be more or less profound and has been shown to change only minimally in a select group of patients.[5] The difference in diastolic blood pressure response is probably due to the state of the cardiovascular system. An increase of more than 10 mm Hg has been implicated as being suggestive of cardiovascular disease, primarily atherosclerotic cardiovascular disease.[88] Atherosclerotic coronary disease prevents the adequate return of blood to the heart (venous and coronary), which decreases the cardiac output and causes a reflexive peripheral vasoconstriction that increases TPR and in many instances the diastolic blood pressure.

It is evident from the preceding discussion and from the equation for systolic blood pressure (systolic blood pressure = TRP × CO) that change in systolic blood pressure is not only the result of alterations in TPR but also depends on *central* adaptation, specifically, cardiac output. Cardiac output is the product of heart rate (HR) and stroke volume (SV) (CO = HR × SV) and depends on both values, although the heart rate is of greater importance at greater levels of exertion. The cardiac output is the amount of blood pumped from the heart during each minute, and the *heart rate* component is frequently referred to as the *chronotropic* response, whereas the force of myocardial contraction (which increases or decreases the *stroke volume*) is referred to as the *inotropic* response.[49] The stroke volume therefore depends on the inotropic response, as well as several important processes. These processes can be best explained by discussing the Frank Starling law and its effect on stroke volume and the inotropic response of the heart. It appears that "an optimal range of left ventricular filling pressure exists which, when exceeded, decreases the left ventricular stroke work considerably."[17] Therefore the primary point of the Frank Starling law is that an increase in the left ventricular filling pressure is accompanied by a subsequent increase in left ventricular muscle fiber stretch during diastole (when blood is ejected from the left atrium into the left ventricle). The variables that determine the magnitude of myocardial stretch include the atrial contribution to ventricular filling, total blood volume, body position, intrathoracic pressure, intrapericardial pressure, venous tone, and pumping action of skeletal muscle.[49]

The magnitude of stretch on the left ventricle during diastole (as blood fills the left ventricle) greatly determines the stroke volume and is analogous to pulling backward on a slingshot. The farther the rubber band of a slingshot is pulled back, the greater will be the force and distance at which the object travels on release. In much the same way, increased left ventricular filling pressure increases the stretch on myocardial muscle fibers in the left ventricle, which enhances the inotropic response (increases the force of myocardial contraction) as long as the left ventricular filling pressure is not extreme. Extreme left ventricular filling pressure *decreases* myocardial efficiency and the inotropic response. This is a problem in many patients with myocardial infarction, cardiomyopathy, and valvular heart disease and is discussed later in this chapter.

As depicted in Fig. 7-2, stroke volume can increase from 100 to 150 ml (by approximately 50%), whereas heart rate increases by as much as 50 to 200 beats per min (an increase of approximately 300%).[5] These changes produce an increase in cardiac output from 5.0 to 30.0 L per min (or six times the resting level).[5] This sixfold increase in cardiac output is often associated with a *20-fold* increase in oxygen consumption, which is due primarily to increased extraction of oxygen from active skeletal muscles and is evident in a widened arteriovenous difference in oxygen (a-Vo_2 difference).[5] This difference is expressed in the following equation:

$$oxygen\ consumption = CO \times a\text{-}Vo_2\ difference$$

The expected increase in a-Vo_2 difference is from 50 to 165 ml per L of blood (3.3 times the resting level). This improved a-Vo_2 difference occurs because the blood flow is redistributed during exercise so that skeletal muscles, with their pronounced ability to extract oxygen, may receive 80% to 85% of the cardiac output, as compared with some 15% at rest and because the oxygen dissociation curve is shifted so that more oxyhemoglobin is reduced than normally at a given pressure for oxygen, that is, the percentage of saturation is less.[5]

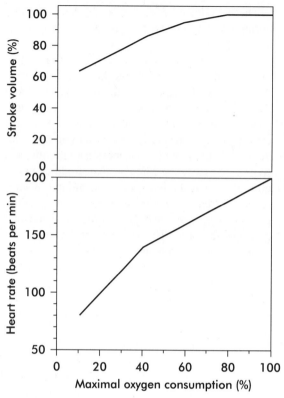

Fig. 7-2 Heart rate increases linearly during exercise, whereas maximal stroke volume is achieved at approximately 50% of the maximal exercise capacity (oxygen consumption).

EXERCISE TOLERANCE AND CARDIAC PERFORMANCE IN PATIENTS WITH CARDIOVASCULAR DISEASE
Peripheral Adaptations

The previously described reasons for improved oxygen extraction (and widening of the A-Vo$_2$ difference) are compromised in cardiovascular disease. Atherosclerotic cardiovascular disease of the coronary arteries or large peripheral arteries can severely limit the redistribution of blood to active muscles, which are often functioning at a level of near-maximal capacity during exercise of minimal to moderate intensity. The limited redistribution of blood to active muscles and subsequent lack of improvement in a-Vo$_2$ difference result from the right-

ward or leftward shift of the oxyhemoglobin dissociation curve that results from increased levels of lactic acid[5] (which may profoundly limit functional work capacity) and the abnormal skeletal muscle of many patients with cardiovascular disease. Abnormalities of skeletal muscle include increased intracellular phosphatase acid activity and intracellular lipid accumulation, as well as atrophy of types 1 and 2 muscle fibers.[63] The limitations that result from these pathologic processes can be assessed and categorized by means of the cardiopulmonary responses and subsequent work performance during graded exercise testing. The cardiopulmonary responses to functional testing are discussed in the following section.

Functional assessment. A classification scheme for functional limitations in patients with cardiovascular disease was introduced by the New York Heart Association in 1954. Limitations were classified into functional classes 1 through 4,[72] depending on signs and symptoms in the patient (Table 7-1). This classification system crudely identified the functional status of patients with cardiovascular disease and only recently has been reassessed for its lack of objective measurement. The classification system of the Canadian Cardiovascular Society[22] is similar (Table 7-1) and may, along with the New York Heart Association system, be replaced by a more objective system based on data obtained from exercise testing, respiratory gas analysis, and other noninvasive and invasive assessments.[68]

However, the specific functional activity scale (Table 7-2) proposed by Goldman et al.[43] may be the most appropriate and effective method for objectively assessing functional status when more objective tests (such as respiratory gas analysis) cannot be employed.[68] Functional activities (such as climbing stairs or performing specific tasks) are *directly* evaluated during patient assessment, and the specific activity scale has been observed to have greater validity and reliability than the New York Heart Association or the Canadian system.[43] The specific activities of daily living are observed, and a rating of the patient's performance is documented. The functional activity scale has also been tested in a nonphysician group (a variety of healthcare professionals), and high levels of validity and

Table 7-1 Three methods used to assess cardiovascular disability

Class	New York Heart Association	Canadian Cardiovascular Society	Specific functional activity scale
1	Patients with cardiac disease but without resulting limitations of physical activity; ordinary physical activity does not cause undue fatigue, palpitation, dyspnea, or anginal pain	Ordinary physical activity, such as walking and climbing stairs, does not cause angina; angina results from strenuous, rapid, or prolonged exertion at work or recreation	Patients can perform to completion any activity requiring 7 METS or more; e.g., can carry 24 lb up eight steps, carry objects that weigh 80 lb, do outdoor work (shovel snow), do recreational activity (such as skiing)
2	Patients with cardiac disease resulting in slight limitation of physical activity; they are comfortable at rest; ordinary physical activity results in fatigue, palpitation, dyspnea, or anginal pain	Slight limitation of ordinary activity: Walking or climbing stairs rapidly, uphill, after meals, in cold, in wind, when under stress, or only during the few hours after awakening; walking more than 2 blocks on level or climbing more than 1 flight of stairs at a normal pace	Patient can perform to completion any activity requiring 5 METS or more but cannot perform to completion activities requiring 7 METS or more, e.g., sexual intercourse without stopping; gardening; dancing; or walking at 4 mph on level ground
3	Patients with cardiac disease resulting in marked limitation of physical activity; they are comfortable at rest; less than ordinary physical activity causes fatigue, dyspnea, or anginal pain	Marked limitations of ordinary physical activity: Walking 1 or 2 blocks on the level and climbing more than 1 flight of stairs	Patient can perform to completion any activity requiring 2 METS or more but cannot perform to completion activities requiring 5 METS or more, e.g., showering without stopping; cleaning windows; walking at 2.5 mph; bowling; golfing; or dressing without stopping
4	Patients with cardiac disease resulting in inability to carry on any physical activity without discomfort; symptoms of cardiac insufficiency or anginal syndrome may be present at rest; if activity is undertaken, discomfort is increased	Inability to carry on any physical activity without discomfort; anginal syndrome may be present at rest	Patient cannot perform to completion activities requiring 2 METS or more; cannot carry out activities listed for class III

METS, Metabolic equivalents of oxygen consumption.

reliability were demonstrated.[43] Thus the functional activity scale may be appropriate for allied health professionals as well as physicians.

Patient function can also be assessed objectively via exercise performance during treadmill testing,[15] as was demonstrated by Robert Bruce (the person responsible for the Bruce protocol). Although this work was performed approximately 20 years ago, it still provides an objective assessment of exercise tolerance insofar as a patient's age and

---

PRIMARY CARDIOVASCULAR DISORDERS

Atherosclerotic heart disease
Valvular heart disease
Cardiomyopathy
Congestive heart failure
Peripheral vascular disease

---

duration of exercise during a multistage treadmill exercise test are plotted on a nomogram. Although nomograms were constructed for men with coronary artery disease and men and women without coronary artery disease, a nomogram for women with coronary artery disease does not exist. Despite this shortcoming, the nomograms of Bruce provide an estimated Vo_2 max and conversely, a functional aerobic impairment (FAI) value. The nomograms of Bruce are effective for clinical examination but cannot directly *identify* the primary cardiovascular disorders, which include atherosclerotic heart disease, valvular heart disease, cardiomyopathy, congestive heart failure, and peripheral vascular disease[49] (see the box on p. 128). Recent contributions from Wasserman et al.[95] have provided a battery of clinical tests in which such measures as respiratory gas analysis, ECG monitoring, oxygen saturation level, hematologic evaluation, and exercise performance are used to identify the primary cardiovascular disorder and to enhance the overall assessment and treatment of patients with cardiopulmonary disease.

Surgical versus medical treatment. The identification and treatment of patients with the previously mentioned cardiovascular disorders is important. The treatment, however, is controversial, as, for example, in the clinical decision to treat atherosclerotic heart disease by means of medications or coronary artery surgery. A review follows of the primary investigations evaluating the effects of medical therapy versus surgical intervention in the treatment of atherosclerotic heart disease.

The multicenter Veterans Administration (VA) study[75] was most recently performed and evaluated the effects of medical versus surgical treatment af-

ter 5 years in patients with atherosclerotic heart disease. In this review of 468 patients no significant difference in mortality or morbidity was observed between most patients receiving medicine and those who had coronary artery bypass graft surgery. However, patients with three-vessel coronary artery disease did benefit from surgical intervention. Another VA study[50] evaluated the effects of medical versus surgical therapy after 10 years (n = 42) and found that surgery significantly accelerated the atherosclerotic progression in the grafted vessels.

Although the results of the previously mentioned studies were recently documented, the beneficial effects of surgery for patients with three-vessel disease and poor ejection fractions were also previously observed in the Coronary Artery Surgery Study,[71] which likewise evaluated the effects of surgical versus medical therapy in patients with atherosclerotic heart disease. Analysis of the 10-year survival data identified a similar subgroup of patients who benefited significantly from coronary artery bypass graft surgery. These patients had poor left ventricular function and multivessel coronary artery disease.[24] However, in patients *without* multivessel disease and poor left ventricular function the comparison of survival data showed no statistically significant difference between the surgical and medical intervention groups. The quality (measured via questionnaire) of the patients' lives in the surgical intervention group was only slightly better than that of the patients in the group receiving medical treatment (that is, less angina). However, 10 years after coronary artery bypass graft surgery, the difference in quality of life between the groups was insignificant.[24] Neither therapeutic exercise training nor cardiac rehabilitation was given to either group. To determine the effect of such training was not the purpose of the study, but it may have been beneficial in improving quality of patient life (that is, less angina and increased endurance) for members of both groups.

The five primary cardiovascular disease processes listed in the box on p. 128 can profoundly limit exercise tolerance. They can also alter the normal physiologic response to exercise because of severely deconditioned and glycolytic skeletal muscle, reduced blood flow to active muscles, and a reduced cardiac output. The effects of a reduced cardiac output are discussed in the following section.

Central Adaptations

Patients with atherosclerotic heart disease, valvular heart disease, cardiomyopathy, congestive heart failure, and peripheral vascular disease all have a similar condition, a reduced cardiac output during exercise.[14] Patients with peripheral vascular disease frequently demonstrate a reduced cardiac output because of increased afterload (the peripheral resistance that the left ventricle must work against) and decreased preload (the volume and subsequent pressure in the ventricles before ventricular contraction).[24] Patients with atherosclerotic heart disease, valvular heart disease, cardiomyopathy, and congestive heart failure frequently have an increased preload and occasionally have an increased afterload.

In peripheral vascular disease the atherosclerotic occlusions in the peripheral vessels increase the peripheral resistance, which increases the afterload and potentially decreases the cardiac output. In addition, in patients with peripheral vascular disease less blood than normal is moved through the peripheral vessels, which subsequently reduces the venous return to the heart and decreases the amount of blood in the heart (decreasing the preload), thereby reducing the cardiac output.[14] In diseased states other than peripheral vascular disease (that is, atherosclerotic heart disease and congestive heart failure), the increased preload and, occasionally, increased afterload occur because of an inadequate stroke volume that "leaves behind" an increased amount of blood in the left or right ventricles, or both, thus increasing the left (and, possibly, right) ventricular end-diastolic volume and pressure (preload).[14] Because of the decreased stroke volume and subsequent decrease in cardiac output, the pressoreceptors and chemoreceptors increase the vasomotor tone of the peripheral vessels (increasing the peripheral vascular resistance) to augment the return of blood to the heart and improve the cardiac output.[14] This response, of course, is ineffective in improving the cardiac out-

put and further increases the preload, which continues to *reduce* the cardiac output. Thus a vicious cycle ensues.

The effects of the primary cardiovascular disorders on physiologic response to exercise include the following:

1. More easily provoked subjective complaints of dyspnea and fatigue and higher ratings of perceived exertion
2. Greater heart rate response than during comparable work in healthy persons, but chronotropic incompetence (inability of the heart rate to increase during progressive exercise) may occur, which produces lower heart rates than those expected in a healthy person during specific exercise workloads
3. Frequently a blunted, flat (no increase in systolic blood pressure during progressive exercise), or hypoadaptive (decreasing) systolic blood pressure response to exercise that appears to depend on the degree of cardiovascular disease
4. Possible symptoms and signs of myocardial ischemia on ECG for patients with atherosclerotic heart disease
5. Possibly, increased ectopy (premature ventricular or atrial contractions and the like)
6. Decreased levels of oxygen consumption

The magnitude of the previously listed effects frequently depends on the degree of reduction in cardiac output. Patients with a markedly reduced cardiac output have the most profound signs and symptoms, and their conditions are likely to be classified as New York Heart Association class 3 or 4 (with significant functional limitations).

The classic work of Wasserman and Whipp[94] in 1975 indirectly identified the important role of the heart rate and stroke volume in maintaining cardiac output, oxygen consumption, and exercise performance. During maximal work patients with cardiac disease had higher heart rates and lower levels of oxygen consumption than those of patients with respiratory disease, octogenarians, and healthy persons because the reduced stroke volume that results from cardiovascular disease (that is, myocardial infarction, valvular heart disease, or cardiomyopathy) decreases the cardiac output and adequate delivery of oxygen to exercising muscles (thus lowering the oxygen consumption).

The 1987 textbook of Wasserman et al.[95] provided specific information on exercise testing by evaluating and comparing the physiologic responses of cardiac patients to the responses of others. Respiratory gas analysis provided clinically discernible data that were used to identify specific disease processes. During exercise, patients with heart disease were often observed to have the following:

1. Low value plateau of the oxygen pulse
2. Low Vo_2 max that failed to rise with continued exercise
3. Steep heart rate-Vo_2 relationship
4. Low anaerobic threshold
5. Low oxygen uptake–work relationship during incremental exercise

In contrast, patients with chronic obstructive pulmonary disease were observed to have the following:

1. Anaerobic threshold in the normal range or at a higher percentage of the a-Vo_2max than in healthy persons
2. Increased alveolar-arterial Po_2 difference
3. Increased arterial–end tidal Pco_2 difference that remains relatively constant and elevated as exercise is increased, rather that decreasing as in healthy persons
4. Decreased Vo_2max
5. Hypoxemia with ensuing dypsnea and fatigue

The preceding findings reinforce the importance and usefulness of cardiopulmonary assessment, which can enhance the understanding of physiologic response to exercise and effects of exercise training. The effects of exercise training on cardiopulmonary response in both the absence and the presence of cardiovascular disease are discussed in the following section.

EFFECTS OF EXERCISE TRAINING AND CARDIAC PERFORMANCE IN THE ABSENCE OF CARDIOVASCULAR DISEASE
Peripheral Adaptations

From the earlier discussion of peripheral versus central adaptation during exercise it is apparent that the peripheral changes are frequently quite profound and often produce substantial increases in oxygen consumption and physical work performance. The same are true for regular exercise training and are the primary reasons that trained athletes attain higher levels of oxygen consumption and physical work than do untrained individuals. The effects of central adaptation are often less profound because of the smaller range available for improvement, since "myocardial oxygen extraction is reported to be approximately the same at rest"[5] as during exercise and increase in cardiac performance depends on high-intensity exercise, which few individuals are likely to undertake.[14,46] Therefore the peripheral changes associated with regular exercise training[5] are the most profound and include the following:

1. Increase in the number and size of mitochondria
2. Improved extraction of oxygen from circulating blood to the exercising muscles
3. Increased muscle strength
4. Two- to threefold increase in mitochondrel enzyme activity
5. Proliferation of capillaries
6. Increase in the mean transit time of blood through the muscle capillaries
7. Lowering of peripheral vascular resistance
8. Increased arteriovenous oxygen (A-Vo_2) difference
9. Increased parasympathetic nervous system activity

The increase in parasympathetic nervous system activity is a poorly understood phenomenon, but the often dramatic reduction in resting heart rate (and exercise heart rates during specific work loads) and blood pressure in trained individuals is thought to be due to *more effective and efficient* skeletal muscle (with its increased number and size of capillaries and mitochondria).[5,56,83] The increased number and size of capillaries and mitochondria increase the supply and extraction of oxygen and require the heart to beat less often to deliver needed blood and its oxygen supply. Despite this beneficial effect of regular exercise training, there also appears to be a complex interaction between the peripheral skeletal muscles' decrease in peripheral vascular resistance and the central nervous system activity on the heart.[33,56,83] This interaction can best be understood by reviewing the literature on the effects of *regular* exercise training on central adaptation and the heart's response to the previously described peripheral adaptations. The lowering of peripheral vascular resistance in response to regular exercise training is an important adaptation and one deserving of further discussion, since it undoubtedly affects the central adaptations associated with regular exercise training.

Central Adaptations

The most frequently cited central adaptations to regular exercise training include improved lung function (a decrease in the transit time index [TTI] during submaximal-intensity exercise and improved heart performance (increased stroke volume and cardiac output, increased parasympathetic activity that decreases resting and exercise heart rates, improved myocardial metabolic response, and decreased myocardial oxygen consumption during submaximal-intensity exercise).[5] These central changes produce what many refer to as an "athlete's heart," which is characterized by left ventricular hypertrophy, very low resting heart rates, lower-than-normal exercise heart rates, ventricular dilation with preserved fractional shortening, and faster myocardial relaxation.[37] Regular exercise training at the appropriate intensity, duration, and frequency increases the number and size of myocardial cells, thus increasing the size of the heart (left ventricular hypertrophy) and the force of myocardial contraction, which subsequently increases the stroke volume and cardiac output. However, these changes can potentially decrease the "*efficiency*" of the heart. That is, as the heart enlarges, contraction of the hypertrophied ventricle requires more energy and for each contraction (despite it being more powerful and ejecting a greater volume) the additional energy cost decreases the efficiency of cardiac performance.[14]

Although the previously described changes are often of no apparent consequence for healthy individuals, such adaptations could be detrimental for individuals with cardiovascular disease. In addition, even in apparently healthy individuals, recent research questions the magnitude of improved heart performance as a result of regular exercise training and suggests that "*cardiac fatigue*," which previously had been thought to occur only in persons with coronary heart disease, may accompany prolonged exercise sessions in *healthy* individuals.[29] The implications are that such cardiac fatigue in those with heart disease could be serious and in some instances fatal.

The cardiovascular dynamics of healthy athletes appear to differ significantly from those in healthy untrained individuals. Recently Fisman et al.[38] suggested that "the ejection fraction at rest and during exercise is significantly lower in athletes and that some athletes exhibit altered left ventricular volume responses to exercise, accompanied by segmental wall motion abnormalities." The ejection fraction (again, the percentage of blood ejected from the total amount of blood in the left ventricle) of trained athletes (22 professional soccer players with a mean age of 23.1 ± 2.3 years) was significantly lower at rest and during exercise ($65 \pm 4\%$ versus $70 \pm 5\%$ and $73 \pm 5\%$ versus $86 \pm 5\%$, respectively) than that in untrained individuals (22 age-matched men with a mean age of 24.3 ± 2.9 years).[38] The untrained individuals demonstrated *no* abnormalities in left ventricular wall motion at rest or during exercise. At peak exercise, however, eight of the trained athletes were observed to have left ventricular wall motion abnormalities. These abnormalities included the absence of the expected myocardial hyperkinesia (increased heart motion) in seven of the athletes (three of the seven athletes demonstrated no change in the pattern of contraction and four were observed to have symmetric *hypokinesia*) and marked dyskinesia of the anterior wall of the left ventricle in one athlete.

In addition, the left ventricular end-systolic and end-diastolic volumes at rest and during supine bicycle exercise were greater in the trained athletes than in the healthy untrained individuals.[38] The larger end-systolic volume is somewhat surprising in view of the previous discussions regarding the reduction of TPR and increased cardiac output in trained individuals. Both the increased cardiac output and the decreased TPR normally produce a smaller end-systolic volume because of less peripheral vascular resistance and because a presumably greater cardiac output is ejected. These changes normally decrease the volume of blood remaining in the left ventricle at the end of systole and produce a smaller end-systolic volume.

In contrast, the greater end-diastolic volume in trained athletes is in keeping with previous studies that show increases in end-diastolic volume at *higher levels* of exercise whereas a mild or moderate level of supine exercise produces no change or even decreases in end-diastolic volume). These results are also in keeping with the previous discussion of increased exertion, which increases the amount of vasoconstriction in nonactive muscles so that active muscles can be supplied with an adequate amount of blood. The increased vasoconstriction of inactive muscles during higher levels of exertion therefore increases the venous return to the heart and ultimately increases the amount of blood in the left ventricle at the end of diastole, which increases the cardiac output that is desperately needed by *maximally* exercising muscles.

However, mild to moderate levels of exercise may decrease the end-diastolic volume because of the aforementioned decrease in TPR, which redistributes the blood supply throughout a larger portion of the peripheral system and ultimately may reduce venous return. This mechanism could potentially decrease the volume of blood in the left ventricle at the end of diastole and may be one reason why six of the athletes were observed to have *no* change or a decrease in the end-diastolic volume, as compared with an increase in the end-diastolic volume in *all* of the untrained individuals. That is, the maximal exercise performed by the trained athletes produced cardiovascular changes *suggestive of mildly or moderately intense exercise*.

Whatever the mechanism for the altered left ventricular volumes and ejection fractions in trained athletes as compared with untrained individuals, perhaps the most important and crucial aspect, as previously noted, is the intensity of the exercise performed. This aspect was evident when the echocardiographic findings observed before and after prolonged bicycling performed at approximately 66% of the maximum heart rate (Race Across America participants) were compared with those associated with prolonged exercise (Ironman Triathlon) performed at 80% or more of the maximal heart rate.[20] No evidence of *profound* cardiac abnormality was observed after the exercise that was performed at 66% of maximal heart rate, but significant reductions in cardiac motion and ejection fraction were observed in the athletes exercising at 80% or more of maximal heart rate.

Several interesting papers have been published recently about cardiac performance before and after the Hawaii Ironman Triathlon (3.9-km swim, 180.2-km bicycle ride, and 42.2-km run).[29-31,37] Approximately 40 athletes have been evaluated over a 6-year period via two-dimensional echocardiography or Doppler echocardiography, or both. The triathlon has been completed in an average time of 12 hours 21 minutes (ranging from 9 to 16 hours) and, as mentioned earlier, at an intensity of 80% or more of maximal heart rate.

Analysis of the before-and-after echocardiograms[29,30,37] revealed the following:

1. Reduction in the left ventricular and left and right atrial sizes, whereas the right ventricular size increased (possibly because of changes in right ventricular function, shape, or compliance)
2. Regional left ventricular wall motion abnormalities (midseptal and apical-septal motion)
3. Lower ejection fractions immediately after the triathlon (46% versus 51%), which increased to 54% one day after the triathlon

These findings are suggestive of a type of *cardiac fatigue* that appears to be associated with higher intensities of exercise.[31] No evidence of such profound cardiac fatigue was observed when we analyzed the echocardiograms of four ultramarathon athletes who bicycled from the West Coast to the East Coast of the United States during the

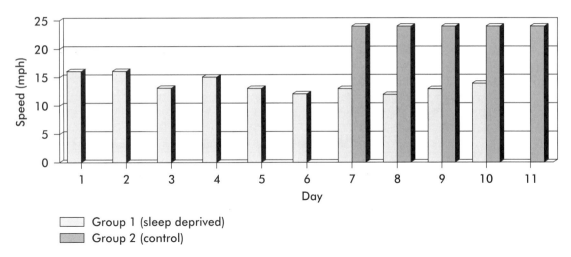

Fig. 7-3 Exercise performance (average daily cycling speed) during the Race Across America. Performance remained much the same from day to day in both groups. The average daily distance traveled was 293 miles for group 1 and 580 miles for group 2.

Race Across America.[20] The exercise of the four athletes participating in the Race Across America was performed for approximately 22 hours per day for a period of 7.5 to 12.25 days (two athletes completed the race in 7.5 days, one in 9 days, and one in 12.25 days) at an intensity of approximately 66% of maximal heart rate. The echocardiograms obtained after the Race Across America revealed slight decreases in ejection fraction (0.04%) and left ventricular diameter percentage of shortening (0.05%) (an important measurement of myocardial muscle performance and the ability of the myocardial fibers to shorten).[20] Therefore it appears that an exercise intensity threshold may exist which, if exceeded, may impair cardiac performance.

However, the maintenance of cardiac performance during the Race Across America may also be due to sleep deprivation. Previous results suggest that an inverse relationship may exist between sleep deprivation and cardiopulmonary function (exercise heart rate and Vo_2).[19] As sleep deprivation increases, exercise heart rates and Vo_2 have been observed to decrease. These effects were seen in six ultramarathon bicyclists during the 1989 Race Across America. Three of the athletes bicycled individually and were significantly deprived of sleep (average sleep of 2 hours per night), competing the race in 9 days (group 1). The other three athletes bicycled 4 to 6 hours per day, participating on a relay team of four and completing the Race Across America in 5 days with approximately 6 hours of sleep per night (group 2). Exercise performance during the Race Across America decreased only slightly in both groups (Fig. 7-3), and in group 1 the mean exercise heart rate and Vo_2 decreased 24% and 39%, respectively, whereas group 2 exhibited an 11% and a 13% reduction in mean exercise heart rate and Vo_2, respectively (Figs. 7-4 and 7-5).[19] Also of interest were the results of maximal bicycle ergometry exercise tests that were performed immediately after the Race Across America, demonstrating (1) attainment of 75% to 96% of prerace maximal workloads, (2) lower heart rates and blood pressure in general during each work load, as compared with the values demonstrated in prerace tests, (3) lower maximal heart rates than those during prerace tests (4% to 11%), and (4) in several athletes a more rapid recovery with lower recovery heart rates after exercise testing.

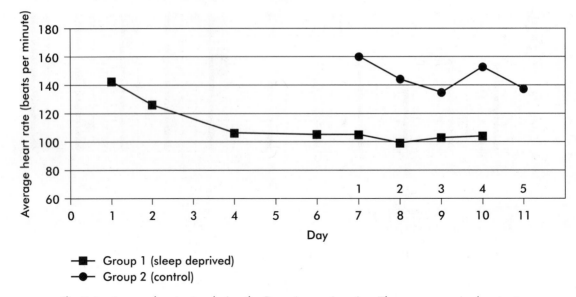

Fig. 7-4   Average heart rates during the Race Across America. The mean exercise heart rate declined from day 1 to day 3 and then remained relatively stable for both groups.

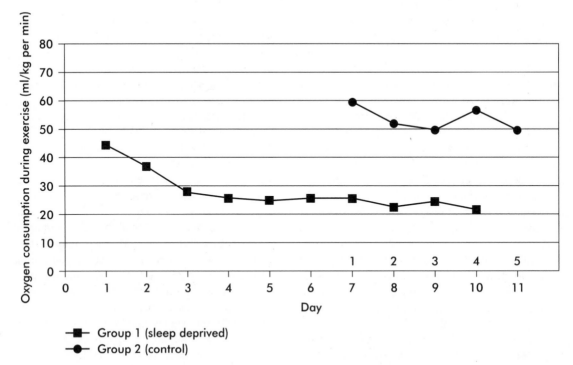

Fig. 7-5   Predicted oxygen consumption and heart rate showed the same responses during the Race Across America.

The changes described in the preceding paragraph appear to be partly due to sleep deprivation, which may increase parasympathetic nervous system activity, but the magnitude of reduction in exercise heart rates and oxygen consumption during ultramarathon bicycling, as well as several of the previously described observations during maximal exercise testing after the Race Across America, suggest that a profound training effect may also be responsible. This hypothesis is reinforced by the findings of Sarnoff et al.,[86] who observed in 1958 that marked increases in cardiac output during physical exercise are not necessarily accompanied by increased levels of myocardial oxygen consumption. The authors concluded their classic paper by stating that "it might be that the heart demands a progressively smaller fraction of the total oxygen utilized by the organism as physical activity increases, especially when the heart rate is maintained at low levels as in well-trained athletes."

Of particular importance are the echocardiographic findings in one of the 1990 Race Across America research participants, who demonstrated an increased stroke volume (7.15 ml) and left ventricular mass (8.71 g), both of which are suggestive of specific *training adaptations*.[21] These findings demonstrate that although the exercise duration in the Race Across America is longer than that in the Ironman Triathlon, the lower exercise intensity appears to maintain and may possibly enhance cardiac performance rather than impair it, as has been observed after the shorter but more intense Ironman Triathlon. However, 24 hours after the Ironman Triathlon the average ejection fraction increased to 54%, which before the triathlon was 51% (and immediately afterward decreased to 46%).[29] The initial decrease in ejection fraction immediately after the Ironman Triathlon does suggest "cardiac fatigue," but the increase 24 hours later to a value greater than that before the triathlon (54% versus 51%) demonstrates that although the heart may have been fatigued, the fatigue was not long-lasting and, in fact, a training stimulus apparently accompanied the cardiac fatigue. Although the effects of such cardiac fatigue seemed to promote central training effects, the patient with cardiovascular disease may not tolerate such "cardiac fatigue" as well as athletes do.

EFFECTS OF EXERCISE TRAINING AND CARDIAC PERFORMANCE IN PATIENTS WITH CARDIOVASCULAR DISEASE
Peripheral Adaptations

The peripheral adaptations accompanying exercise and regular exercise training in the patient with cardiovascular disease can be either more or less profound than those in the healthy individual because the patient's initial level of fitness appears to determine (perhaps more so than in the healthy person) the respective cardiopulmonary response and the adaptation to regular exercise training.[25,26] Patients with poor levels of physical fitness are most likely to make impressive cardiovascular adaptations, whereas patients in relatively good shape demonstrate less cardiovascular change but tolerate work loads more effectively and efficiently as exercise training is continued. Thus the American College of Physicians strongly recommends exercise training for patients with impaired left ventricular function and an initially poor physical work capacity.[44] The physicians state that "patients with cardiac disease with significant limitation of maximal work capacity, for example, less than 7 METS soon after infarction, may expect to achieve meaningful improvement in work capacity by participating in an exercise training program. The 15% to 25% greater improvement in work capacity that may be expected to occur in an exercise program is likely to be of greatest clinical benefit in such patients."

All the adaptations to regular exercise training in the healthy individual should be expected to occur in the patient with cardiovascular disease, but the peripheral adaptations to exercise training in individuals with cardiovascular disease depend much more on the central adaptations to exercise. This was demonstrated by Wassermann and Whipp,[94] who stated that "diseases that limit the output of the cardiac pump may result in an inadequate oxygen delivery to muscles at a relatively low work rate.'' Such conditions may occur with myocardial infarction, valvular heart disease, or cardiomyopathy. In addition, although Bruce, Kusumi, and Hosmer[15] have provided a detailed assessment of Vo_2max and FAI in heathy individuals and patients with cardiac disease during incremental exercise tests, in the study sedentary and active patients with cardiac disease were not separately studied, whereas the healthy men and women were. It is my opinion that trained cardiac patients have a much different cardiovascular profile than that portrayed by Bruce, Kusumi, and Hosmer[15] and Wasserman and Whipp.[94] The FAI of endurance-trained cardiac patients (participants in the Specialized Coronary Outpatient Rehabilitation (SCOR) cardiac cycling and jogging clubs) appears to follow a pattern similar to that for the normal men and women described by Bruce, Kusumi, and Hosmer.[15] Therefore the submaximal work of trained cardiac patients requires less of the Vo_2max and provides the trained cardiac patient an *oxygen reserve.*[18]

The lower oxygen consumption of patients with cardiac disease (because of less oxygen delivery and uptake in peripheral skeletal muscles) is closely related to cardiac performance. Cardiac performance depends on the stroke volume and heart rate, which in patients with cardiovascular disease are frequently altered.[94] The stroke volume tends to be reduced and patients with heart disease, although having an equally low maximal Vo_2, have a relatively high heart rate. [94] These relationships therefore demonstrate the importance of assessing the central adaptations to exercise and regular exercise training so that a thorough understanding of cardiac performance can be obtained.

Central Adaptations

The primary central adaptations to regular exercise training include a decrease in resting and exercise heart rates and an increase in stroke volume and myocardial blood supply (resulting from myocardial collateralization, that is, increased blood supply to heart muscle via increased number and size of arteries in the heart).[40] The reduction in heart rate that was discussed in the section on exercise tolerance for healthy persons appears to be more profound the longer exercise training is performed. This is also true for patients with heart disease, but the role of the heart rate in maintaining cardiac output is much more important because of the frequent decrease in stroke volume associated with cardiovascular disease.[94] Therefore a reduction in *resting* heart rate can be expected in patients with cardiovascular disease, but the reduction in *exercise* heart rate during progressive exercise is often less pronounced because of the need to maintain or increase cardiac output in the presence of a limited stroke volume, that is, because of damaged myocardium caused by a myocardial infarction.[94] Again, the equation for cardiac output ($CO = HR \times SV$) is helpful in better understanding this concept, since cardiac output is the product of heart rate and stroke volume and a decrease in stroke volume must be matched by an increase in heart rate to maintain the necessary cardiac output. The importance of the stroke volume is evident from the preceding discussion, and the effects of regular exercise training on stroke volume are equally important. The effects of exercise training on stroke volume are still controversial, despite several well-performed studies showing that stroke volume *can* be increased in patients with cardiovascular disease (primarily patients who have had myocardial infarction) by means of aggressive, regular exercise training.

In 1984 Froelicher et al.[40] demonstrated that 1 year of exercise training (at 60% to 85% of estimated Vo_2max for 45 minutes, three times per week) in patients with coronary heart disease could produce many of the aforementioned training effects commonly observed in healthy individuals performing regular exercise training. These effects included significant reductions in resting and exercise heart rates, submaximal rate-pressure product, and change in percentage of end-systolic volume. In addition, significant increases in Vo_2max, maximal rate-pressure product, stroke volume, cardiac output (in patients without angina), and thallium perfusion (suggesting increased blood flow to the myocardium) were observed.

A particular concern of Froelicher et al.[40] in assessing the decrease in end-systolic volume and increase in stroke volume was the effect of TPR (afterload) in the trained cardiac patients. The authors stated that "there were no significant differences in blood pressure at any stage of bicycle exercise so there is no evidence that decreased afterload would explain this." "This" refers to the decrease in end-systolic volume or conversely, an increase in stroke volume. As previously mentioned, the measurement of blood pressure can provide important indirect information about the status of the cardiovascular system (as is evident in the preceding quotation). The absence of lower blood pressure (suggesting a decreased afterload) during incremental exercise in the previously mentioned study confirms that a greater amount of blood was ejected from the left ventricle during systole, not because of a lower TPR (again, because of the absence of lower blood pressure) but because of the improved contraction of the heart.

Increases in stroke volume and cardiac output in patients with documented coronary artery disease have also been observed by Ehsani[33] and Ehsani et al.,[34,35] who observed many of the training adaptations documented by Froelicher et al.,[40] as well as several other adaptations. These included an increase in ejection fraction and a decrease in end-systolic volume, despite a larger increase in systolic blood pressure (suggesting an increased afterload).[33] *All these adaptations demonstrate that cardiac performance (specifically, left ventricular contractile function) can be improved by means of properly progressed exercise training in patients with coronary artery disease. The consensus of many is that improved cardiac performance has been hypothesized "to be due to a reduction of myocardial ischemia."*[33]

ALTERED CARDIOVASCULAR PERFORMANCE

Cardiovascular performance can be altered in many ways other than those just discussed for patients with cardiovascular disease. The most common causes of altered cardiovascular performance are discussed in this section, including the effects

---

> **COMMON CAUSES OF ALTERED CARDIOVASCULAR PERFORMANCE**
>
> Hypertension
> Medications
> Cardiac arrhythmias
> Myocardial infarction
> Congestive heart failure
> Renal failure (multiple organ involvement)
> Peripheral vascular disease
> Diabetes mellitus
> Cardiac surgery and procedures

of hypertension, medications, cardiac arrhythmias, myocardial infarction, congestive heart failure, renal failure (and its multiorgan involvement), peripheral vascular disease, diabetes mellitus, and cardiac surgery and procedures (see the box on p. 137). The effects of exercise training on each of these are reviewed, and the implications for exercise training are emphasized.

Hypertension

Hypertension is an extremely common medical disorder affecting approximately one third of all persons over 65 years of age.[32] Individuals with hypertension have significant alterations in the cardiovascular system when compared to normotensive individuals; the major distinction is that those with hypertension have reduced vasodilating capacity.[94] This reduced capacity may have profound effects on the following:

1. Active musculature, by limiting necessary blood flow to exercising muscles
2. Inactive musculature, by impairing the interplay between vasoconstriction and vasodilation that is necessary for the redistribution of blood during submaximal to maximal levels of exercise
3. Cardiac performance, by potentially decreasing the stroke volume because of an increased afterload

An increased afterload requires a more forceful myocardial contraction to maintain the cardiac output and frequently results in left ventricular hypertrophy. As left ventricular hypertrophy ensues, the increased oxygen requirement of the heart may induce myocardial ischemia and subsequently further impair cardiac performance.

In patients with hypertension, easily provoked dyspnea and a limited physical work capacity may develop as consequences of the previously listed effects. Patients with marked hypertension may have a variety of cardiopulmonary abnormalities, and pulmonary vascular congestion is common.[94] Properly prescribed exercise training has been shown to be beneficial for patients with hypertension. Three important studies evaluating the effects of exercise on hypertension demonstrated a 7- 13-mm Hg decrease in systolic blood pressure and a 4- 7-mm Hg reduction in diastolic blood pressure after 4 to 16 weeks of aerobic exercise training.[32,51,92]

Of additional concern in patients with hypertension is the effect of medications on cardiopulmonary dynamics. The effects of β blockers and calcium-channel blockers on cardiovascular dynamics are reviewed in the following section.

Medications

β Blockers. β-adrenergic receptor-blocking agents compete with β-adrenergic agonists for available β-receptor sites. Some β blockers are selective (blocking only β_1-receptor sites), and others are nonselective (blocking both β_1 and β_2 receptors). β-adrenergic blockade of β_1-receptor sites reduces heart rate, myocardial force of contraction, lipolysis, and plasma values of nonesterified free fatty acids. Nonselective β blockade produces the preceding effects and *inhibits* vasodilation in capillary beds, muscle relaxation in the bronchial tracts, glycogenolysis in the liver and muscles, and the release of insulin from the pancreas.[16]

The effects of the previously mentioned medications on cardiovascular, pulmonary, muscular, and metabolic function can be profound. "Reductions have been observed in (1) resting and exercise heart rates, (2) blood pressure, (3) skeletal muscle and coronary blood flow, (4) cardiac output at rest and during exercise, (5) myocardial oxygen requirements, (6) exercise-induced lipolysis, (7) translocation of lactate from the muscle cell to the blood, (8) peripheral blood flow, and (9) carbon dioxide production."[16]

Of particular interest is the suggestion that β blockade may lead to a reduction in the number of slow-twitch muscle fibers (type 2 fibers, which are necessary for endurance and capable of high levels of oxygen consumption) because of a reduction or loss of sympathetic nervous system activity in the specific muscles.[58] If such a reduction occurs, it must be minimal, since many studies evaluating the effects of β blockade on exercise training have shown improved Vo_2max.[73,81,93] However, in some studies patients have shown minimal or no improvement in Vo_2max,[66,84] and the underlying reason may be that the majority of the patients could have had a greater percentage of slow-twitch muscle fibers, which, because of β blockade, would have decreased the ability of the muscles to utilize delivered oxygen supplies (decreasing the Vo_2max). This may also explain why well-trained *endurance* athletes have dramatic reductions in Vo_2max when administered even low doses of β blockers.[3]

Nonetheless, cardiovascular performance is markedly altered as a result of β blockade. However, in view of the available data, specific training effects (both central and peripheral) can occur in those with or without coronary artery disease (1) when the training stimulus is appropriate (adequate frequency, intensity, and duration), (2) when dosages of β blockers are not extreme (when the peak heart rate is reduced by less than 40 beats per minute), (3) when the initial cardiorespiratory fitness is not extreme, as suggested by Davies and Knibbs,[27] who stated that the magnitude of Vo_2max increase during training depends on its starting value, and (4) when the percentages of slow-twitch muscle fibers and fast-twitch muscle fibers are relatively equal.[16]

Calcium-channel blockers. The calcium-channel blockers block (to varying degrees) the slow calcium channels from the sarcoplasmic reticulum of primarily smooth muscle. However, the effects of calcium-channel blockade appear to affect skeletal and cardiac muscle in much the same way that smooth muscle is affected.[10] The effects of calcium-channel blockade on cardiac performance appear to be variable and are probably due to differing patient response to different calcium-channel blockers, thus exerting "confounding effects on preload, afterload, and heart rate, all of which can artificially change the systolic and diastolic properties of the myocardium."[10] However, the following effects of calcium-channel blockers at rest and during exercise[3,10,16] appear to be well accepted:

1. Dilation of peripheral arterioles, which reduces total peripheral vascular resistance and systolic wall tension
2. Alteration of the cardiac action potential (initiating each heart beat) by depressing phase 4 depolarization and lengthening phases 1 and 2 of repolarization, thus decreasing sinoatrial and atrioventricular node conduction and prolonging the atrioventricular node effective and functional refractory periods
3. Dilation of the coronary arteries and arterioles, thus inhibiting coronary spasm and maintaining myocardial oxygen supply (reducing myocardial ischemia) while providing substantial antianginal effects
4. Decreased resting end-diastolic and end-systolic volumes
5. Increased ejection fraction
6. Increased levels of plasma noradrenaline, adrenaline, and renin activity
7. Improved recovery of systolic and diastolic ventricular function after various durations of ischemia

"Calcium-channel blockers are generally indicated for supraventricular dysrhythmias and are used only occasionally for ventricular dysrhythmias."[16]

The previously listed actions improve cardiac efficiency in much the same way that β blockers do, but without the concomitant decrease in myocardial force of contraction that frequently accompanies β blockade (except for β blockers such as pindolol and acebutolol, which have an inherent inotropic effect that is referred to as *intrinsic sympathomimetic activity*).[16] Calcium-channel blockers are common drugs of choice, since they allow the heart to contract more freely against a lower peripheral resistance without decreasing the force of myocardial contraction. In addition, calcium-channel blockade may even improve abnormal cardiovascular dynamics resulting from left ventricular hypertrophy (by actually decreasing the magnitude of left ventricular hypertrophy).[64] Hypertensive patients who have received several months of calcium-channel blockade have demonstrated *less* abnormality in left ventricular filling (allowing the myocardial fibers to stretch, whereas stretching was previously limited because of hypertrophied heart muscle) and emptying (requiring less energy cost because of less cardiac muscle mass).[64] Improved cardiovascular dynamics after prolonged calcium-channel blockade may reverse left ventricular hypertrophy, as demonstrated by Saragoca et al.,[85] and improve the efficiency of each heart beat. Cardiovascular efficiency occurs because the reduction in cardiac muscle mass allows the myocardium to stretch more (filling with more blood as the Frank-Starling mechanism is increasingly utilized) and to contract more efficiently at a lower energy cost because of less muscle mass and less total peripheral resistance. The cardiovascular dynamics therefore become more effective, which improves overall cardiac efficiency at rest and during exercise. However, the overall improved efficiency resulting from the use of calcium-channel blockers may be limited or short-lived; one recent study[28] observed a progression in cardiac hypertrophy during long-term therapy with the calcium-channel blocker Tiapamil.

Cardiac Arrhythmias

Cardiac function is intimately related to cardiac rhythm. Heart rhythms that are abnormally slow, fast, or unsynchronized can quickly impair ventricular and atrial performance and can produce a distinct type of cardiac muscle dysfunction. Although this type of cardiac muscle dysfunction can be

Table 7-2 Significant cardiac arrhythmias and contraindications for exercise training

Arrythmia	Contraindications
Ventricular	
Unifocal PVC	None
Multifocal PVCs	Relative
Coupled PVCs (R-on-T)	Relative
Tachycardia	Absolute
Fibrillation	Absolute
Atrial	
PAC	None
PNC	None
Fibrillation	Relative
Paroxysmal tachycardia	Absolute
Flutter	Absolute
Other	
Bundle-branch block	None
AV node block	Relative

AV, Atrioventricular; *PAC,* premature atrial contraction; *PNC,* premature nodal contraction; *PVC,* premature ventricular contraction.

reversed by means of medication, cardioversion, or defibrillation, if left untreated, profound complications such as syncope, congestive heart failure, and death may occur.[13] The effects of cardiac arrhythmias on exercise training are detrimental, and cautious assessment and monitoring must be employed when assessing and training patients with significant cardiac arrhythmias. Absolute and relative contraindications to exercise training for specific arrhythmias are given in Table 7-2.

The effects of exercise training on cardiac arrhythmias are questionable, but regular exercise training may decrease the incidence and severity of cardiac arrhythmias caused by coronary artery disease.[8] In contrast, arrhythmias unrelated to coronary artery disease appear to decrease during bouts of exercise, probably because of the increased sympathetic drive of the sinoatrial node to increase the heart rate during progressive work or exercise.[8]

Cardiac arrhythmias, whether fast or slow, can

significantly alter cardiac performance. The primary alteration associated with rapid or slow heart rates is the inability of the heart to maintain an adequate cardiac output. Once again, the equation for cardiac output (CO = HR × SV) applies. When the heart rate decreases to less than 30 or 40 beats per min, a linear decrease in cardiac output occurs. The threshold for decreasing cardiac output depends on the patient's level of physical fitness and age and the presence of any other disease processes.

Rapid heart rates impair cardiac performance in much the same way that slow heart rates do, but the primary effect of rapid heart rate activity is that the left ventricle is not allowed enough time to fill with blood. This can severely limit the left ventricular end-diastolic volume (preload), which can significantly decrease the cardiac output.

Thus both rapid and slow heart rates produce ineffective pumping. Rapid heart rates decrease the stroke volume and cardiac output, whereas slow heart rates maintain an adequate stroke volume but limit the amount of blood expelled in 1 minute, which decreases the cardiac output.

Myocardial Infarction

It is apparent from earlier discussion that the effects of myocardial infarction on cardiovascular performance can be marked. In some instances, however, the degree of myocardial damage may be minimal, in which case the effects on cardiovascular performance may be insignificant. Minimal effects are frequently associated with inferior wall myocardial infarctions.[49] Myocardial damage to the anterior, lateral, or inferoposterior walls, or a combination of these, seems to produce more significant cardiovascular changes, most commonly a decreased force of myocardial contraction (reducing the cardiac output) and impaired filling of the left and right ventricles (with blood from each respective atrium).[49] The latter effect has recently been of great concern, both at the time of an infarction and long after an infarction has occurred. Long after an infarction has occurred, left and right ventricular filling can decrease because of the ineffective stretch of the fibrous scar formed at the site of the myocardial infarction, which increases the end-diastolic pressure. If the stretch on the heart that results from increased left or right ventricular end-diastolic volume and pressure is too great or too little, cardiac performance deteriorates, resulting in a low and ineffective stroke volume and cardiac output. Therefore the primary cause of such an ineffective stroke volume and cardiac output is poor filling of the heart's ventricles during diastole or, as recently described in the literature, "*diastolic dysfunction.*" Diastolic dysfunction may also be responsible for impaired ventricular performance at the time of an acute myocardial infarction, but systolic dysfunction (poor contractility) is primarily responsible.

It is well documented that the effects of diastolic dysfunction are as important as those of systolic dysfunction.[54] Thus cardiovascular performance, as well as physical work performance, may be more appropriately assessed and predicted by determination of the left ventricular end-diastolic pressure (and other diastolic indices) than by determination of the ejection fraction and other systolic variables (which have been proven to be poor predictors of exercise performance).

Whether systolic or diastolic dysfunction (or both) occurs after a myocardial infarction, the *end result* is a reduction in cardiac output accompanied by an increased work load and increased myocardial oxygen cost for the remaining (living) myocardium.[76] Cardiac output is *usually* maintained at rest and during submaximal exercise after a myocardial infarction. However, in a patient with an extensive myocardial infarction or in a patient with a minor or moderate-sized infarction who is in poor physical condition the cardiac output at rest and during submaximal exercise can be significantly compromised. In such patients minimal exertion may place a greater demand on the heart than it can tolerate, because of a reduced stroke volume that decreases the cardiac output. The decreased cardiac output can produce significant lactic acidosis[94] (see the earlier discussion), and if exercise is prolonged (or even minimal in the patient with extensive myocardial damage), congestive heart failure may ensue.[49] In this situation congestive heartfailure is the result

of a "backing up of blood" into the lungs because of inefficient, ineffective myocardial pumping or filling, or both. Thus, exercise sessions and regular exercise training for patients with *extensive anterior myocardial infarctions* and *severe multiple coronary artery disease* should be cautiously progressed.[1] The goal of such exercise training is to prevent the cardiac muscle dysfunction that may lead to congestive heart failure while improving musculoskeletal performance. The manner of progression and key clinical criteria for exercise training in these patients are discussed in the section on exercise training.

Congestive Heart Failure

The effects of congestive heart failure on cardiovascular performance are truly profound.[49] As previously noted, the most common cause of congestive heart failure (whether precipitated by exertion or not) is the systolic or diastolic dysfunction that results from myocardial infarction.[57] The decreased cardiac output that results from systolic or diastolic dysfunction is sensed by the neuroreceptors and chemoreceptors of the body (that is, carotid bodies of the carotid arteries and the like), which incorrectly interpret a decreased volume of blood because of the decreased cardiac output. In response to this interpretation a message is sent to the kidneys to retain fluid so that a greater volume of blood can be pumped to the necessary tissues and organs. However, hypovolemia is not the cause of the sensed decrease in vascular volume. Rather, the impaired pumping ability of the left ventricle or the inability of the left ventricle to adequately accept enough blood, or both, causes the decrease in cardiac output and prevents the necessary volume of blood from reaching the peripheral tissues. In extreme cases certain central organs, including myocardial tissue, may receive less oxygenated blood than normal.

A decrease in oxygenated blood can further impair cardiac performance and produce a type of "ischemic cardiac muscle dysfunction." Such a decreased supply of oxygenated blood to the myocardium and peripheral tissues is caused not only

---

CHARACTERISTIC SIGNS AND SYMPTOMS OF CONGESTIVE HEART FAILURE

Dyspnea
Tachypnea
Paroxysmal nocturnal dyspnea
Orthopnea
Peripheral edema
Weight gain
Hepatomegaly
Jugular venous distention
Rales
Tubular breath sounds and consolidation
Presence of third heart sound (S_3)
Sinus tachycardia
Decreased exercise tolerance or
   physical work capacity

---

by the poor systolic and diastolic function but also by the decreased oxygenation in the lungs, which in congestive heart failure are filled with fluid (to varying degrees, depending on the severity of the congestive failure). This decreases the effective diffusion of oxygen and carbon dioxide and produces a scenario similar to that in obstructive lung disease, in which a decrease in adequate ventilatory space occurs. Therefore patients with congestive heart failure frequently have *dyspnea* (sometimes even at rest) and may demonstrate other signs characteristic of chronic obstructive pulmonary disease, such as the following:

Tachypnea (rapid breathing)
Paroxysmal nocturnal dyspnea
Orthopnea
Abnormal breath and heart sounds (that is, rales, rhonchi, and the third heart sound [S_3])
Sinus tachycardia
Decreased exercise tolerance or physical work capacity
Characteristic signs and symptoms of congestive heart failure are listed in the box on p. 142.

The consequences of congestive heart failure include increased myocardial work, decreased levels of oxygenated blood, and abnormal function of

one or more of the following systems: renal, hepatic, neurohumoral, hematologic, musculoskeletal, nutritional, and pancreatic. When the preceding conditions exist concomitantly, exercise prescription can be most helpful—and most dangerous. Improper exercise prescription for patients with congestive heart failure can have serious side effects, and a worsening of symptoms or bodily function is not uncommon in patients with *multisystem disease*.

Renal Failure

Renal failure is a disease process that can impair cardiovascular function; conversely renal function can be markedly impaired as a consequence of cardiovascular disease, as previously discussed. Congestive heart failure and a decreased cardiac output ultimately decrease peripheral and even central vascular perfusion. In this type of disease process (that of a fluid overload resulting from cardiovascular disease), which is characterized by an exaggerated vascular vasoconstriction (both peripheral and central) that redistributes the body's blood supply to the heart to increase the cardiac output, central renal function is taxed when it attempts to retain more fluid.[14] Fluid retention is accomplished via augmented α-adrenergic neural activity, circulating catecholamines, and increased circulating and locally produced angiotensin II, all of which produce renal vasoconstriction that decreases the glomerular filtration rate (GFR) and renal blood flow.[14] These cardiovascular changes produce renal ischemia that, if left untreated, irreversibly impairs renal function and is likely to necessitate peritoneal dialysis or ultrafiltration.[14]

In addition, patients with most end-stage organ diseases such as liver and heart failure often have a certain degree of renal insufficiency because of abnormal hemodynamic and multisystem complications. Thus patients with end-stage organ disease must be assessed for signs and symptoms of congestive heart failure (see the box on p. 142) and receive appropriate treatment.

Different levels of exercise produce differing effects on normal renal function; nonetheless, individuals with compromised (perhaps even mildly impaired) renal performance appear to have a pronounced redistribution of blood to the exercising muscles. This redistribution of blood includes the shunting of central blood from the kidneys to the exercising musculature. The renal ischemia previously discussed is thus accelerated, causing further deterioration in kidney function.[14]

In addition, the cardiovascular response to exercise in patients with renal failure is difficult to interpret because individuals with renal failure *frequently* demonstrate a blunted heart rate response during exercise.[47,59] This feature may partly result from a *specific autonomic dysfunction*,[91] but the exact mechanism is unknown. Consequently, alternative methods should probably be employed to judge exercise response. The following methods have been suggested:

Dyspnea indices

Blood pressure response (although it, too, appears to be blunted during exercise)

Electrocardiogram for heart rate and rhythm as well as ischemia

Ratings of perceived exertion

Oxygen saturation level

Respiratory rate

Pattern of breathing

Probably the most useful, accurate way to evaluate cardiovascular performance is to use a combination of the previously listed methods; of these, ratings of perceived exertion, oxygen saturation monitors, and ECG may be the most effective. However, if peripheral vascular disease is present, the use of oxygen saturation monitors is at least questionable, since decreased oxygen saturation levels could be the result of peripheral vascular occlusion.[23]

Peripheral Vascular Disease

The deposition of lipids and other substances (such as calcium) often occurs in response to trauma resulting from cigarette smoke (because of less oxygenated blood and greater levels of the irritant carbon monoxide in circulating blood), hypertension (because of increased pressures on the peripheral vasculature, which is analogous to a bi-cycle tire inner tube that is inflated beyond its means, producing weakened areas, leaks, cracks, and fissures), and diabetes mellitus (decreasing needed energy to peripheral tissues). Lipid accumulation can severely limit blood flow through damaged arteries, which not only promotes muscular ischemia (or intermittent claudication) but also in its advanced form could produce myocardial ischemia and markedly reduce the cardiac output. Both of the latter effects result from an inadequate supply of blood to the heart. Although the coronary circulation is fed via the left and right main coronary arteries arising from the aorta, the inefficient movement of blood through the peripheral vessels decreases venous return to the heart and essentially decreases the available blood supply for myocardial and skeletal muscle activity. During exercise a volume- and pressure-sensed feedback mechanism produces a profound redistribution of blood that provides the myocardium with a blood supply that is increased but not of the magnitude of the supply distributed to skeletal muscle (Fig. 7-1).[5] Because of peripheral vascular disease, however, the redistribution of blood is impaired, which in effect can lower the threshold for myocardial ischemia. If coronary artery disease is present and this threshold is exceeded, cardiac performance is further impaired. This situation results in a reduction in the force of myocardial contraction, which is already compromised by reduced blood supply because of decreased venous return. In addition to the previously mentioned consequences of peripheral vascular disease, the specific effects of exercise on the treatment of peripheral vascular disease are discussed in the following paragraphs.

Although it is difficult to investigate the preventive role of exercise in persons with peripheral vascular disease, the therapeutic effects of exercise on peripheral vascular disease may be substantial.[6,87] In the initial assessment of patients with peripheral vascular disease the Winsor and Heyman scale (see the box on p.144) can be used to classify patients according to functional status.[97] Patients can be graded from 1 to 4; grade 1 patients demonstrate

---

WINSOR AND HEYMAN SCALE

Grade 1 No functional limits

Grade 2 Ambulatory for a distance of more than 4 blocks before onset of claudication

Grade 3 Ambulatory for a distance of less than 4 blocks

Grade 4 Nonambulatory because of ischemic pain at rest

---

no functional limits, and grade 4 patients are non-ambulatory because of ischemic pain at rest.[97] For patients in grades 1, 2, and, occasionally, 3 a therapeutic walking exercise program that involves walking continuously to the point of mild to moderate pain is frequently prescribed. Rest periods are then provided until the pain subsides. Repeated walk-rest sessions are performed to the patient's level of tolerance for 20 to 30 minutes, and such therapy has proved beneficial.[6,87] The primary benefit appears to be improved muscular efficiency, probably the result of enhanced energy-producing systems (aerobic and anaerobic), and possible collateralization to the ischemic muscles.[6,87] However, the latter has not been observed in humans, and a recent study[53] suggested that an observed increase in total walking distance was not due to increased common femoral artery blood flow. This conclusion was based on insignificant increases in common femoral artery blood flow measurements obtained 3 months after an exercise training program.[53] However, these findings must be cautiously interpreted, since the changes resulting from exercise training may occur more distally in the peripheral arterial tree and because 7 of the 10 persons studied continued to smoke.[53]

Patients with grades 3 and 4 peripheral vascular disease may benefit from *properly* prescribed exercise. Often these patients have had aortofemoral bypass graft surgery, after which exercise is crucial. Therefore the use of electrical stimulation, Jobst garments, and cautiously prescribed exercise (gentle, active, and active-assisted range of motion) *before* and *after* such surgery may be indicated for selected patients. Such a prescription may condition skeletal muscles and improve blood flow through the peripheral vessels during minimal to moderate muscle contraction (thus improving the pumping action).[82] Also of prime importance is the cessation of smoking (as was evident in the previously cited study[53]).

The treatment of peripheral vascular disease is an important and a necessary therapy, since intermittent claudication has been recognized as an independent risk factor for increased mortality and since the treatment and assessment of peripheral vascular disease have benefited from a new enthusiasm.[41,90] A significant aspect of this renewed interest is the development of changing perspectives on the vascular component of heart disease that can be simply and effectively evaluated.[69,78] The evaluation should include not only the physician's assessment but also the patient's interpretation of his or her condition, which has been shown to be extremely helpful in cardiovascular risk assessment and screening programs.[90]

Diabetes Mellitus

Screening of patients for peripheral vascular disease involves the assessment of diabetes mellitus, which can potentially alter cardiovascular performance substantially. Not only does diabetes mellitus affect the peripheral vasculature (as was previously implied), but also it appears to be related to a specific type of cardiac muscle dysfunction.[52,98] In fact, the term *diabetic cardiomyopathy* has been used in the literature and refers to many of the pathophysiologic processes of a cardiomyopathy that eventually leads to congestive heart failure.

Diabetes mellitus is also associated with an autonomic nervous system dysfunction,[74] which can impair much of the sympathetic nervous system information that is so important for the maintenance of proper cardiopulmonary function (that is, increased heart rate, blood pressure, and respiratory rate). Thus patients with diabetes mellitus may have inappropriate exercise responses not only because of a "diabetic cardiomyopathy" but also because of impaired autonomic nervous system activity.[74] The resultant heart rate and blood pressure, as well as central adaptations to exercise (that is, force of myocardial contraction to increase stroke volume and cardiac output) may be less than expected and may lead to potentially dangerous and even fatal situations.

Cardiac Surgery and Procedures

Although cardiac performance is frequently improved because of surgical procedures, many deleterious effects result from any cardiovascular procedure. These include "organ and subsystem dysfunction,"[60] abnormal bleeding, inflammatory reactions, renal dysfunction, hemodynamic and metabolic problems (resulting from peripheral and possibly central vasoconstriction), breakdown of red blood cells, and increased susceptibility to infection.[60]

The following quote clarifies the effects that such "dysfunction" could have on patient response to exercise (especially in the early treatment of patients immediately after cardiovascular surgical procedures): "The fact that most patients convalesce normally after cardiopulmonary bypass attests only to patients' abilities to compensate for these damaging effects and not to their absence."[60]

In view of clinical experience patients *without* additional disease processes appear to convalesce normally, adapting to the previously mentioned abnormalities. However, patients *with* other disease processes appear to convalesce poorly and are often unable to adequately adapt to the damaging effects of cardiovascular surgical procedures (primarily those involving cardiopulmonary bypass surgery).[60] Although relatively few patients have complications resulting from surgical intervention, it is important to be aware of the complications and risk factors of surgery and the interrelationships of additional disease processes. Therefore a complete and thorough chart review is essential in better understanding the physiologic responses of patients to prescribed exercise.

Several important risk factors for complications after cardiovascular surgical procedures have been identified in association with what some call the "postpump syndrome,"[60] including the following:

1. Duration of cardiopulmonary bypass surgery (if longer than 90 to 120 minutes for young infants or 150 minutes for adults)
2. Patient age
3. Presence of cyanosis after surgery
4. Perfusion flow rate
5. Composition of the perfusate
6. Oxygenating surface
7. Patient temperature during the perfusion

EXERCISE TRAINING
Effects of Exercise Training in the Absence of Cardiovascular Disease

Since the fundamentals of exercise training in individuals without cardiovascular disease have previously been presented, only a few aspects are discussed in this section. The most recent general exercise training guidelines presented by the American College of Sports Medicine (ACSM), suggest that the duration, frequency, and intensity of exercise be implemented in a specific manner depending on patient status (symptomatic or nonsymptomatic) and level of fitness (initial, improvement, or maintenance stage).[2] Past and recent investigations fully support these guidelines,[79,80] and Blair et al.[9] have shown that for sedentary patients, as little as 10 or 15 minutes of exercise performed three times a week at a low intensity (40% to 50%) produces many beneficial effects (increased physical work capacity, weight loss, decreased resting and exercise heart rates, and the like). The benefits may not be as great for active or trained individuals and, paraphrasing the words of Davies, exercise response and benefit depend on the initial level of cardiorespiratory fitness.[27]

Because exercise response and benefit depend on the initial level of fitness, the use of steady-state exercise to assess the exercise performance of elite athletes and individuals with heart disease may be somewhat limiting. The principle of steady-state exercise "denotes a work situation where oxygen uptake equals the oxygen requirement of the tissues; consequently, there is no accumulation of lactic acid in the body."[5] At such times the heart rate and stroke volume (thus the cardiac output), as well as pulmonary ventilation, have adapted to the gentler *steady states* of exercise. Therefore during steady-state exercise the efficiency of the exercise performed can be assessed. The clinical application of such testing is questionable however, (1) since the threshold for non–steady-state exercise has been hypothesized to be at approximately 50% of an individual's Vo_2 max (2) since exercise or work performed for a prolonged period, such as during *a whole working day,* may have a non–steady-state threshold of less than 50% of Vo_2max (as suggested by Astrand and Rodahl[5]); and (3) since athletes and laborers often work at exercise levels greater than or equal to 50% of Vo_2max.[5] Thus the clinical application of data obtained during steady-state exercise appears to be both variable and nonrepresentative of functional activities in athletes and laborers, and possibly even in patients with cardiovascular disease. The effects of such exercise and exercise testing must be further investigated because of the preceding considerations and because levels of exercise greater than or equal to 50% of Vo_2max appear to increase the concentration of lactic acid in the blood, which decreases the body's pH and affects muscular tissue, respiration, and other functions.[5] This information is probably most important in the clinical assessment of patient response to physical work. However, the efficiency of exercise in healthy individuals at levels lower or higher than 50% of Vo_2max may be more representative of functional capacity than similar levels of exercise in patients with cardiac disease or well-trained athletes.

In view of the preceding observations steady-state exercise testing may limit the assessment of total exercise or work performance, since the anaerobic bodily processes (utilized at greater levels of exercise requiring increased power) are frequently not evaluated (except when prolonged work or exercise is performed). This limitation is unfortunate, since elite athletes significantly depend on anaerobic processes to win events. Likewise, patients with cardiovascular disease also depend on anaerobic processes, since patients with congestive heart failure and peripheral vascular disease function at exercise levels that are accompanied by increased levels of lactic acid.[65] There-

fore the assessment of steady-state exercise and the efficiency of specific types of exercise in patients with cardiovascular disease is difficult when the purest definition of steady-state exercise is used.

Although the level of Vo_2max can be obtained during "nonmaximal" steady-state exercise, a *thorough and necessary* assessment of an individual's physiologic response to increasing work loads can probably provide more objective information concerning the following:

1. Heart rate
2. Blood pressure
3. Rate-pressure product
4. Duration necessary to attain the Vo_2max
5. Maximal work load at Vo_2max
6. Ratio of maximal work load to Vo_2max
7. Identification of the anaerobic threshold
8. Magnitude of the aerobic to anaerobic contributions in performing physical work and exercise
9. Amount of time necessary for recovery of heart rate, blood pressure, and other cardiopulmonary variables (i.e., respiratory rate)
10. Safety of exercise or work for specific patients

Maximal incremental exercise testing before and after an exercise training program (from days to months in duration) can be incorporated into clinical patient treatment sessions and can be used to plot patient progress or deterioration.

Elite Training

The "cardiac fatigue" previously discussed and its implications for exercise training are areas of concern. It appears that although cardiac fatigue may exist in healthy individuals participating in prolonged exercise, the effects are not long-lasting. In fact, beneficial effects of cardiac training were observed 24 hours after the Ironman Triathlon, since the mean stroke volume was increased by 4%.[30]

The effect of sleep deprivation or prolonged exercise, or both, on cardiopulmonary performance in highly trained athletes is an area of concern. Many elite athletes are strict disciples of heart rate monitoring. In view of our findings that exercise heart rates decreased during prolonged bicycling (either because of a training effect or because of sleep deprivation), we have discouraged the role of the target heart rate and heart rate monitoring in ultramarathon athletes participating in prolonged exercise (more than 2 or 3 days in duration). Attempts by ultramarathon bicyclists to maintain target heart rates have frequently been unsuccessful and in some instances have been debilitating. Although the mechanism of heart rate reduction in training and the altered heart rates observed in many disease states are poorly understood, the heart rate is a relatively good indicator of physiologic stress in healthy individuals. However, in highly trained individuals and in persons with disease it may not be as good of an indicator. These individuals may benefit from other measurements used to determine exercise intensity, such as the respiratory rate, rating of perceived exertion, or level of dyspnea. Individuals with cardiovascular disease may find greater benefit in using one (or a combination) of these variables, since heart rate changes may be less apparent in such patients and the work they perform (frequently assessed by radial or carotid pulse monitoring) may be inaccurately measured.

Effects of Exercise Training in Patients with Cardiovascular Disease

The previous discussion has briefly reviewed the heart rate–exercise relationship, which may be abnormal in patients with cardiovascular disease. Methods other than heart rate monitoring (target heart rate) during exercise training in patients with heart disease have been used and appear to be useful measures of exercise or work performance. For example, patients with congestive heart failure have benefited from the investigation of dyspnea indices during progressive exercise testing and training.[89]

In addition, thorough assessment of selected patients via ECG monitoring and occasional echocardiographic evaluation can identify those likely to have a detrimental response to exercise training. This recommendation is made in view of studies conducted by Arvan[4] and Jugdutt et al.[55] Arvan observed that to obtain training effects, patients with left ventricular dysfunction (mean ejection fraction of 24%) must *not* demonstrate signs of myocardial ischemia (on ECG). In a study with a similar focus Jugdutt evaluated which patients with left ventricular dysfunction would benefit most from exercise training and discovered that if left ventricular function were below a specific echocardiographic index of contractility, left ventricular function (that is, the ejection fraction) deteriorated, as did functional capacity. These two studies demonstrated the important role of cautious, gradual exercise progression, which should be thoroughly monitored and individually prescribed, keeping the exercise stimulus (intensity, frequency, duration, and mode of exercise) in proper perspective for each individual patient. Fig. 7–6 portrays a method of training to which patients appear to adhere without complication.

According to the American College of Physicians,[1] thorough cardiopulmonary assessment is necessary for patients with any of the following:

1. Severely depressed left ventricular function (ejection fraction of less than 30%)
2. Resting complex ventricular arrhythmias (Lown type IV or V)
3. Ventricular arrhythmias appearing or increasing with exercise
4. Decrease in systolic blood pressure of 15 mm Hg or more with exercise
5. Recent myocardial infarction (within the preceding 6 months) complicated by serious ventricular arrhythmias
6. Marked exercise-induced ischemia, as indicated either by anginal pain or by an ST depression of 2 mm or more on ECG
7. Survival of sudden cardiac arrest.

CLINICAL APPLICATION OF METABOLIC EQUIVALENTS

It is important to discuss the application of metabolic equivalents of oxygen consumption (METS) in view of the previously mentioned recommendations for proper exercise prescription and the earlier discussion of the benefits of exercise training

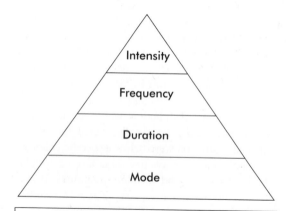

Fundamentals of exercise training

The pyramidal structure of exercise training is important in ensuring safe, effective exercise (beginning with the appropriate mode of exercise and progressing to the proper prescription of exercise duration, frequency, and intensity as dictated by patient response). Increasing the duration of exercise to an adequate level (to meet the patient's needs) before increasing the intensity of exercise helps to enhance patient compliance and decrease cardiopulmonary and musculoskeletal complications.

Fig. 7-6 Schema of multiple factors addressed to ensure patient compliance with exercise training.

for patients with cardiovascular disease, since "patients with cardiac disease with significant limitation of maximal work capacity, for example, less than 7 METS soon after an infarction, may expect to achieve meaningful improvement in work capacity by participating in an exercise training program."[1] The reference to "less than 7 METS" is interesting, since attainment of this level represents a moderately well-conditioned individual who is capable of completing the second stage of the Bruce protocol. It appears that the 7-METS threshold was chosen arbitrarily and conflicts with the observation of a 4-METS level threshold for determining patient deterioration or improvement during exercise testing and train-

ing.[48] In addition, the clinical application of METS for patients with cardiovascular disease seems unfair, since commonly used METS have been obtained from healthy individuals. For these reasons the use of METS in exercise prescription is questionable, and METS may be more appropriately used as a method to assess and compare exercise performance. The metabolic exercise performance of healthy persons and patients with disease can be compared and levels of impairment identified in a manner similar to that for the Bruce nomogram. For example, a patient could be identified as achieving perhaps 80% of the METS level of a healthy individual. In this way METS may have a more meaningful application than at present.

It is also important to mention that METS in patients with cardiopulmonary disease are presently being gathered and are likely to provide a more precise estimate of the metabolic cost of specific exercise and work in persons with cardiovascular and pulmonary complications.[96] However, the use of METS for exercise prescription may remain less patient-specific in view of the more individualized practice of exercise prescription via measures of oxygen consumption, heart rate, respiratory rate, oxygen saturation, work load, and, possibly, ratings of perceived exertion, all of which are obtained from *specific* individual patient assessment and allow for *individualized* exercise prescription. This method of exercise assessment and prescription was suggested as early as 1971[26] and established the need for *individualized* patient assessment and exercise prescription.[39]

RATINGS OF PERCEIVED EXERTION

Ratings of perceived exertion deserve a brief review because of their widespread use. The subjective sensation of physical exertion and the numbering from 6 to 20 or from 0 to 10 may seem peculiar, but the purpose of the ratings was to correlate heart rate with specific numbers that represented a patient's sensation of physical exertion. For example, to the number 9 was ascribed the sensation of "very light exertion," and the number

CASE STUDY 1

Mr. L. P. is a 58-year-old man who recently had coronary artery bypass graft surgery. The surgery was performed because of unstable angina and multivessel coronary artery disease (70% to 90% blockage of the left anterior descending artery, right coronary artery, and circumflex and diagonal arteries) that was unresponsive to medical management (β blockade, calcium-channel blockade, and nitrates). The surgery was uncomplicated and consisted of the left internal mammary artery being grafted to the left anterior descending artery and three saphenous vein grafts to the right coronary artery, circumflex artery, and a large diagonal artery off the circumflex artery. Days 1 and 2 after surgery were also uncomplicated, and the patient began gaining independence in functional activities of daily living.

However, on the third day after surgery the patient passed out and collapsed while changing from a sitting to a standing position. Fortunately the only injuries he sustained were slight abrasions on his forehead and left elbow. The patient was evaluated during gradual progressive exercise. During the assessment the patient was observed to be moderately agitated and to have a rapid respiratory rate (38 breaths per minute), pericardial friction rub, and distant heart sounds. The patient also demonstrated a pulsus paradoxis (a marked reduction in systolic blood pressure, usually of 20 mm Hg or more, and in strength of the arterial pulse during *inspiration*) and a dramatic decrease in systolic blood pressure when changing position from sitting to standing (from 140/80 to 100/70 mm Hg), at which time the patient complained of moderate dizziness.

In view of the preceding observations the patient was returned to a sitting position and instructed to perform active lower-extremity exercise (bilateral ankle pumping and knee flexion-extension) in an attempt to increase the systolic blood pressure. Although the patient actively performed these exercises, it took approximately 5 minutes for the dizziness and blood pressure to improve.

The following day the patient's blood pressure during positional change was slightly improved, but during ambulation of approximately 5 feet the patient's systolic blood pressure decreased from a standing value of 110/70 to 70/50 mm Hg. At that time the patient complained of moderate to severe dizziness and was observed to be very short of breath (respiratory rate of 46 breaths per minute). The patient was returned to his bed and placed in a semisupine position, where his status slowly improved but a pronounced pulsus paradoxus persisted.

The results of the repeated assessments and treatment were discussed with the patient's primary physician, who ordered a stat chest radiograph and an echocardiogram, both of which revealed a moderate to severe pericardial effusion with cardiac compression (cardiac tamponade). Compression on the heart from increased fluid in the pericardial sac (pericarditis secondary to bypass graft surgery) prevented adequate filling of the left ventricle. This limited the amount of blood in the left ventricle and the stretch imposed on it, limiting the beneficial effects of Starling's law. As a result the patient's cardiac output and stroke volume were markedly reduced, and the reductions were accentuated during positional change or minimal bouts of exercise. The patient was immediately started on a regimen of prednisone, and exercise was carefully and gradually initiated in the sitting and semisupine positions. The patient responded well, and exercise was progressed after the signs and symptoms of cardiac tamponade were reduced.

Important points

1. Surgical intervention can improve cardiac function, but unwanted adverse effects can occasionally occur, such as cardiac tamponade resulting from pericarditis.
2. Compression on the heart caused by an inflamed, heavy pericardial sac prevented adequate filling of the left ventricle, which

---

CASE STUDY 1 — cont'd

subsequently reduced the stroke volume and cardiac output and produced a hypoadaptive systolic blood pressure response to exercise.

3. The pulsus paradoxis was the result of an exaggerated increase in right ventricular dimension (caused by increased venous return) that displaced the interventricular septum *into* the left ventricle. This decreased the amount of blood able to fill the left ventricle and the amount of blood ejected from it.

4. Objective assessment of the patient's signs and symptoms identified pathophysiologic processes on day 1 of treatment, thus exemplifying the importance of an objective cardiopulmonary assessment.

Table 7-3 Borg linear and ratio scales for perceived exertion

Linear scale (related to heart rate and Vo_2 responses to aerobic exercise)		Ratio scale (related to effort during anaerobic exercise)	
Valve	**Description**	**Valve**	**Description**
6	No exertion at all	0	Nothing at all
7		0.5	Extremely weak (just noticeable)
	Extremely light		
8		1	Very weak
9	Very light	2	Weak (light)
10		3	Moderate
11	Light	4	Somewhat strong
12		5	Strong (heavy)
13	Somewhat hard	6	
14		7	Very strong
15	Hard (heavy)	8	
16		9	
17	Very hard	10	Extremely strong (almost maximal)
18			
19	Extremely hard		
20	Maximal exertion	—	Maximal

9 was originally correlated with a heart rate of 90 beats per minute (Table 7–3). Each consecutive number from 6 to 20 therefore represents a specific heart rate. The heart rates obtained by Borg and Ottoson[11] (from healthy, middle-aged, male participants) correlated well with the numbering scale.

Although the rating system correlated highly with the heart rates of Borg's initial study participants, several subsequent investigations have found much lower correlation coefficients and have questioned the use of the Borg scale for other types of patients.[11] Despite this major problem, *the Borg rating system does allow a subjective (and possibly objective) assessment of physical exertion that also provides important information about an individual's performance of exercise or work.*

Thirty-two-year-old SN has been an ultramarathon bicyclist for 10 years. She has no significant medical history except for a grade 1-2/5 midsystolic murmur that is due to mild regurgitant blood flow into the left atrium during systole, which is characteristic of mitral insufficiency. She has completed four separate 10- to 12-day transcontinental crossings on a bicycle. During the last crossing, the 1989 Race Across America (RAAM), extensive medical testing was performed. Exercise tests were administered before and immediately after RAAM and during the post-RAAM test, and a reduction in exercise heart rates during most work loads was observed (Fig. 7-7). In addition, the post-RAAM maximal heart rate and maximal work load were decreased (by 9% and 26%, respectively), and the blood pressure measurements were blunted.

The preceding responses were surprising, not only because the woman had bicycled across the United States in 10 days (sleeping only 2 to 4 hours per night), but also because midway through RAAM she demonstrated signs and symptoms suggestive of congestiveheart failure. The woman had gained 16 pounds (7.3 kg), complained of moderate to severe dyspnea and fatigue, andwas observed to have a rapid resting respiratory rate (34 breaths per minute), a 3+

level of pitting edema, and fine crackles in the lower lobes bilaterally.

The athlete's primary physician was contacted, and administration of a diuretic was started, which quickly improved her status and allowed her to win the women's division of the RAAM. Echocardiography could not be performed at the end of the 1989 RAAM, and although marked "cardiac fatigue" has not been observed in other ultramarathon bicyclists, the signs and symptoms of the woman in Case Study 2 certainly suggest that "cardiac fatigue" and cardiac muscle dysfunction (CMD) occurred. Further research in this area is needed.

Important points

1. Many athletes appear to have heart murmurs, possibly resulting from valvular insufficiency caused by left ventricular hypertrophy.
2. The exercise tests before and after RAAM are analogous to the tests before and after treatment that are used in clinical patient care.
3. Ultramarathon bicycling appears to be associated with a reduction in cardiopulmonary function.
4. Specific signs and symptoms can identify congestive heart failure.
5. "Cardiac fatigue" and CMD may occur during prolonged physical exertion.

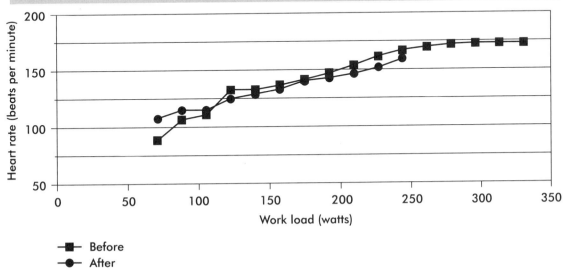

Fig. 7-7 Effects of exercise testing on one athlete's heart rate response before and after the Race Across America. Heart rate response at any given work load was usually lower after completion of the event.

CASE STUDY 3

Mr. L. B. is an 84-year-old man with a 38-year history of diabetes mellitus. He also had a large anterior myocardial infarction 3 years ago, approximately 6 months after an above-knee amputation was performed for severe peripheral vascular disease. The patient convalesced slowly after the myocardial infarction and since then has had a rapid, shallow breathing pattern. This breathing pattern was observed during the initial *physical therapy home visit* and subsequent physical examination revealed moderate crackles in the lower lobes bilaterally with a resting respiratory rate of 34 breaths per minute. In addition, the patient's resting heart rate and blood pressure were 82 beats per minute and 140/80 mm Hg, respectively. Attempts were made to put on the patient's prosthetic leg but were discontinued after the patient's respiratory rate and blood pressure increased to 44 breaths per minute and 208/90 mm Hg, respectively. Mr. L. B. also complained of extreme fatigue, and for all these reasons physical therapy was discontinued on that day.

Consultation with the patient's primary physician resulted in a medication change to better treat the patient's chronic congestive heart failure (which was not documented in the physical therapy referral) and increased knowledge of the patient and his condition. Mr. L. B. gradually progressed from minimal active upper- and lower-extremity exercise to independent donning of his prosthesis. Other functional activities and short ambulation distances were initiated, which the patient tolerated well and independently assessed by using the Borg scale of perceived exertion (6 to 20).

However, the increased blood pressure response that was previously observed during prosthetic donning continued. Frequently blood pressure readings of 200/94 mm Hg were obtained during ambulation or functional activities, whereas the heart rate remained relatively unchanged at 84 beats per minute. The patient was *not* taking a β blocker and therefore probably had an autonomic nervous system dysfunc-

tion because of the diabetes mellitus. Nonetheless, blood pressure measurements did increase significantly, probably because of an imbalance of the necessary vasoconstriction and vasodilation in skeletal musculature. Reduced muscle mass in the left leg (because of the amputation) and an abnormal vasodilation and constriction of the skeletal muscles probably contributed to the high blood pressure response during minimal physical exertion. In addition, Mr. L. B.'s ambulation consisted of both a dynamic and a strong static component. During ambulation a great deal of cocontracture was necessary to stabilize the torso, trunk, and lower extremities. The specific static components consisted of maximal hand grip on the walker and rigid bilateral arm support, as well as rigid stabilization of the lower extremities during prosthetic gait training. The inefficient gait and the pathophysiologic processes of diabetes and heart disease (with congestive heart failure) produced the described cardiopulmonary responses.

Important points

1. In the growing practice of home health care cardiopulmonary assessments and prescribed treatments are necessary.
2. Chronic congestive heart failure can occur and most likely represents ineffective cardiac performance resulting from systolic or diastolic dysfunction.
3. Exercise prescription must be based on cardiopulmonary response to exercise, which is determined by means of appropriate methods of assessment (such as respiratory rate and Borg ratings of perceived exertion).
4. Diabetes mellitus may produce an autonomic nervous system dysfunction that apparently can impair cardiovascular performance (that is, unchanged heart rate with exercise and proper vasodilation and vasoconstriction of skeletal musculature).
5. The redistribution of available blood volume during various types of physical activity (static and dynamic) dictates the cardiopulmonary response.

A later scale from 1 to 10 was also developed by Borg (Table 7-3). Whatever method is used, *it is important that all individuals be educated in the proper use of either of the Borg scales so that ratings are valid and reliable. These scales are likely to provide an additional tool to better assess physical response to exercise. Of course, individuals interpret pain and discomfort in different ways, but attempts to objectively interpret a subjective variable should be encouraged and further researched.*

SUMMARY

Many aspects of cardiovascular and pulmonary rehabilitation are in evolutionary stages and are in critical need of clinical investigation based on cardiopulmonary assessment of patient performance. "Recent advances in technology and medical therapy have demonstrated other indications for routine cardiovascular assessments, including but not limited to the prevalence of silent ischemia in patients with coronary artery disease, potential need for percutaneous transluminal coronary angioplasty soon after an acute myocardial infarction, continued evidence supporting atherosclerotic regression, evaluating and reprogramming pacemakers, mild to moderate congestive heart failure, poor left ventricular function, and heart transplantation. Such treatment provides primary physicians with information necessary for the management of their patients. . . ."[18] Through such individualized assessment and treatment high-risk and low-risk patients alike will receive quality patient care.

The effects of exercise on cardiac performance are substantial. Physical performance depends on proper cardiopulmonary function, which can be assessed by evaluating symptoms, heart rate, blood pressure, and respiratory rate and by analyzing other respiratory measurements (such as oxygen consumption, oxygen saturation, and anaerobic threshold). Evaluation of other cardiopulmonary variables such as the ECG, rate-pressure product, tension-time index, stroke volume, cardiac output, and left ventricular end-diastolic pressure can enhance the assessment and interpretation of exercise performance. In addition, these variables provide

---

CLINICAL VARIABLES COMMONLY USED TO ASSESS PHYSICAL EXERCISE AND CARDIAC PERFORMANCE

Symptoms (ratings of perceived exertion and level of dyspnea)
Electrocardiogram
Ventilatory rate
Auscultation of the heart and lungs
Heart rate
Blood pressure
Rate-pressure product (heart rate × blood pressure)
Tension-time index (heart rate × blood pressure × QT interval)
Stroke volume
Cardiac output
Ejection fraction of left and right ventricles
Left ventricular end-systolic and end-diastolic volumes
Left ventricular end-systolic and end-diastolic pressures
Respiratory gas analysis (Vo_2max and anaerobic threshold)

---

important diagnostic and prognostic information that can be used to prescribe appropriate, effective treatment. Clinical variables that may be helpful in assessing exercise and cardiac performance are listed in the box on p. 153. These variables can provide diagnostic and prognostic information about cardiopulmonary function during physical exertion, or more specifically, the effects of exercise on cardiac performance. The case studies demonstrate how the clinical assessment of cardiopulmonary function and subsequent treatment prescribed in view of the cardiopulmonary response enhance exercise and cardiac performance.

REFERENCES

1. American College of Physicians Health and Public Policy Committee: Cardiac rehabilitation services, *Ann Intern Med* 1:671, 1988.
2. American College of Sports Medicine: *Guidelines for exercise testing and prescription,* ed 4, Philadelphia, 1991, Lea & Febiger.

3. Anderson RL et al: Effects of cardioselective and nonselective beta-adrenergic blockade on the performance of highly trained runners, *Am J Cardiol* 55:149D, 1985.

4. Arvan S: Exercise performance of the high risk acute myocardial infarction patients after cardiac rehabilitation, *Am J Cardiol* 62:197, 1988.

5. Astrand P, Rodahl K: *Textbook of work physiology: physiological bases of exercise,* New York, 1977, McGraw-Hill.

6. Barnard RJ, Hall JA: Patients with peripheral vascular disease. In Franklin BA, Gordon S, Timmis GC, editors: *Exercise in modern medicine,* Baltimore, 1989, Williams & Wilkins.

7. Beaver WL, Wasserman K, Whipp BJ: Improved detection of lactate threshold during exercise using a log-log transformation, *J Appl Physiol* 59:1936, 1985.

8. Blackburn H et al: Premature ventricular complexes induced by stress testing: their frequency and response to physical conditioning, *Am J Cardiol* 31:441, 1973.

9. Blair SN et al: Physical fitness and all-cause mortality: a prospective study of healthy men and women, *JAMA* 262:2395, 1989.

10. Bolli R, Triana F, Jeroudi MO: Postischemic mechanical and vascular dysfunction (myocardial "stunning" and microvascular "stunning") and the effects of calcium-channel blockers on ischemia-reperfusion injury, *Clin Cardiol* 12(3):16, 1989.

11. Borg G, Ottoson D: *The perception of exertion in physical work,* London, 1986, Macmillan.

12. Braunwald E: Assessment of cardiac function. In Braunwald E, editor: *Heart disease: a textbook of cardiovascular medicine,* vol 1, Philadelphia, 1988, WB Saunders.

13. Braunwald E: Clinical manifestations of heart failure. In Braunwald E, editor: *Heart disease: a textbook of cardiovascular medicine,* vol 1, Philadelphia, 1988, WB Saunders.

14. Braunwald E: Pathophysiology of heart failure. In Braunwald E, editor: *Heart disease: a textbook of cardiovascular medicine,* vol 1, Philadelphia, 1988, WB Saunders.

15. Bruce RA, Kusumi F, Hosmer D: Maximal oxygen intake and nomographic assessment of functional aerobic impairment in cardiovascular disease, *Am Heart J* 85:546, 1973.

16. Cahalin LP: Cardiovascular medications. In Mallone T, editor: *Physical and occupational therapy: drug implications for practice,* Philadelphia, 1989, JB Lippincott.

17. Cahalin LP: Cardiac muscle dysfunction. In Hillegass E, Sadowsky SH, editors: *Textbook of cardiopulmonary physical therapy,* Philadelphia, WB Saunders (in press).

18. Cahalin LP, Ice RG, Irwin S: Program planning and implementation. In Irwin S, Tecklin JS, editors: *Cardiopulmonary physical therapy,* St Louis, 1990, Mosby.

19. Cahalin LP et al: The effects of sleep deprivation and ultramarathon exercise upon exercise heart rates and oxygen consumption during the Race Across America, American Physical Therapy Association Annual Conference, 1990 (abstract).

20. Cahalin LP et al: Cardiac performance during ultramarathon bicycling, *Phys Ther* 71:527, 1991 (abstract).

21. Cahalin LP et al: Cardiovascular adaptations to ultramarathon bicycling. Proceedings of the American College of Sports Medicine Midwest Winter Meeting, Boyne Mountain, In, February 1991, p 18 (abstract).

22. Campeau L: Grading of angina pectoris, *Circulation* 54:522, 1975.

23. Cecil WT et al: A clinical evaluation of the accuracy of the Nellcor N-100 and Ohmeda 3700 pulse oximeters, *J Clin Monit* 4:31, 1988.

24. Chaitman BR et al: Coronary Artery Surgery Study: comparability of 10 year survival in randomized and randomizable patients, *J Am Coll Cardiol* 16:1071, 1990.

25. Clausen JP: Circulatory adjustment to dynamic exercise and effect of exercise training in normal subjects and patients with ischaemic heart disease, *Prog Cardiovasc Dis* 18:459, 1976.

26. Reference deleted in proofs.

27. Davies CTM, Knibbs AV: The training stimulus: the effects of intensity, duration, and frequency of effort on maximum aerobic power output, *Int Z Angew Physiol* 5:29, 1971.

28. Ding YA et al: Progression of cardiac hypertrophy during long-term calcium antagonist treatment with tiapamil, *J Hum Hypertension* 3:239, 1989.

29. Douglas PS, O'Toole ML, Woolard J: Regional wall motion abnormalities after prolonged exercise in the normal left ventricle, *Circulation* 82:2108, 1990.

30. Douglas PS et al: Different effects of prolonged exercise on the right and left ventricles, *J Am Coll Cardiol* 15:64, 1990.

31. Douglas PS et al: Determinants of reduced left ventricular function following prolonged exercise, *J Am Coll Cardiol* 17:353A, 1991 (abstract).

32. Duncan JJ et al: The effects of aerobic exercise on plasma catecholamines and blood pressure in patients with mild essential hypertension, *JAMA* 254:2609, 1985.

33. Ehsani AA: Mechanisms responsible for enhanced stroke volume after exercise training in coronary heart disease, *Eur Heart J* 8:9, 1987.

34. Ehsani AA et al: Cardiac effects of prolonged and intense exercise training in patients with coronary artery disease, *Am J Cardiol* 50:246, 1982.

35. Ehsani AA et al: Improvement in left ventricular contractile function by exercise training in patients with coronary artery disease, *Circulation* 74:350, 1986.

36. Ellestad MH: *Stress testing: principles and practice,* ed 2, Philadelphia, 1980, FA Davis.

37. Fagard R, van den Broeke C, Amery A: Left ventricular dynamics during exercise in elite marathon runners, *J Am Coll Cardiol* 14:112, 1989.

38. Fisman EZ et al: Altered left ventricular volume and ejection fraction responses to supine dynamic exercise in athletes, *J Am Coll Cardiol* 15:582, 1990.

39. Fox SM III, Naughton JP, Haskell WL: Physical activity and the prevention of coronary heart disease, *Ann Clin Res* 3:404, 1981.

40. Froelicher V et al: A randomized trial of exercise training in patients with coronary heart disease, *JAMA* 252:1291, 1984.

41. Frye RL: President's Page: role of the cardiologist in peripheral vascular disease, *J Am Coll Cardiol* 18:641, 1991.

42. Garber AV et al: The myocardial efficacy index: correlation with ejection fraction during exercise, *J Cardiac Rehabil* 3:857, 1983.

43. Goldman L et al: Comparative reproducibility and validity of systems for assessing cardiovascular functional class: advantages of a new specific activity scale, *Circulation* 64:1227, 1981.

44. Greenland P, Chu JS: Efficacy of cardiac rehabilitation services with emphasis on patients after myocardial infarction, *Ann Intern Med* 109:650, 1988.

45. Greer M, Dimick S, Burns S: Heart rate and blood pressure response to several methods of strength training, *Phys Ther* 64:179, 1984.

46. Guyton AC: The relationship of cardiac output and arterial pressure control, *Circulation* 64:1079, 1981.

47. Hagberg JM: Patients with end-stage renal disease. In Franklin BA, Gordon S, Timmis GC, editors: *Exercise in modern medicine,* Baltimore, 1989, Williams & Wilkins.

48. Hislop HJ et al: Exercise testing soon after myocardial infarction. Proceedings of the eleventh international congress of the World Confederation for Physical Therapy. II. London, 1991.

49. Holman BL: Nuclear cardiology. In Braunwald E, editor: *Heart disease: a textbook of cardiovascular medicine,* vol 1, Philadelphia, 1988, WB Saunders.

50. Hwang MH et al: Progression of native coronary artery disease at 10 years: insights from a randomized study of medical versus surgical therapy for angina, *J Am Coll Cardiol* 16:1066, 1990.

51. Jennings G et al: The effects of changes in physical activity on major cardiovascular risk factors, hemodynamics, sympathetic function, and glucose utilization in man: a controlled study of four levels of activity, *Circulation* 73:30, 1986.

52. Jermendy G et al: Left ventricular diastolic dysfunction in type 1 (insulin-dependent) diabetic patients during dynamic exercise, *Cardiology* 77:9, 1990.

53. Johnson EC et al: Effects of exercise training on common femoral artery blood flow in patients with intermittent claudication, *Circulation* 80(suppl 3):59, 1989.

54. Judge KW et al: Congestive heart failure symptoms in patients with preserved left ventricular systolic function: analysis of the CASS Registry, *J Am Coll Cardiol* 18:377, 1991.

55. Jugdutt BI et al: Exercise training after anterior Q wave myocardial infarction: importance of regional left ventricular function and topography, *J Am Coll Cardiol* 12:362, 1988.

56. Kamath MV, Fallen EL, McKelvie R: Effects of steady state exercise on the power spectrum of heart rate variability, *Med Sci Sports Exerc* 23:428, 1991.

57. Kannel WB, Belanger AJ: Epidemiology of heart failure, *Am Heart J* 121:951, 1991.

58. Karlsson J et al: Muscle metabolism, regulation of circulation and beta blockade, *J Cardiac Rehabil* 3:404, 1983.

59. Kettner A et al: Cardiovascular and metabolic responses to submaximal exercise in hemodialysis patients, *Kidney Int* 26:66, 1984.

60. Kirklin JW, Blackstone EH, Kirklin JK: Cardiac surgery. In Braunwald E, editor: Heart disease: a textbook of cardiovascular medicine, vol 2, Philadelphia, 1988, WBSaunders.

61. Kitamura K et al: Hemodynamic correlates of myocardial oxygen consumption during upright exercise, *J Appl Physiol* 32:516, 1972.

62. Kuipers H et al: Comparison of heart rate as a non-invasive determinant of anaerobic threshold with the lactate threshold when cycling, *Eur J Appl Physiol* 58:303, 1988.

63. Lipkin DP et al: Abnormalities of skeletal muscle in patients with chronic heart failure, *Int J Cardiol* 18:187, 1988.

64. Lund-Johansen P: Age hemodynamics and exercise in essential hypertension: difference between beta blockers and dihydropyridine calcium antagonists, *J Cardiovasc Pharmacol* 14(suppl 10):S7, 1989.

65. Mancini DM et al: Contribution of intrinsic skeletal muscle changes to ^{31}P NMR skeletal muscle metabolic abnormalities in patients with chronic heart failure, *Circulation* 80:1338, 1989.

66. Marsh RC et al: Attenuation of exercise conditioning by low-dose beta-adrenergic receptor blockade, *J Am Coll Cardiol* 2:551, 1983.

67. Martin DE, Benario HW, Gynn RWH: Development of the marathon from Pheidippides to the present: with statistics of significant races, *Ann N Y Acad Sci* 301:820, 1977.

68. Matsumura N et al: Determination of anaerobic threshold for assessment of functional state in patients with chronic heart failure, *Circulation* 68:360, 1983.

69. McCulloch Jr JM: Examination procedure for patients with vascular system problems, *Clin Management* 1:17, 1981.

70. McMeeken J et al: Effects of isokinetic assessment regimes on cardiovascular parameters. Proceedings of the eleventh international congress of the World Confederation for Physical Therapy. III. London, 1991.

71. National Heart, Lung, and Blood Institute Coronary Artery Surgery Study: American Heart Association Monograph, No 79, *Circulation* 63(2),1981.

72. New York Heart Association Criteria Committee: *Diseases of the heart and blood vessels: nomenclature and criteria for diagnosis,* ed 6, Boston, 1964, Little, Brown.

73. Obma RT et al: Effect of conditioning program in patients taking propranolol for angina pectoris, *Cardiology* 64:365, 1979.

74. Page M, Watkins PG: Cardiorespiratory arrest and diabetic autonomic neuropathy, *Lancet* 1:14, 1978.

75. Parisi AF et al: Medical compared with surgical management of unstable angina: five-year mortality and morbidity in the Veterans Administration study, *Circulation* 80:1176, 1989.

76. Pasternak RC, Braunwald E, Sobel BE: Acute myocardial infarction. In Braunwald E, editor: *Heart disease: a textbook of cardiovascular medicine,* vol 2, Philadelphia, 1988, WB Saunders.

77. Peduzzi P et al: Ten-year effect of medical and surgical therapy on quality of life: Veterans Administration Cooperative Study of Coronary Artery Surgery, *Am J Cardiol* 59:1017, 1987.

78. Peripheral vascular disease, *Circulation* 83(suppl):106, 1991.

79. Pollack ML: How much exercise is enough? *Phys Sports Med* 6:4, 1978.

80. Pollock ML et al: Effects of training two days per week at different intensities on middle-aged men, *Med Sci Sports* 4:192, 1972.

81. Pratt CM et al: Demonstration of training effect during chronic beta-adrenergic blockade in patients with coronary artery disease, *Circulation* 64:1125, 1981.

82. Reed BF: The peripheral vascular effects of electrical stimulation. In Currier DP, Nelson RM, editors: Excitable and connective tissue: recent advances and clinical concepts, Philadelphia, FA Davis (in press).

83. Richard CA et al: The nucleus reticularis gigantocellularis modulates the cardiopulmonary responses to central and peripheral drives related to exercise, *Brain Res* 483:49, 1989.

84. Sable DL et al: Attenuation of exercise conditioning by beta-adrenergic blockade, *Circulation* 65:679, 1982.

85. Saragoca MA et al: Pump performance after regression of cardiac hypertrophy following treatment of hypertension with isradipine, *J Hypertension* 7(suppl 6):S288, 1989.

86. Sarnoff SJ et al: Hemodynamic determinants of oxygen consumption of the heart with special reference to the tension-time index, *Am J Physiol* 192:148, 1958.

87. Scheel KW: The stimulus for coronary collateral growth: ischemia or mechanical factors? *J Cardiac Rehabil* 1:149, 1981.

88. Sheps DS et al: Exercise-induced increase in diastolic pressure: indicator of severe coronary artery disease, *Am J Cardiol* 43:708, 1979.

89. Simon PM et al: Distinguishable types of dyspnea in patients with shortness of breath, *Am Rev Respir Dis* 142:1009, 1990.

90. Smith GD, Shipley MJ, Rose G: Intermittent claudication, heart disease risk factors, and mortality: the Whilehall Study, *Circulation* 82:1925, 1990.

91. Tyler HR: Neurological aspects of dialysis patients. In Drukker W, Parsons FM, Maher JF, editors: *Replacement of renal function by dialysis,* The Hague, 1978, Martinus Nijhoff.

92. Urata H et al: Antihypertensive and volume-depleting effects of mild exercise on essential hypertension, *Hypertension* 9:245, 1987.

93. Vanhees J, Eagard R, Amery A: Influence of beta-adrenergic blockade on effects of physical training in patients with ischaemic heart disease, *Br Heart J* 48:33, 1982.

94. Wasserman K, Whipp BJ: Exercise physiology in health and disease, *Am Rev Respir Dis* 112:219, 1975.

95. Wasserman K et al: Principles of exercise testing and interpretation, Philadelphia, 1987, Lea & Febiger.

96. Wilke NA: Letter from Wilke NA, OTR, Clement J Zablocki Medical Center, Veterans Administration, Milwaukee, Wisconsin, to Truman Wilkin, LPT, St Luke's Hospital, Cedar Rapids, IA Sept 1989.

97. Winsor T, Hyman C: *A primer of peripheral vascular diseases,* Philadelphia, 1965, Lea & Febiger.

98. Zarich SW, Nesto RW: Diabetic cardiomyopathy, *Am Heart J* 118:1000, 1989.

99. Zetterquist S: The effect of active training on the nutritive blood flow in exercising ischemic legs, *Scand J Clin Lab Invest* 25:101, 1970.

STUDY QUESTIONS

■ Describe the causes of and risk factors for cardiovascular disease.

■ Describe the differences in the origin of myocardial infarction, congestive heart failure, and peripheral vascular disease.

■ Describe exercise tolerance and the effects of exercise training in patients with myocardial infarction, peripheral vascular disease, and congestive heart failure.

■ Describe the effect of exercise training on plasma lipids, blood pressure and cardiac output in patients with cardiovascular disease.

PART IV

EXERCISE AND THE MUSCULOSKELETAL AND NEUROMUSCULAR SYSTEMS

■ **KEEP IN MIND WHILE YOU READ** . . . *Jay Williams and Lewis Nashner, in Chapters 8 and 10, respectively, describe the musculoskeletal and neuromuscular cellular anatomy and physiology for healthy individuals. In Chapter 9 Scott Hasson describes how progressive and degenerative neuromuscular diseases affect function and the impact of exercise training on these conditions. In addition, factors that affect muscle mass are described, and the effect of exercise training is explored for patients who are traditionally weak and highly detrained. In Chapter 10 Lewis Nashner reviews neuromuscular aspects of normal posture and movement. Balance training and evaluation are explored in depth. Balance training as a form of exercise training is described, and its effect on various patients is discussed. Assessment of functional outcome by means of posturography is one future evaluation tool that is gaining popularity. Balance exercise training is becoming incorporated within many clinical and hospital settings. Please focus on indications and contraindications for exercise training.* ■

CHAPTER 8

NORMAL MUSCULOSKELETAL AND NEUROMUSCULAR ANATOMY, PHYSIOLOGY, AND RESPONSES TO TRAINING

Jay H. Williams

Skeletal muscles are responsible for performing movements as precise and delicate as positioning of the eye or as forceful as those of a weight lifter lifting a massive weight. The force-producing tissue makes up approximately 40% to 45% of the body's weight in men and about 23% to 25% of the weight in women.[15,21] The functions of skeletal muscle are manifold and include production of locomotion, postural support, maintenance of body temperature by means of shivering, and assisting the return of venous blood to the heart by means of vascular compression. The most obvious and possibly the most important of these functions is the ability of skeletal muscle to support movement of the limbs. In mass, muscle is the most abundant tissue in the body, and in function it is one of the most important; thus a thorough understanding of its structure and function is essential for researcher and clinician alike. The purpose of this chapter is to examine both the structure and the function of skeletal muscle.

ANATOMY OF MUSCLE

Skeletal muscle is composed of several types of tissues, including neural, vascular, and connective tissue and the muscle cells themselves. To control contractions of individual muscle cells or muscle fibers, each is innervated by a motor neuron. Similarly, to ensure an adequate supply of nutrients and an adequate means of waste removal, each fiber is innervated by arterial and venous blood supplies.

Connective Tissue

Connective tissue is an important structural and mechanical constituent of skeletal muscle. Each whole muscle is attached to the skeleton by tough connective tissue called *tendons*. In general a proximal tendon attaches one end of the muscle to a stationary bone (*origin*), the other end is attached to a bone that is freely moved during contraction (*insertion*) via a distal tendon.

Fig. 8-1 shows the relationships of the various connective tissues within a whole muscle. Individual

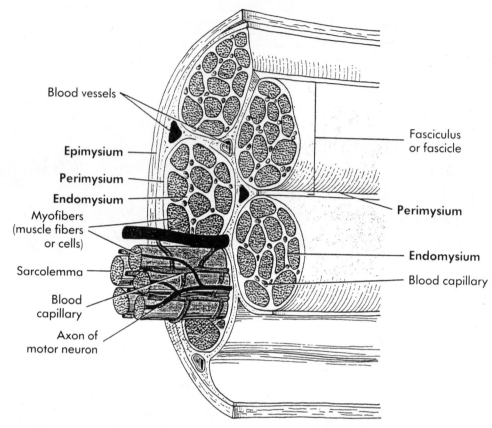

Fig. 8-1 Relationships of connective tissue within skeletal muscle, indicating the relative positions of the epimysium, perimysium, and endomysium. (From Tortora GJ, Anagnostakos NP: *Principles of anatomy and physiology,* New York, 1990, Harper & Row.)

muscles are separated and held in place by *fascial sheaths*. Each whole skeletal muscle is surrounded by a sheath of connective tissue called the *epimysium*. The epimysium is actually located between the fascial sheath and the muscle itself. Located within the whole muscle are a number of muscle fiber bundles called *fasciculi*. Each fascicle is surrounded by a layer of connective tissue called the *perimysium*. Within each fascicle are individual muscle fibers that are surrounded by connective tissue called *endomysium*.

Muscle Fiber Structure

Individual muscle fibers or muscle cells are cylindric, ranging from 10 to 60 μm in diameter and from 1 to 400 mm in length. The membrane that encases the muscle fiber is the *sarcolemma* (Fig. 8-2). This membrane lies directly underneath the endomysium. Because the sarcolemma is a plasma membrane, it provides active and selective transport of ions and nutrients. It is also an excitable membrane, possessing a resting potential of about -70 mV. The fluid encased by the sarcolemma is called the *myoplasm* or *sarcoplasm*, which contains fuel sources (such as lipids, glycogen, phosphagen, and adenosine triphosphate [ATP]), various ions (for example, potassium and magnesium), and several enzymes (such as myosin adenosine triphosphatase [M-ATPase] and phosphorylase). Despite the unique shape of muscle fibers, many of the same organelles that are found in other cells are also found in muscle cells. These include mitochondria, nuclei, and lysozomes. Unlike most other cells in the body, however, skeletal muscle cells are multinucleated, that is, they possess more than one nucleus. This structure appears to be necessary for the high rate of protein synthesis required by the muscle cell.

In addition to the sarcolemma, two other membrane systems are important contributors to the functional abilities of skeletal muscle. A membranous structure known as the *transverse tubule* (T tubule) runs perpendicular to the long axis of the fiber. The T-tubule network is also continuous with the sarcolemma and provides a means by which the extracellular fluid can be in close proximity to the interior of the fiber. Also located in the fiber's intracellular space is a membrane structure known as the *sarcoplasmic reticulum*, which runs mostly parallel to the long axis of the fiber. The middle portion of the sarcoplasmic reticulum is known as the *longitudinal* sarcoplasmic reticulum; the ends are known as the *terminal cisternae*. The primary function of the sarcoplasmic reticulum is to regulate the intracellular concentration of calcium ions (Ca^{2+}), an important role in the contractile process. The sarcoplasmic reticulum spans the space between adjacent T tubules. It comes into close contact with the T tubules, although the physical connection between the two membranes is not well understood. The junction between the T tubule and the sarcoplasmic reticulum terminal cisternae located on either side is known as the *triad*.

From a mechanical viewpoint the most important component of the sarcoplasm is the contractile apparatus, which is made up of bundles of *myofilaments* arranged into *myofibrils*. These myofibrils run the entire length of the muscle fiber, hence the entire length of the muscle. One of the most striking features of the skeletal muscle myofibril is the microscopic appearance of striations. These striations are produced by repeating light and dark bands (Fig. 8-2). The dark bands, known as the *A bands*, are anisotropic to, or do not pass, polarized light. The *I bands*, which are isotropic

to, or do pass, polarized light, appear lighter than the A bands. A dark line known as the *Z line* (Zwischenscheibe, or between disk) can be seen bisecting the I bands. In addition to the I and A bands, a light region is located in the center of the sarcomere. This region is known as the *H zone* (Hellerscheibe, or clear disk) and is bisected by a dark line known as the *M line* (Mittelscheibe, or middle disk). On histologic study the portion of a myofibril located between the Z line is a *sarcomere* and is the basic contractile unit of skeletal muscle. A single myofibril comprises many sarcomeres arranged in series. Thus a sarcomere with a resting length of about 2.5 μm located in a 20-mm myofibril represents approximately 8000 sarcomeres attached end to end.

The striations evident in the microscopic images represent the different protein structures present on the muscle tissue. These structures can be divided into two main constituents, thick and thin myofilaments. The thin myofilaments are attached to the Z lines and are found in the I band and in the part of the A band that excludes the H zone (Fig. 8-2). The structure of the thin myofilament is dominated by the protein *actin* but also includes the proteins *troponin* and *tropomyosin* (Fig. 8-3). Each thin myofilament is composed of two strands of *F-actin* (fibrous) that are wound in an α-helix. Each F-actin strand is composed of *G-actin* (globular) monomers. Located within each groove of the F-actin helix are two strands of tropomyosin. Located at the end of each F-actin strand is the *troponin molecule* (TN). This TN contains three subunits, *TN-T*, which binds the molecule to tropomyosin, *TN-C*, which has binding sites for Ca^{2+}, and *TN-I*, which inhibits G-actin from binding to the thick myofilament. Located on each actin molecule is an *active site*, which allows for the formation of cross-bridges with the thick myofilament during contraction. During rest these active sites are somehow blocked or inhibited by the troponin-tropomyosin complex. Specifically, the tropomyosin molecule seems to be situated over the active site so that it is covered. Thus the troponin-tropomyosin complex prevents the formation of myofilament cross-bridges and subsequent contraction.

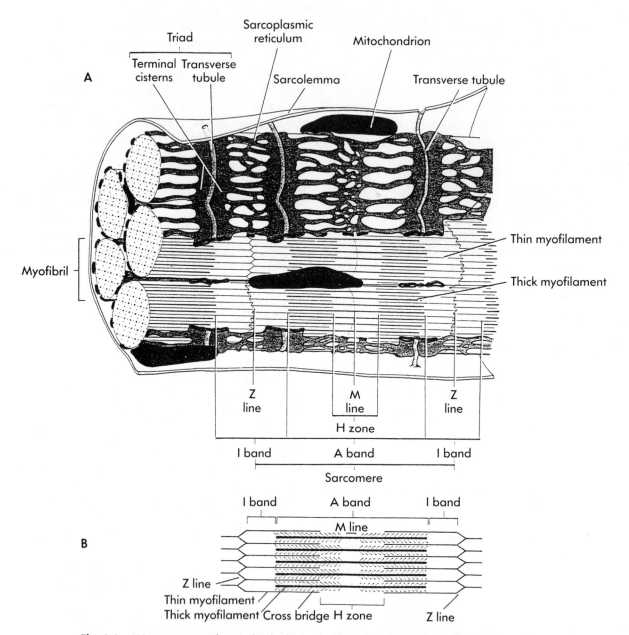

Fig. 8-2 Microstructure of an individual muscle fiber. **A,** A three-dimensional view of the myofibrils and membrane structures. **B,** Schematic diagram of an individual myofibril showing the relative positions of the thick and thin myofilaments. (From Tortora GJ, Anagnostakos NP: *Principles of anatomy and physiology,* New York, 1990, Harper & Row.)

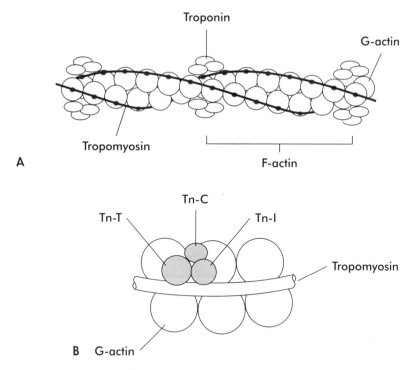

Fig. 8-3 Arrangement of the thin myofilament proteins. **A,** Location of actin, troponin, and tropomyosin along the thin myofilament. **B,** Detail of the troponin-tropomyosin complex. *Tn = C,* Troponin C; *Tn = I,* troponin I; *Tn = T,* troponin T.

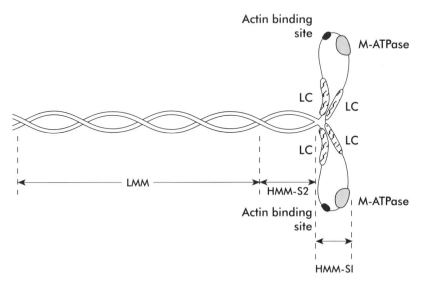

Fig. 8-4 Structure of the myosin molecule showing the location of the light and heavy meromyosin subunits (LMM, HMM-S1, and HMM-S2), the light chain (LC) subunits, myosin ATPase (M-ATPase) enzyme, and the actin binding sites.

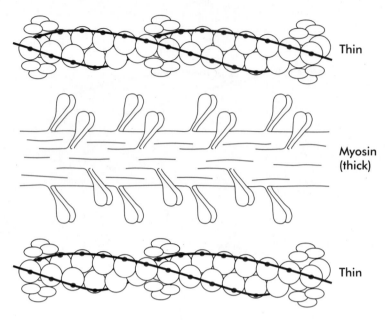

Fig. 8-5 Arrangement of the thick and thin myofilaments.

The thick myofilament is located in the A band of the sarcomere and is composed of the protein *myosin* (Fig. 8-4). Each myosin molecule has a long, double-helical tail that terminates in two large, globular heads. The myosin molecule can be decomposed by enzymatic cleavage into *light mero-myosin* (LMM) and *heavy meromyosin* (HMM). The HMM can be further decomposed into *sub-fragments 1* and *2* (S1 and S2). By a different enzymatic cleavage process the myosin molecule can be broken down into two *heavy chains,* each located in the tail and in part of the head, and four *light chains,* which are located within the head. The exact functions of the myosin molecule sub-units are discussed later. The myosin heads also contain the enzyme *M-ATPase,* which is responsible for catalyzing the breakdown of ATP into energy, and a site that binds the head to the actin molecule active site during contraction.

The thick and thin myofilaments are arranged so that some overlap exists between them (Fig. 8-2). This area of overlap can be found in the portion of the A band that does not include the H zone. When viewed in cross-section, each thick myofilament is surrounded by six thin myofilaments, whereas each thin myofilament is adjacent to three thick myofilaments. Fig. 8-5 shows that in the area of myofilament overlap the HMM heads project away from the backbone of the thick myofilament and toward the thin. Although not firmly established, it is thought that at rest no physical connection exists between the two myofilaments. As discussed later, for contraction of the sarcomere to occur, a physical connection between the myosin head (S1 HMM) and the actin molecules of the thin myofilament is required.

Motor Neuron and Neuromuscular Junction

Activation of skeletal muscle is controlled by an *α-motoneuron* that originates within the cell body (*soma*) in the spinal cord and terminates at the muscle fibers (Fig. 8-6). The soma resides in the spinal cord gray matter, with the remainder of the neuron exiting from the ventral portion of the spinal cord. The portion that connects the soma to the distal end of the neuron is called the *axon.* Toward the distal end the α-motoneuron branches into several

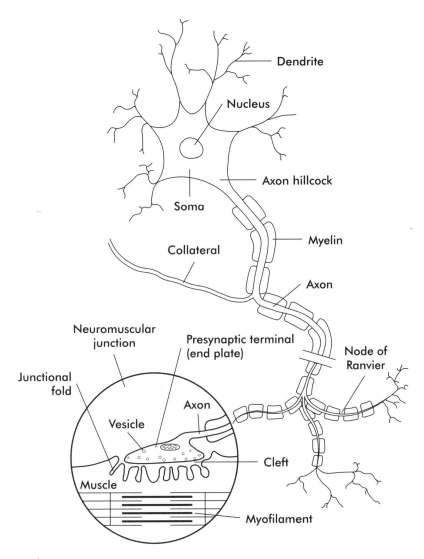

Fig. 8-6 The α-motoneuron, showing the following morphologic regions: dendrites, soma, axon, and motor end plate. (From Enoka RM: *Neuromechanical basis of kinesiology,* Champaign, Ill, 1988, Human Kinetics.)

collaterals; each collateral innervates a single muscle fiber. Thus a single α-motoneuron may innervate many muscle fibers. However, a single muscle fiber is innervated by only one α-motoneuron collateral. An individual α-motoneuron, all its collateral branches, and all the muscle fibers that the branches innervate are termed a *motor unit.* The number of muscle fibers within a single motor unit may vary from as few as 15 or 20 in the case of the ocular muscles to as many as 2000 in the case of the large locomotor muscles (such as gastrocnemius and vastus lateralis). This innervation ratio is related to the function of the muscle: the lower innervation ratios are found in muscles that control fine movements.

Surrounding the axon of each α-motoneuron are *Schwann's cells,* which form sheaths of *myelin.*

These myelin sheaths are continuous along the length of the neuron but are separated by small gaps called *nodes of Ranvier*. These nodes facilitate the passing of an impulse from the soma along the axon by a process called *saltatory conduction*. Instead of having to travel along the entire length of the α-motoneuron, saltatory conduction allows the impulse to ''jump'' from node to node, a much faster means of conduction.

The distal ends of each α-motoneuron (*motor end plates*) never actually come into physical contact with the muscle membrane but are surrounded by *junctional folds* in the sarcolemma and separated by the *synaptic cleft*. This area in which the neuron and muscle fiber are found is known as the *neuromuscular junction,* and the space between the nerve terminal and sarcolemma is called the *synapse*. Stored inside the nerve terminal are approximately 300,000 synaptic vesicles that contain the neurotransmitter (*acetylcholine* (ACh).

PHYSIOLOGY OF MUSCLE CONTRACTION
Energy for Contraction

Energy is required in a number of the steps in the excitation and contraction processes. These include restoration of the resting membrane potential, force generation by individual cross-bridges, and Ca^{2+} reuptake by the sarcoplasmic reticulum. In addition, the presence of ATP is required for the dissociation of actin and myosin. Energy required by these processes is derived from the breakdown of ATP by a specific *ATPase* enzyme. As mentioned earlier, the ATPase that breaks ATP attached to the myosin head is known as M-ATPase. In addition, the enzyme that provides energy for the reuptake of Ca^{2+} by the sarcoplasmic reticulum is called the *sarcoplasmic reticulum ATPase* (SR-ATPase). Each of these enzymes hydrolyzes ATP into adenosine diphosphate plus inorganic phosphate ($ADP + P_i$) and energy.[27] As discussed later, the rates at which these ATPases hydrolyze ATP determine the rates at which the fiber shortens and relaxes.

Excitation

The initiation of muscle contraction can occur at the level of the brain or as the result of feedback from one of many sensory receptors. In either case the α-motoneuron is activated in the spinal cord at its soma. This activation generates an electrical impulse that travels the length of the neuron and along each of its collaterals. At the nerve terminal the α-motoneuron mobilizes between 250 and 300 vesicles and releases ACh into the synaptic cleft (Fig. 8-7). This release of ACh depends on the entry of extracellular Ca^{2+} into the nerve terminal. The ACh then binds to specific receptors located on the sarcolemma (the postsynaptic membrane). This in turn causes depolarization of the sarcolemma and initiates an action potential. The communication between the α-motoneuron and the sarcolemma involves both electrical and chemical processes. The stimulus for ACh release is the α-motoneuron action potential, an electrical event, whereas depolarization of the sarcolemma is initiated by ACh binding, a chemical process. Immediately after the sarcolemma action potential has been generated, ACh remaining in the synapse is degraded by *acetylcholinesterase* into acetate and choline.

Contraction Process

Ca^{2+} activation of the contractile apparatus. Once an action potential has been initiated at the neuromuscular junction, it propagates along the long axis of the fiber. This depolarization also travels laterally into the fiber along the T-tubule network toward the triad region (Fig. 8-7). By a process that is not fully understood[10,11,13], depolarization of the T tubule activates the release of Ca^{2+} from the terminal cisternae of the sarcoplasmic reticulum. The Ca^{2+} diffuses into the sarcoplasm and into the region of the contractile apparatus. Once a threshold level is reached (approximately 10^{-7} M), Ca^{2+} binds to the C subunit of troponin, which causes a conformational change in the actin-troponin-tropomyosin complex. This conformational change results in force generation by the contractile apparatus (discussed

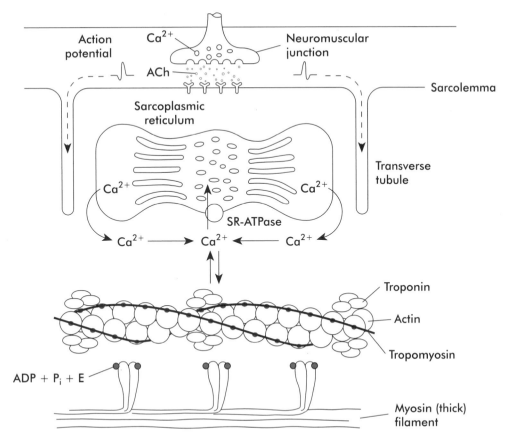

Fig. 8-7 Schematic diagram of the excitation and contraction processes, showing the role of Ca^{2+}. (Adapted from Vander AJ, Sherman JH, Luciano DS: *Human physiology,* New York, 1980, McGraw-Hill.)

later), which continues as long as sufficient Ca^{2+} is present in the sarcoplasm. Once activation of the fiber is terminated and the sarcolemma has returned to its resting polarity, Ca^{2+} is actively resequestered by the longitudinal portion of the sarcoplasmic reticulum. This is accomplished by an energy dependent "Ca^{2+} pump" called the *SR-ATPase*. During this time, Ca^{2+} concentration in the myoplasm declines and Ca^{2+} dissociates from TN-C. This in turn causes the actin-troponin-tropomyosin complex to return to its resting conformation, and force generation by the contractile apparatus ceases. Elastic forces then return the sarcomere to its resting length. In addition to force

generation, the reuptake of Ca^{2+} requires energy in the form of ATP hydrolysis.

Biochemistry of force generation. The myosin heads project away from the thick filament and toward the thin. This arrangement allows the myosin heads to form *cross-bridges* with the actin molecules. These cross-bridges exist in two states, *weak binding states,* which do not contribute to force production, and *strong binding states,* which result in force generation by the contractile apparatus (Fig. 8-8).[3,5,8,9] At rest the cross-bridges are in the weak binding states. Also, one ATP molecule is bound to the myosin head and may be hydrolyzed so that ADP + P_i is bound (Fig. 8-9).

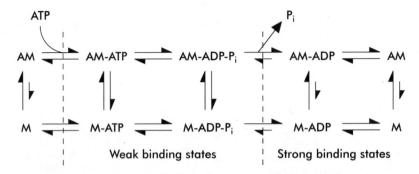

Fig. 8-8 Partial scheme of the cross-bridge cycle, showing force production as a function of the transition from weak binding states to the strong binding states. (From Chalovich JM, Yu LC, Brenner B: *J Muscle Res Cell Motil* 12:503, 1991.)

Under these resting conditions actin and myosin reversibly associate but with very low affinity (Fig. 8-8). Calcium ion binding to the TN-C causes all the troponin subunits to bind less tightly to actin and tropomyosin. This in turn causes an alteration in the binding of tropomyosin to actin. The result of these changes in the thin filament are threefold: the affinity of myosin for actin is increased, the kinetic aspect of ATP hydrolysis is increased, and the release of P_i from the myosin head is facilitated. Thus Ca^{2+} activation of the thin filament causes a transition of the cross-bridges from a

weak to a strong binding state. In this strong binding state the affinity of myosin for actin increases 1500-fold.

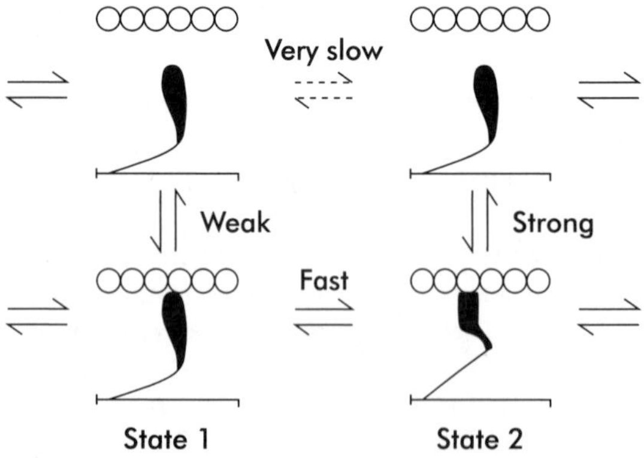

In the strong binding state energy from the hydrolyzed ATP molecule causes the myosin head (specifically the S1 HMM) to rotate toward the center of the thick myofilament. This cross-bridge force pulls the thin myofilament across the thick, causing the sarcomere to shorten. In this process the Z lines move closer together and the I band disappears. The process of the thin filament being pulled across the thick is known as the *Huxley sliding myofilament theory* and is the most widely accepted explanation of the contraction process.[23-25]

In the strong binding states ADP is released, and a "new" ATP molecule is required for the cross-bridges to return to the weak binding states. Once ATP binds to the myosin head and the affinity between actin and myosin is reduced, the myosin head returns to its resting conformation. Without sufficient ATP the fiber fails to relax, and a condition known as *rigor mortis* occurs. Although ATP is required to return the cross-bridges to their resting state, its hydrolysis and the release of energy are *not*. If activation of the fiber persists and Ca^{2+} concentration in the myoplasm remains elevated, the M-ATPase hydrolyzes the ATP and the cross-bridges once again move to the strong binding states and cause additional force production and sarcomere shortening. This process continues

Fig. 8-9 Biochemical steps involved in the cross-bridge cycle. A-actin, M-myosin, AM-bound actin, and myosin. (Adapted from Brenner B: Proc Natl Acad Sci USA 85:3265, 1988; Chalovich JM: *Pharmacol Ther* 55:95, 1992.)

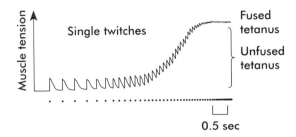

Fig. 8-10 Changes in muscle force as a function of stimulation frequency. Stimulation of a muscle fiber at progressively higher frequencies (*dots below trace*) elicits progressively greater force. (From Carew TJ, Ghez C. In Kandel ER, Schwartz JH; editors: *Principles of neural science,* New York, 1985, Elsevier.)

as long as stimuli are present, myoplasmic Ca^{2+} concentration is elevated, and ATP is available.

During normal muscular contraction many cross-bridges cycle between the strong and the weak binding states. While some cross-bridges are generating force and causing the sarcomere to shorten, others are forming bonds between adjacent actin and myosin molecules. This repetitive process of cross-bridge cycling causes the thin myofilament to be "ratcheted" or "walked across" the thick myofilament. By means of this mechanism each sarcomere shortens, and the muscle fiber contracts.

Types of Contraction

When a muscle receives a single stimulus, the muscle fiber responds with a single, brief *twitch* contraction (Fig. 8-10). A twitch can be divided into three phases. First, immediately after the stimulus there is a short *latent period* (of 2 to 5 msec) during which no measurable force is developed. During this time Ca^{2+} is being released from the sarcoplasmic reticulum, cross-bridges are beginning to cycle, and the elastic components are being stretched. During the second period, the *contraction phase*, force increases until peak force is reached. *Contraction time* (CT) usually lasts for 30 to 40 msec. Once the peak force is reached, it declines exponentially during the third period, the

relaxation phase (of 60 to 90 msec). This relaxation phase is characterized by the *half-relaxation time* (HRT), that is, the time required for the fiber to relax to half of its peak tension. The muscle's HRT seems to be determined by the SR-ATPase activity and the rate at which Ca^{2+} is resequestered by the sarcoplasmic reticulum.

If a second stimulus is given before the fiber fully relaxes, peak force of the subsequent twitch is somewhat larger than that of the first (Fig. 8-10). Likewise, additional stimuli also increase peak force of each twitch until a plateau is reached. This process, known as *twitch summation*, produces an *unfused tetanus*. The plateau, or peak force reached during summation, depends on the frequency of stimulation. At stimulation frequencies below about 4 Hz (4 stimuli per sec), little summation occurs. At stimulation frequencies between 10 and 25 Hz a direct relationship exists between frequency and force. At stimulation frequencies above 60 Hz full summation, or a *fused tetanus*, occurs and maximal force output or tetanic force of the fiber is reached.

Taxonomy of Contraction

Traditionally skeletal muscle performance has been characterized by the term "strength." However, this term is inappropriate, since it is extremely nonspecific, has no inherent definition, and has no unit of measure. Thus contraction *force* is most often used to assess the muscle's performance and is quantified by the Newton (N). The appropriateness of the term "muscle contraction" has also been questioned.[7] Because *contraction* connotes muscle fiber shortening and because some muscle activity may involve force production without shortening or force production with lengthening, the terms *action, exertion,* and *effort* have been introduced. A detailed discussion of the appropriateness of these terms is beyond the scope of this text. For simplicity, however, the conventional term, *muscle contraction,* has been used.

The contraction of muscle is typically characterized in terms of three variables, time or duration of the contraction (and its derivative velocity), displacement of the muscle (length change), and force produced or the mass (or moment of inertia) of the object moved. Under experimental conditions one or more of these variables are controlled and the others measured. To describe contractions in terms of these variables, the following terms have been traditionally used: (1) *isometric,* in which the degree of displacement is 0 (that is, no shortening), (2) *isokinetic,* in which the rate of displacement is constant (that is, constant velocity of lengthening or shortening), and (3) *isotonic,* in which force production is constant. In experimental circumstances it is not difficult to produce true isometric, isotonic, or isokinetic contractions. In the human body, however, it is often difficult or impossible to produce contractions of these types. Thus these terms may be applicable to experimental study of isolated whole muscle or of single muscle fibers but may be inappropriate for describing human muscle performance.

When human performance is examined, the term *isometric* is used to describe a condition in which the degree of displacement of a limb or rotation of a joint is 0. Because of the elastic properties of the muscle connective tissue and the joint involved, however, the muscle fibers shorten to some extent. Nonetheless, the term *isometric* still has wide use in the field of human performance. However, its definition has been modified to characterize contractions in which the degree of limb displacement is 0.

In the human body true isokinetic contractions rarely if ever occur. However, conditions in which the rate of limb displacement or joint rotation is constant do occur. Thus the terms *isovelocity* and *isokinematic* have replaced *isokinetic*.[28] This is an important concept, since maintenance of constant limb velocity while joint muscle insertion angles change requires quite varied velocities of muscle fiber shortening.

It is nearly impossible to maintain a constant force output by the muscle during normal, everyday movement. Typically the external load lifted by the individual is held constant. Under such conditions muscle force must vary considerably to account for changes in muscle length and joint biomechanics during movement. Thus the terms *isoinertial* and *isotorque* have replaced *isotonic* in

the description of conditions in which mass and force are held constant.[28]

MUSCLE TYPES
Functional, Structural, and Biochemical Characteristics

The maximal amount of force produced by different muscle fibers can vary considerably. In addition, the time course of contractions and the fatigability of individual fibers also vary. These variations have led to the classification of muscle into different *fiber types* or *motor unit types* (Fig. 8-11; Table 8-1). Human muscle is generally classified into two broad types based on contraction characteristics: slow-twitch (type 1) and fast-twitch (type 2). As would be expected, slow, or type 1, fibers contract slowly, having CTs and HRTs of approximately 100 msec. Although these fibers contract slowly, they have little fatigue when subjected to repetitive stimulation, since their energy needs are met primarily by aerobic metabolism. Type 1 fibers are also small in diameter and can generate only a small amount of absolute force. Type 1 fibers are also termed slow oxidative (SO) fibers.[30,31]

Fast-twitch, or type 2, fibers contract rapidly and have CTs and HRTs that are approximately 75% lower than those of type 1 fibers. However, type 2 fibers show rapid, marked fatigue during repetitive stimulation and rely primarily on anaerobic metabolism. These fibers are large in diameter and generate a large amount of absolute force. Interestingly, when the amount of force is expressed in relation to cross-sectional areas, types 1 and 2 fibers generate nearly equal amounts of force. Because of different contraction kinetics and biochemical capacities, type 2 fibers are also described as fast glycolytic (FG) or fast fatigable (FF) fibers.

Differences in biochemical properties and endurance characteristics have led to subclassifications of the type 2 fibers into type 2a, or intermediate, fibers and type 2b, or fast, fibers. Type 2a fibers are characterized by slightly slower contraction and relaxation times and slightly lower force output than those for type 2b fibers, a marked resistance to fatigue, and the ability to utilize both

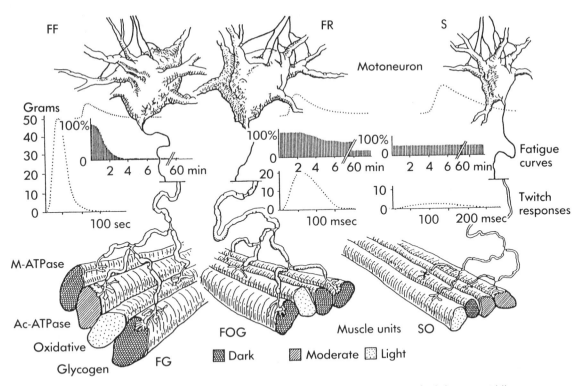

Fig. 8-11 Structural, functional, and biochemical differences in types 2b (*left*), 2a (*middle*), and 1 (*right*) motor units. (From Edington DW, Edgerton VR: *The biology of physical activity,* Boston, 1986, Houghton Mifflin.)

aerobic and anaerobic energy systems. Type 2a fibers are also termed *fast, oxidative, glycolytic* (FOG) fibers or *fast fatigue-resistant* (FR) fibers.

Fig. 8-11 shows some of the differences in the structural, physiologic and biochemical properties of types 1, 2a, and 2b fibers. Specific differences among fiber types are described in detail in Table 8-1. Within an individual motor unit all the fibers are of the same type. In addition, fast and slow motor units also vary in α-motoneuron soma size, axon size, degree of branching, and conduction velocity.[35] The latter properties, as discussed later, determine which motor units are activated during various types of activity.

Fiber Type Distributions and Training

In humans the relative proportion of fiber types varies greatly among individuals. In the average sedentary individual about 45% to 55% of fibers are type 1. This distribution does not seem to be a factor of age or sex. The percentage of types 1, 2a, and 2b fibers, however, varies widely across and within different athletic populations. For example, in trained distance runners the percentage of type 1 fibers may be as high as 90% and as low as 60%; in trained sprinters the proportion of type 1 fibers may range from 25% to 45%. Large proportions of type 1 fibers also exist in other types of athletes who engage in endurance events (such as cross-country skiing, cycling, and swimming), whereas small proportions can be found in power athletes such as weight lifters, and shot-putters.[30,32] Some overlap in relative distribution of fiber types exists among many groups of athletes, especially in the distribution of type 2a fibers.

The most recent research indicates that training can do little to change the relative proportions of fast and slow fiber types. For example, endurance

Table 8-1   Motor unit characteristics

Characteristic	Muscle fiber (type)		
	1	**2a**	**2b**
Nomenclature	S; SO; red	Intermediate; FOG; FR	Fast; FG; FF; white
α-Motoneuron properties			
Cell body size	Small	Medium	Large
Axon diameter	Small	Medium	Large
Threshold for recruitment	Low	Moderate	High
Conduction velocity	Slow	Fast	Fast
Physiologic properties			
Shortening velocity	Slow	Moderate	Fast
Rate of force development	Slow	Moderate	Fast
Absolute force output	Low	Moderate	High
Resistance to fatigue	High	Moderate	Low
Structure			
Diameter	Small	Moderate	Large
Z-line thickness	Wide	Moderate	Narrow
T-tubule surface area	Small	Large	Large
Terminal cisternae surface area	Small	Moderate	Large
Myosin light-chain type	Slow	Fast	Fast
Biochemical properties			
Ca^{2+} sensitivity of the contractile apparatus	High	Low	Low
Myosin ATPase activity	Low	High	High
Mitochondrial density	High	High	Low
Aerobic capacity	High	High	Low
Glycolytic (anaerobic) capacity	Low	High	High
Glycogen content	Low	High	High
Myoglobin content	High	High	Low
Capillary density	High	High	Low
Predominant energy system	Aerobic	Combination	Anaerobic

FF, Fast fatigable; *FG,* fast glycolytic; *FOG,* fast oxidative glycolytic; *FR,* fast fatigue-resistant; *S,* slow-twitch; *SO,* slow oxidative.

training does not increase the percentage of type 1 fibers, nor does weight lifting increase the percentage of type 2 fibers. It is possible, however, to alter some of the biochemical and structural properties of both fiber types with training. Endurance training increases the oxidative capacity of type 2 fibers, whereas sprint training increases the anaerobic capacity and diameter of type 1 fibers. However, conversion of type 1 fibers into type 2 fibers or vice versa does not occur, even with severe training regimens.[2,16,22,26] It appears that the large proportion of type 1 fibers in endurance athletes is not a function of training but probably results from genetic factors.

REGULATION OF MUSCLE FORCE

The force output by the whole muscle is influenced by a number of physiologic and mechanical factors. In this section these factors have been divided into neural factors, that is, activation patterns, and mechanical factors, which include length-tension and force-velocity relationships.

Motor Unit Activation Patterns

When activated, all the fibers of a given motor unit contract. As discussed earlier, the frequency at which a muscle fiber or a motor unit is activated markedly influences the force of contraction. For example, in humans a single stimulus elicits twitch responses, whereas multiple stimuli delivered at a rate of 30 to 40 Hz elicit tetanic contractions.[14,19] Normally the force of a twitch contraction is approximately 33% of tetanic force. Contractions evoked via stimulation frequencies of 5 to 40 Hz evoke force output somewhere between twitch and tetanic forces. Thus force output of a motor unit and a whole muscle can be regulated by the frequency at which they are activated. This concept has been called *rate coding*.[14]

A second means of increasing force output of a whole muscle is to activate more motor units. As the force exerted by the muscle increases, additional motor units are recruited. Once an additional motor unit is activated, it remains active until the force declines. As the force declines, motor units are sequentially derecruited or deactivated in reverse order of their recruitment. The relative contribution of motor unit recruitment to muscle force varies among different muscles. For example, in some muscles additional motor units are recruited until force reaches about 85% of maximal force. In other muscles all motor units may be activated when force reaches about 30% of maximal force.[14]

The recruitment of additional motor units for increased force production follows a set pattern that is based on the ''size'' of the motor unit. As discussed earlier, there are differences in the sizes of the α-motoneuron soma and axon. In fast motor units all these structures are larger than those of slow motor units. Thus fast motor units are often referred to as large and slow units, small. As noted in Table 8-1, the threshold for recruitment of small motor units is low. Thus when a muscle is required to exert a small amount of force, the low-threshold

or small motor units are activated. As the force requirement increases, higher-threshold or larger motor units are sequentially recruited. When force output of the whole muscle declines, the motor units are derecruited in reverse order, large first and small last. This orderly recruitment pattern is known as the *size principle*.[14,20]

The size principle suggests that during low-intensity activities such as jogging, which require low force output by the active muscles, small, slow motor units are recruited. On the other hand, high-intensity exercises such as sprinting or weight lifting are supported by the recruitment of both small and large motor units. According to the size principle, high-intensity exercises involve activation of both large and small motor units because the small units must be activated before the large units can be recruited.

During normal muscle contraction, changes in rate coding and motor unit recruitment occur simultaneously. That is, as larger motor units are being activated, the activation frequency of previously recruited motor units is increasing. Thus regulation of force by varying the pattern of activation involves both rate coding and application of the size principle.

Length-Tension Relationships

In addition to the previously described neural factors, several mechanical factors such as the initial length of the fiber and the velocity of shortening can influence force output of muscle fiber.

At rest the muscle fiber acts somewhat like a spring, that is, as the fiber is stretched, passive force is generated. In the case of an ideal spring the amount of resting or passive force produced is linearly related to its length. However, this concept, known as Hook's law, does not directly apply to skeletal muscle. Although the resting force of a muscle fiber increases with stretch, the relationship between these two variables is not linear. At near-resting lengths the relationship is somewhat flat, whereas at excessive lengths the relationship becomes much more steep (Fig. 8-12). The causes of this *resting length-tension* relationship reside in the elastic components of the fiber. As noted previously, skeletal muscle contains a large amount of

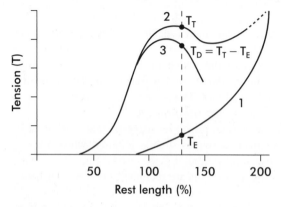

Fig. 8-12 Length-tension relationships of skeletal muscle. *Curve 1,* Passive tension (T_E). *Curve 2,* Total tension (T_T). *Curve 3,* Developed tension (T_D), computed by subtracting curve 1 from curve 2 ($T_D = T_T - T_E$). (From Gowitzke BA, Milner M: *Scientific basis of human movement,* Baltimore, 1988, Williams & Wilkins.)

connective tissue, the elastic properties of which account for this relationship.

Not only does the muscle develop more resting force as its length changes, but also the amount of developed force varies with length (Fig. 8-12). The mechanisms that underlie this *active length-tension* relationship are somewhat different from those that influence the resting relationship (Fig. 8-13). At long lengths the fiber is stretched to the point that little myofilament overlap occurs. Under this condition it is difficult for cross-bridges to form and for subsequent force to be developed. On the other hand, at short fiber lengths the myofilaments are so compressed between adjacent Z lines that when cross-bridges are formed, there is no room left for the sarcomere to shorten. In this case the thin myofilaments may even bump into the Z lines. At an optimal muscle length there is plenty of myofilament overlap, so a maximal number of cross-bridges and force can be generated. In addition, there is adequate room for the thin myofilament to be pulled across the thick and for the sarcomere to fully shorten.[17]

In humans a resting length-tension relationship is difficult to assess because mechanical limits are imposed by various joint structures. However, active length-tension relationships can be constructed, typically by varying the angle of the joint across which the muscle group of interest acts. For the most part the typical length-tension relationship exists between joint angle and torque, since when the joint is fully flexed or extended (short and long muscle lengths), little joint torque is produced. Peak torque is produced when the joint is somewhere between full flexion and extension and the muscle is at a moderate length.

Force-Velocity Relationship

When the force that is generated by a skeletal muscle overcomes a resistance that is to be lifted, the muscle shortens and the load is lifted. The velocity at which the muscle is able to shorten and the rate at which the load is moved are influenced by the force output required to overcome the resting inertia of the object. The *force-velocity relationship* during contractions in which the muscle is shortening, holds that as the load is increased, velocity of shortening is decreased. That is, high muscular force outputs are associated with slow shortening velocities, and vice versa. Fig. 8-14 shows the relationship between force and velocity for shortening (*concentric*), lengthening (*eccentric*), and isometric contractions. Maximal shortening velocity (Vmax) occurs only in a muscle that is allowed to contract against a load of 0. The mechanisms by which a muscle produces Vmax appear to reside in the contractile apparatus and the rate of cross-bridge cycling.[4,29] For a muscle to rapidly shorten, cross-bridges must be formed, broken, and reformed quickly. Thus the rates at which ADP + P_i is released from the myosin head and the "new" ATP is hydrolyzed by the M-ATPase have a large influence on Vmax. When the cross-bridge turnover rate is high, the force generated by individual cross-bridges may decrease and fewer cross-bridges may be formed. In addition, the rate of Ca^{2+} release from the sarcoplasmic reticulum may influence the maximal rate of muscle shortening.[29] By using isolated muscle preparations, it is possible to obtain a measure of Vmax. However, measuring Vmax is impossible in humans, since contracting muscle

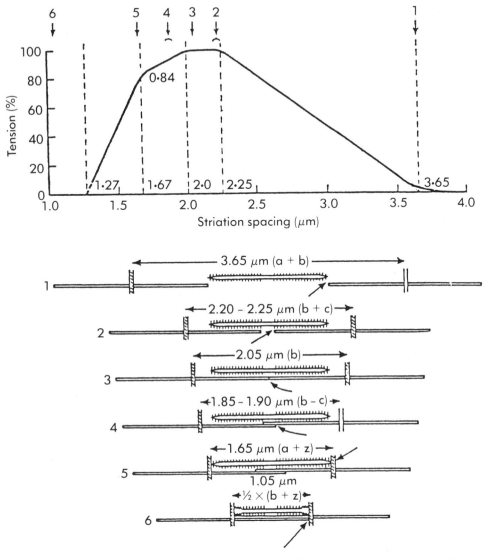

Fig. 8-13 Relationships of sarcomere length (a), myofilament overlap (c), and developed force (b). (From Gordon AM, Huxley AF, Julian FJ: *J Physiol [Lond]*, 184:170, 1966.)

must always move one of the limb segments to which it is attached.

Traditionally, maximal force output of a muscle (P_O) has been defined as that produced during an isometric contraction (that is, maximal isometric force). As can be seen in Fig. 8-14, however, force output of a muscle actually increases above P_O during eccentric contractions. Currently the expla-

nation for this phenomenon is unclear. It is possible that during an eccentric contraction the force required to break cross-bridges is greater than that required to hold an isometric contraction. Alternatively, stretching the muscle fiber may either increase the amount of Ca^{2+} released from the sarcoplasmic reticulum or stretch incompletely activated sarcomeres within each myofibril. An

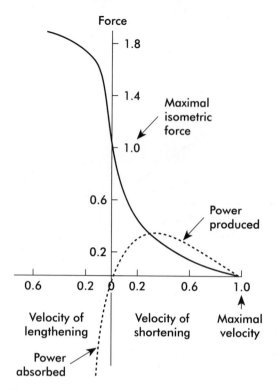

Fig. 8-14 Force-velocity relationship of skeletal muscle. Concentric, isometric, and eccentric contractions are shown. Also shown is the relationship between power and shortening velocity. (From Åstrand P-O, Rodahl K: *Textbook of work physiology,* New York, 1977, McGraw-Hill.)

important concept is that in either case eccentric contractions are more forceful than isometric or concentric contractions. Also of interest is that eccentric contractions are typically associated with delayed-onset muscle soreness and, possibly, with structural damage.

The product of force and velocity is *power*. The relationship between force application and power output is shown in Fig. 8-14. As can be seen, power output is low for slow or near-static contractions, despite high force output. Also, when shortening velocity is high, power output is again low. Peak power output is obtained at a moderate force output and shortening velocity. Specifically, peak power occurs when the force being exerted is about one third of P_O.

As noted previously, some differences exist between the force-velocity-power relationships in isolated muscles and in muscles of intact humans. In humans the force-velocity curve has the same general shape as that shown in Fig. 8-14. However, the curve for humans typically shows a slight plateau at slow contractile velocities. This may be a function of limitations on activation of the musculature or may be due to changes that occur in the mechanical arrangements between the joint system and muscle when the limb moves, or both may apply.

REFERENCES

1. Åstrand P-O, Rodahl K: *Textbook of work physiology,* New York, 1977, McGraw-Hill.
2. Bagby G, Sembrowich W, Gollnick P: Myosin ATPase and fiber type composition from trained and untrained rat skeletal muscle, *J Appl Physiol* 223:1415, 1972.
3. Brenner B: Mechanical and structural approaches to correlation of cross-bridge action in muscle with actomyosin ATPase in solution, *Ann Rev Physiol* 49:655, 1987.
4. Brenner B: Effect of Ca^{2+} on cross-bridge turnover kinetics in skinned single rabbit psoas fibers: implications for regulation of muscle contraction, *Proc Natl Acad Sci USA* 85:3265, 1988.
5. Brenner B: Rapid dissociation and reassociation of actomyosin cross-bridges during force generation: a newly observed facet of cross-bridge action in muscle, *Proc Natl Acad Sci* 88:10490, 1991.
6. Carew TJ, Ghez C: Muscles and muscle receptors. In Kandel ER, Schwartz JH, editors: *Principles of neural science,* New York, 1985, Elsevier.
7. Cavanagh PR: On ''muscle action'' vs. ''muscle contraction'' *Biomechanics* 21:69, 1988.
8. Chalovich JM: Actin-mediated regulation of muscle contraction, *Pharmacol Ther* 55:95, 1992.
9. Chalovich JM, Yu LC, Brenner B: Involvement of weak binding cross-bridges in force production in muscle, *J Muscle Res Cell Motil* 12:503, 1991.
10. Ebashi S: Excitation-contraction coupling, *Ann Rev Physiol* 38:293, 1976.
11. Ebashi S: Excitation-contraction coupling and the mechanism of muscle contraction, *Ann Rev Physiol* 53:1, 1991.
12. Edington DW, Edgerton VR: *The biology of physical activity,* Boston, 1976, Houghton Mifflin.
13. Endo M: Calcium release from the sarcoplasmic reticulum, *Physiol Rev* 57:71, 1977.
14. Enoka RM: *Neuromechanical basis of kinesiology,* Champaign, Ill, 1988, Ill, Human Kinetics.
15. Fox S: *Human physiology,* Dubuque, IA, 1987, William C Brown.

16. Gollnick P, Saltin B: Hypothesis: significance of skeletal muscle oxidative capacity with endurance training, *Clin Physiol* 2:1, 1983.

17. Gordon AM, Huxley AF, Julian FJ: The variation in isometric tension with sarcomere length in vertebrate muscle fibers, *J Physiol (Lond)* 184:170, 1966.

18. Gowitzke BA, Milner M: *Scientific basis of human movement,* Baltimore, 1988, Williams & Wilkins.

19. Gydikov A, Kosarov D: Some features of different motor units in human biceps brachii, *Pflügers Arch* 347:75, 1974.

20. Henneman E: Relation between size of neurons and their susceptibility to discharge, *Science* 126:1345, 1957.

21. Hole J: *Human anatomy and physiology,* Dubuque, IA, 1987, William C Brown.

22. Hoppler H: Exercise-induced ultrastructure changes in skeletal muscle, *Int J Sports Med* 7:187, 1986.

23. Huxley AF: Review lecture: muscular contraction, *J Physiol (Lond)* 243:1, 1974.

24. Huxley HE: The structural basis of muscular contraction, *Proc Royal Soc Med* 178:131, 1971.

25. Huxley HE, Hanson J: Changes in the cross-striations of muscle during contraction and stretch and their structural interpretation, *Nature* 173:973, 1954.

26. Jansson E, Kaijser L: Muscle adaptation to extreme endurance training in man, *Acta Physiol Scand* 100:315, 1977.

27. Kodama T: Thermodynamic analysis of muscle ATPase mechanisms, *Physiol Rev* 65:468, 1985.

28. Kroemer KHE: A taxonomy of dynamic muscle exertions, *J Hum Muscle Perform* 1:1, 1991.

29. Metzger JM, Moss RL: Calcium-sensitive cross-bridge transitions in mammalian fast and slow skeletal muscle fibers, *Science* 247:1088, 1990.

30. Pette D: *Plasticity of muscle,* New York, 1980, Walter de Gruyter.

31. Pette D, Spamer C: Metabolic properties of muscle fibers, *Fed Proc* 45:2910, 1986.

32. Tesch PA, Thorsson A, Kaiser P: Muscle capillary supply and fiber type characteristics in weight and power lifters, *J Appl Physiol* 56:35, 1984.

33. Tortora GJ, Anagnostakos NP: *Principles of anatomy and physiology,* New York, 1990, Harper & Row.

34. Vander AJ, Sherman JH, Luciano DS: *Human physiology,* New York, 1980, McGraw-Hill.

35. Vrbova G: Influence of activity on some characteristic properties of slow and fast mammalian muscles, *Exerc Sport Sci Rev* 7:181, 1979.

STUDY QUESTIONS

- Describe the structure of the motor neuron, skeletal muscle, and connective tissue.
- Describe the muscle contraction process.
- Compare and contrast types 1 and 2 muscle fibers and motor units.
- Describe the processes of motor unit recruitment and muscle force development.
- Describe the length-tension and force-velocity relationships.

CHAPTER 9

PROGRESSIVE AND DEGENERATIVE NEUROMUSCULAR DISEASES AND SEVERE MUSCULAR ATROPHY

Scott M. Hasson

The ability to perform work and exercise depends on the integrity of the cardiopulmonary and skeletal muscular systems. As described in Chapter 2, oxygen must be available to perform long-term work. Oxygen is delivered through the cardiopulmonary system, and the oxygen is utilized within the muscle tissue. The inability to oxidize fuels and how this inability affects exercise performance and exercise training are discussed in Chapter 3. Another cause of poor exercise tolerance, besides an inability to regulate, store, and oxidize fuel sources, is muscle weakness that results from muscle necrosis and severe muscular atrophy. The diseases that promote muscle necrosis are classified as muscle dystrophies. Severe muscular atrophy can occur in various patients when muscle activation is threatened, diet is impaired, myopathic drugs are taken, or a cessation of physical activity occurs. Skeletal muscle physiology and function are thoroughly described in Chapter 8. The major emphases in Chapter 9 are (1) to describe briefly some progressive, degenerative-neuromuscular diseases, the effect of decreased-muscle mass on exercise tolerance, and the effect of exercise training, (2) to describe briefly what factors affect muscle mass and exercise performance, and (3) to discuss the effect of exercise

training in patients who have severe muscular atrophy caused by inactivity, impaired diet, myopathic drugs, or a combination of these.

NEUROMUSCULAR DISEASES: EXERCISE TOLERANCE AND EFFECT OF EXERCISE TRAINING

The ability to use oxygen depends on the "quality" as well as the quantity of muscle. In this section the degenerative effect on skeletal muscle in patients with progressive degenerative neuromuscular diseases is briefly described. In addition, the implications of these diseases for exercise tolerance and the effect of exercise training are discussed.

Progressive Degenerative Motor Neuron Disease

Neuromuscular diseases that result in muscular atrophy and necrosis are rare, and the affected area of lesion can be the motor neuron, the neuromuscular junction, or the muscle tissue itself. The typical clinical picture for motor neuron disease is one of severe muscle weakness, fatigue, and atrophy. Motor neuron diseases involve the central nervous system (CNS) and result in impaired activation of the muscle and muscle atrophy caused by disuse and denervation.

Amyotrophic Lateral Sclerosis

The most common neuromuscular disease that affects the motor neuron is amyotrophic lateral sclerosis (ALS).[6] Amyotrophic lateral sclerosis is progressive and degenerative, resulting in irreversible denervation of the neural system. Amyotrophic lateral sclerosis can involve all portions of the CNS but primarily affects muscle function because of specific denervation of the motor neurons.[37] The effect of ALS is profound muscular atrophy, decreased strength, and decreased endurance.

Amyotrophic lateral sclerosis is characterized by destruction of motor neurons and axons.[37] This disease initially affects distal musculature of the appendages but eventually involves the proximal musculature, including the muscles of posture, speech, swallowing, and respiration.[9] The cause is presently unknown, but ALS may be of viral origin.[47,60] The results are a decrease in and, finally, cessation of neural signals to the skeletal muscle.[5,21] Symptoms of the disease may develop rapidly and initially involve the muscles in the hands, forearms, legs, and feet. Severe muscle weakness and fatigability of the affected muscles occur. Eventually gait and balance are affected, since profound weakness occurs in the muscles of the ankles and, later, of the hip and trunk. Generally the course of the disease is rapid, and the final prognosis is death. The usual cause of death is failure of the pulmonary system, since the individual becomes wheelchair bound and sedentary. However, some individuals have lived for more than 5 years after diagnosis of the disease.[10] Although Charcot initially described ALS in the 1870s, there is still no cure for this disease.

Although no cure exists, exercise and physical training have been promoted as a way to treat ALS so that function can be maintained for as long as possible.

Amyotrophic lateral sclerosis has implications for exercise tolerance and the effect of exercise training. Before exercise is promoted for improving function, the major patient problems and causes of disease must be explored fully. In addition it is critical to understand that exercise is not a single entity but a sequence of complex events that place different demands on the muscle. The demand of the exercise activity (aerobic or anaerobic) and types of contractions initiated dictates what fiber types are recruited. Early in the disease process of ALS the major concern is decreased muscle strength and endurance, which impairs gait, balance, and many upper-extremity activities of daily living (such as grooming and feeding). This decline in muscle function occurs because both type I (slow-twitch) and type 2 (fast-twitch) motor units are affected.

During upper-extremity and lower-extremity resistance exercise testing of patients with ALS there is a marked decrease in muscle strength.[7] Depending on the time of testing (early or later in the course of the disease) muscle strength is reduced by 25% to 75% as compared with matched normal muscle strength. In addition, fatigue occurs with anaerobic and aerobic activities. Muscle damage has not been reported to occur during resistance testing or training.[85]

During lower-extremity cycle ergometry testing of ALS patients energy requirements appear to be greater than normal. This appears to be related to a decrease in mechanical efficiency of lower-extremity muscles. Overall work capacity and maximal oxygen consumption (Vo_2max) are reduced by approximately 25% to 40%, but heart rate, blood pressure, and ventilation responses are normal.[86] Therefore the reduction in oxygen consumption appears to be primarily related to utilization at the muscle site and not to delivery of oxygen. Once the disease progresses to later stages and affects muscles of swallowing and ventilation, oxygen delivery does appear to become a problem. Fuel use appears to be affected during exercise, since less free fatty acid (FFA) is mobilized. Other indicators of metabolic activity, blood glucose levels, and lactate responses are normal during exercise testing.[86]

Patients with ALS respond normally to acute exercise but have significantly lowered responses in force production and oxygen use. These lowered responses appear to be primarily due to the decrease in muscle mass. No contraindications to

Table 9-1 Effect of denervation on biochemical properties of skeletal muscle

Property	Range of decline (%)		Duration of denervation
	Type 1	Type 2	
Glycogen	15-25	15-25	24 hours
Glycogen synthetase	70-80	50-60	24 hours
Pyruvate dehydrogenase	35-45	40-50	1 week
Lactate dehydrogenase	40-50	20-30	3 weeks
Palmitate oxidation	No change	No change	1 week
Cytochrome oxidase	No change	35-35-	6 weeks

low- or high-intensity training appear to be present.

In patients with ALS neuromuscular control mechanisms are disrupted by denervation. The results of denervation are decreases in biochemical properties of skeletal muscle (Table 9-1) that are in direct opposition to the effect of exercise training (see Chapter 2). Therefore, since the muscle appears to be normal (only denervated), exercise training to maximize motor unit recruitment may be of benefit. The role of resistance and endurance exercise training for patients with ALS has been reviewed only in case studies.

Anaerobic (resistance-strengthening) and aerobic (endurance) exercise training regimens have some effects in patients with ALS. The result of 10 weeks of resistance training (manual resistance to isolate specific muscles and muscle groups) for patients with ALS appears to be an improvement in strength.[7] In the case study just cited not all muscle groups improved. Of the 18 upper-extremity muscle groups trained and tested, however, 14 demonstrated an ability to increase isometric force production. Improvements in functional activities like clearing the buttocks during transfers and pivoting a wheelchair on carpet also occurred. Bohannon[7] observed that in patients with ALS muscles are affected at varying rates. One difficulty in the study of ALS and other progressive neuromuscular diseases is the inability to distinguish the effect of the disease process from that of the training process. Quantitative electromyography may eventually assist in evaluating the changes that occur in recruitment pat-

terns, thereby allowing for a correlation to changes in strength and function.[24]

Endurance training is important for patients with ALS, since they are easily fatigued. The result of 6 weeks of arm and leg cycle ergometry performed four days a week at an intensity of 50% Vo_2max and a duration of 30 minutes per day (5 minutes of work and 5 minutes of rest) was to improve voluntary and minute ventilation by 20% and 25%, respectively.[86] In addition, the ability to perform upper-extremity work improved, oxygen consumption increased during arm cranking activity, and isometric (static) and isokinetic (dynamic) strength increased. Lower-extremity function and oxygen consumption tested during leg ergometry did not improve, nor did lower-extremity static and dynamic strength. Again, the effect of disease activity during training was unknown, but it was suspected that a more rapid disease process may have been occurring in the lower extremities than in the upper extremities during the evaluation and training session.[86]

On the basis of pilot case studies it appears that exercise training may have a beneficial impact on muscle strength and endurance for patients with ALS. The effect on ventilatory responses during upper-extremity activity is especially promising. Many questions still exist concerning the benefits of exercise training for individuals with progressive neuromuscular disease, but it appears that no negative side effects result from moderate-intensity endurance and resistance exercise for patients with ALS. Prescribing exercise training activities that maximize recruitment of specific muscle groups and fiber types, especially during functional activity, may further optimize beneficial effects.

Muscular Dystrophy

Muscular dystrophy is a neuromuscular disease that specifically affects muscle tissue and results in muscle tissue atrophy and necrosis. The major types of muscular dystrophy are Duchenne's dystrophy, Becker's dystrophy, limb-girdle dystrophy, and facioscapulohumeral (FSH) dystrophy. The typical clinical picture for muscular dystrophy is severe skeletal muscle weakness, fatigue, and muscle atrophy or pseudohypertrophy, or both. Muscular dystrophy is a genetic inherited disease that affects the muscle fiber and directly results in a biochemical deficiency of the muscle membrane. The pathologic sequence of events is muscle fiber necrosis with replacement by fat or connective tissue, or both. The atrophy and pseudohypertrophy depend on the amount of fat and connective tissue that are deposited in replacement of muscle tissue. The disease usually affects proximal musculature (Duchenne's, Becker's and limb-girdle muscular dystrophies), but in FSH muscular dystrophy specific muscles of the face, shoulder girdle, and upper extremity are involved. Eventually distal, ventilatory, and cardiac muscle may become involved, particularly in Duchenne's dystrophy.

Symptoms of *Duchenne's dystrophy* usually become evident in boys from 3 to 4 years of age, although histologic evidence of muscle necrosis exists at birth. Only males are affected. Children with Duchenne's dystrophy become wheelchair bound, usually by 8 to 10 years of age, when physical growth increases and the necessary torque to maintain balance at the hip and ankle is surpassed. Frequent falling results in eventual confinement to the safer environment of the wheelchair. Once wheelchair bound, the child with Duchenne's dystrophy usually has continued physical growth, often has obesity, and has contractures of the joints that prevent normal movement of the extremities. Death usually occurs in the late teens or early twenties as a result of pulmonary complications related to weakness of the muscles of ventilation and swallowing.[90]

Symptoms of *Becker's dystrophy* occur later in adolescence than do those of Duchenne's dystrophy, and Becker's dystrophy has a much longer and milder course. As with Duchenne's dystrophy, only males are affected. Loss of independent ambulation usually occurs in early adulthood and is followed later by pulmonary complications and muscle contractures; death eventually occurs during middle adulthood. Cardiac muscle involvement can also occur, resulting in limitations on physical performance and eventual heart failure.[50]

Symptoms of *limb-girdle dystrophy* usually occur during the second or third decade and affect ambulation and balance. The muscles about the hip and pelvis are usually first affected. Symptoms usually show only mild progression, but weakness does spread to the shoulder girdle region, affecting upper-extremity work and activities of daily living. Eventual confinement to the wheelchair does occur in later middle age, but patients usually have a normal life span.[4] Limb-girdle dystrophy affects men and women equally.

Symptoms of *FSH dystrophy* usually occur at the end of the first decade but may occur within the first 2 years of life. Weakness initially involves muscle of the face, shoulder girdle, and arm. The symptoms progress slowly, and muscles of the pelvic girdle and leg are affected much later than are those in the shoulder girdle and arm. Individuals with FSH usually have only minor disability and have a normal life expectancy.[36] Facioscapulohumeral dystrophy, like limb-girdle dystrophy, affects men and women equally.

Muscular dystrophy is known to be caused by defects in gene expression that are inherited. No cure exists, but isolation of specific genes and abnormal protein expression may soon lead scientists into the development of an effective treatment. There is some debate concerning the role of exercise training for these patients, particularly for patients with Duchenne's dystrophy.

Disuse atrophy coupled with "true" atrophy caused by muscle cell necrosis results in severe decline of functional capacity in patients with muscle disease. To maintain muscle strength and metabolic capacity, patients must perform daily activity involving repetitive muscle contractions. It has been suggested that to maintain strength, contractions stronger than 20% of one repetition maximum (1 RM) must be performed regularly; otherwise, muscle atrophy will occur.[48] To maintain the metabolic and biochemical pathways and mitochondrial density and function for patients with muscular dystrophy, moderate-intensity exercise at more than 40% to 50% of Vo_2max must be performed on a near-daily basis.[89,94] In other words, the expression "use it or lose it" appears to particularly apply to the patient with muscular dystrophy. However, some investigators do not agree that exercise is beneficial for patients with muscular dystrophy and think that exercise may in fact be deleterious.[31,46] The deleterious effects have been described anecdotally as "overwork weakness" and, perhaps, increased muscle damage. Most recent studies have reported the opposite—that a well-controlled exercise program promotes improved strength and endurance in these patients, without inducing short or prolonged periods of muscle weakness.

Studies of exercise tolerance and regular exercise training for patients with muscular dystrophy have been made. During upper-extremity and lower-extremity resistance testing (Wingate anaerobic leg cycling and arm-cranking tests of power and isolated joint static and dynamic dynamometry), a marked decrease in power and strength is evident. Muscle power is approximately 50% of normal for boys and men with Becker's dystrophy and only 25% of normal for boys with Duchenne's dystrophy (ages 8 to 14 years).[61,92] Muscle strength, too, is severely reduced to approximately the same percentages of normal strength (35% for boys with Becker's dystrophy and only 25% for boys with Duchenne's dystrophy).[61,92] Patients with FSH dystrophy are less affected and have approximately 40% to 50% of the strength of age-appropriate normal strength.[61] Testing for power and strength is not well tolerated initially and results in severe fatigability. However, there is no documentation of muscle damage resulting from maximal power and strength testing.

During lower-extremity cycling to determine Vo_2max and cardiac output it was found that boys with Duchenne's dystrophy have only 35% of the normal Vo_2max (14 ml/min per kg versus 40 ml/min per kg).[12,92] Conversely, patients with FSH dystrophy have 50% to 60% of normal Vo_2max, and those with limb-girdle dystrophy have 60% to 70% of normal Vo_2max.[12,30,35] In patients with Duchenne's muscular dystrophy the lowered oxygen consumption appears to be primarily due to a reduction in cardiac output (only 50% to 65% of normal) and in the ability to extract oxygen at the muscle site (50% of normal). Cardiac output is severely reduced because of an inability to sufficiently increase heart rate response. (Maximal heart rate in these children is 135 to 165 beats per minute, whereas a normal maximal heart rate is 190 to 200 beats per minute[92].) The significantly lower maximal heart rate may result from the disease process of the heart or may occur because these children are just unable to continue work because of muscle weakness of the legs.[34,54] Probably both processes affect the heart rate response in these patients. The rate of oxygen extraction decline in patients with Duchenne's dystrophy appears to be primarily related to the decline in overall muscle mass and myoglobin content, not to a decline in the oxidative phosphorylation mechanism (although in deconditioned individuals without atrophy this appears to be an important factor).[34,54] Endurance testing is not well tolerated in these patients, who have severe fatigue of the lower extremities. Muscle damage after short-term testing of Vo_2max has not been reported.

Patients with muscular dystrophy respond normally to exercise but have significantly lowered responses of force production and oxygen utilization. These lowered responses appear to be primarily due to the marked decrease in muscle mass. There appear to be no contraindications to brief periods of low- or high-intensity activity. The accumulation of brief periods of activity into a scheduled, consistent format constitutes exercise training. Exercise training for strength and endurance has been evaluated in patients with muscular dystrophy.

Changes occur as a result of regular strength and endurance training. The result of upper-extremity and lower-extremity muscle strength training (working with free weights four times per week, using a load of 10 RM for five sets) for muscular dystrophy patients appears to be an improvement in muscle strength.[61] The duration of training for the patients with muscular dystrophy ranged from 2 months to 2 years. Weight load was increasingly progressed throughout the training regimen. Upper-extremity and lower-extremity muscle strength improved by approximately 80% in patients who initially had moderately weak muscles (Becker's dystrophy and FSH dystrophy). Patients who were enrolled in resistance training with markedly weak muscles (10% to 20% of normal strength) did not demonstrate a training effect. Some of the patients who had marked muscle weakness indicated subjectively that the resistance training increased their muscle weakness.

An important measure of functioning in patients with muscular dystrophy is endurance, since they become easily fatigued, often as a result *low-intensity* activities of daily living. In normal individuals these activities correspond to less than 30% of Vo_2max, whereas in patients with muscular dystrophy these activities of daily living may correspond to as much as 60% or 70% of Vo_2max, which is not considered a low-intensity level of oxygen consumption. The result of 12 weeks of cycle ergometry (three times per week for 30 minutes [six sets of 5-minute bouts with 2 minutes of rest between sets] at 70% of Vo_2max) for patients with muscular dystrophy appears to be an improvement in oxygen consumption and endurance.[30] Intensity was readjusted at 6 weeks to continue progressive adaptation. Maximal oxygen consumption increased by approximately 25% for patients with limb-girdle muscular dystrophy. The mechanisms for improved oxygen consumption in patients with limb-girdle dystrophy are unknown but probably resulted from an increased cardiac output. Increased utilization of oxygen at the muscle site cannot be dismissed, since dystrophy animal models have demonstrated an increase in capillary and mitochondrial density after endurance training.

Although no muscle damage appears to occur during a bout of exercise, repetitive endurance training of moderate to high intensity (70% of Vo_2max) may result in muscle fiber damage, as indicated by increased creatine kinase and myoglo-

bin concentrations in the blood (30% higher than pretraining values).[30] Comparable and even greater elevations of creatine kinase concentrations do occur in normal individuals who perform training incorporating eccentric muscle action.[1] In normal individuals an elevation of creatine kinase concentration does not indicate irreversible muscle damage.[2] Whether moderate- to high-intensity repetitive exercise training causes a progression of muscle damage in patients with muscular dystrophy is unknown. It is known that this type of exercise training does improve oxygen consumption to within normal ranges for patients with some mild types muscular dystrophy.

It appears that exercise training can improve muscle strength for patients with muscular dystrophy who have minimal to moderate weakness, but exercise training does not appear to be effective for those patients who are "severely weak." Also, oxygen consumption improves with endurance training, but muscle damage may be occurring. The biochemical integrity of the dystrophic muscle appears normal; therefore, as described previously, endurance exercise training may improve the "efficiency" of the muscle. In addition, since training does incorporate motor unit recruitment, it may improve functional muscular performance and reduce deconditioning atrophy.

FACTORS THAT AFFECT MUSCLE MASS, MUSCLE PERFORMANCE, AND EFFECT OF TRAINING

Many factors besides the direct disease process can affect an individual's muscle mass. In the fields of rehabilitation and patient care several factors that can cause muscle atrophy are commonly present in patients. Some of these factors are described here, and the effects of strength and muscle training on several patient groups that commonly have one or more of these "atrophic" factors are discussed. Relevant exercise literature for each patient group and case studies I have performed are included. Patients with the following diseases or disorders are discussed: rheumatoid arthritis, osteoarthritis, renal failure, chronic fatigue syndrome, spinal cord injury (quadriplegia and paraplegia), and mental retardation. In all these patients the untrained state results in levels of muscle strength and oxygen consumption that can be similar to those in individuals with ALS and muscular dystrophy.[40]

Atrophic Factors

The effect of abnormal muscle activation in the motor neuron disease ALS is described earlier in this chapter. Whenever muscle activation is interrupted for a prolonged period, muscle atrophy occurs. Muscle activation can be interrupted not only by a disease process or an injury to the spinal cord and peripheral nerve but also as a result of severe inactivity. Studies of individuals during bed rest have demonstrated that muscle mass is lost when muscle activity becomes restricted.[83,84] Patients with some diseases and disorders have the characteristic of sedentary behavior. In most cases the inactivity is brought about because movement causes discomfort or fatigue, or both. Patients who have pain or severe fatigue during activities of daily living and ambulation, if unsupervised and unmotivated, avoid movement. The result is specific muscle atrophy (that is, decreased mass and metabolic function) that may lead to contractures and biomechanical deformities and, eventually, to physical deformities of the joints and skeleton that may further restrict movement.

A possible cause of muscle atrophy besides sedentary behavior is an impaired diet. Diets that are devoid of protein or total calories, or both, can result in muscle atrophy. Many patients, especially elderly persons and patients receiving chemotherapy, may have restricted diets. An improper diet can affect bone density as well as muscle mass and can lead to osteoporosis and spontaneous fractures. Poor diet can be a result of economic limitations, the inability to perform the meal-making activity of daily living (too much energy is expended or too much pain accompanies the movements), or decreased appetite caused by the disease process or medications, or both. Practitioners must consistently perform nutritional evaluations of patients as part of the evaluation and management plan. In addition, all direct and synergistic actions of medications should be evaluated for the side effect of appetite suppression.

As previously stated, some medications may have the side effect of appetite suppression (for example, many of the chemotherapy agents) and may affect muscle mass indirectly. Other medications have the side effect of muscle catabolism or myopathic action. One commonly prescribed group of medications is corticosteroids, which are used to control inflammation and suppress the immune response. Corticosteroids have a catabolic effect on muscle, bone, and connective tissue if administered in moderate to high dosages.[14]

DISEASE-SPECIFIC BENEFITS OF EXERCISE TRAINING FOR SEVERELY DECONDITIONED PATIENTS

In this section exercise training and manipulation of other factors such as diet and medication use are described for patients with specific diseases who are severely deconditioned.

Rheumatoid Arthritis

Patients with rheumatoid arthritis have markedly reduced maximal aerobic capacity and muscle strength. It is estimated that untrained patients with rheumatoid arthritis have deficits of 40% to 50% in aerobic capacity and have a similar decline in muscle strength of both upper and lower extremities.

Physical activity, specifically exercise involving weight bearing and muscle resistance, is essential either to develop or to maintain muscle strength and cardiorespiratory endurance. Patients with rheumatoid arthritis have often been recommended for participation in exercise programs concentrating on nonresisted active range of motion exercise and "rest therapy."[57,91] This type of medical management is intended to decrease the likelihood of exacerbation of joint inflammation, joint pain, and cartilage destruction while maintaining or improving joint range of motion.[53,72,91]

Recent research has demonstrated that patients with rheumatoid arthritis can participate in partial weight-bearing (cycle ergometry and aquatic aerobics)[25,38,56] and full weight-bearing

CASE STUDY 1

Case Study 1 was designed to evaluate the effectiveness of combining reduced corticosteroid use with a supervised exercise training program for muscular strength and endurance in a severely deconditioned 37-year-old woman with rheumatoid arthritis.

Before initiation of treatment baseline data were obtained, including measures of muscle strength, joint active range of motion, joint circumference, Vo_2max, and functional activity level. The patient came to medical attention with bilateral knee pain and difficulty rising from a chair; she was unable to rise from the floor. It was thought that both muscle weakness and joint pain limited her functional status. The woman had been receiving prednisone therapy (15 to 20 mg per day) for an entire year before initiation of the training study. Prednisone therapy at this dosage controlled inflammation, but at dosages below this level the patient had an increase in inflammatory symptoms. The patient's prednisone dosage was reduced to 2.5 mg per day during the course of the investigation. Before the study the patient had been taking 105 mg of corticosteroid each week (all oral prednisone), and during the study she took an estimated total dose of 25 mg of corticosteroid each week (17.5 mg oral prednisone and approximately 6 to 8 mg iontophoresed dexamethasone). The patient received gold therapy (9 mg per day) and sulindac (Clinoril [200 mg twice a day]) (nonsteroidal antiinflammatory drug [NSAID]) therapy throughout the investigation.

The supervised training program was 12 weeks in duration (three times per week) and consisted of the following:

1. Endurance component: Cycle ergometry at an intensity of 65% of Vo_2max and progressed every 2 weeks; initial duration was 10 minutes, and final duration was 45 minutes
2. Strength component: From initial maximal isokinetic exercise at fast speed and low resistance (240 degrees per sec) to final maximal isokinetic exercise at moderate speed and moderate resistance (120 degrees per sec) for four sets of 20 knee joint flexion and extension repetitions
3. Antiinflammation component: Iontophoresis of both knee joints for 20 minutes three times per week with delivery of approximately 1 to 1.5 mg of dexamethasone sodium phosphate

Results

The patient had a reduction of 10 kg in her body weight. Initially the patient had 35% of normal age-matched strength in her weaker leg and 60% in the stronger leg. At the end of the study muscle strength in her weaker leg had increased and was 55% of normal age- and weight-matched strength; strength in her stronger leg was 80% of normal. Initially the patient had a Vo_2max of 17.8 ml/kg per minute and a ventilatory threshold of 7.2 ml/kg per minute. Her Vo_2max and ventilatory threshold both increased by 50% (up to 26.4 ml/kg per minute) and 130% (up to 16.8 ml/kg per minute), respectively. In addition, her joint active range of motion increased in both knees, and the swelling markedly decreased in both knee joints to the normal circumferences of weight- and age-matched women in good health.

(aerobic dance and walking) aerobic conditioning programs[63,73] without exacerbating the disease. The results of these types of exercise training programs are improvements in aerobic capacity and muscular endurance. In addition, long-term physical training (for more than 4 years) that emphasizes weight-bearing activities actually has resulted in a slowed progression of the destructive changes in the joints, as analyzed by radiograph and compared to the control group of sedentary patients with rheumatoid arthritis.[68,70] Muscle strengthening exercise programs

have not been as well studied. Strengthening programs that have been evaluated are those incorporating isometric (nonmoving) contractions. Many health and medical practitioners do not recommend the use of isotonic (dynamic) strengthening exercise, since an increase in joint stress and exacerbation of joint inflammation may occur. However, movement of the human body requires dynamic muscular contractions.

Drug therapy is currently used in several forms to treat rheumatoid arthritis and is often successful in modulating synovial inflammation. However, when large dosages of corticosteroids are taken, systemic side effects are of concern. Corticosteroid use has been associated with weight gain,[14] muscle weakness and atrophy,[14] and behavioral changes.[88] The observed side effects of corticosteroid use further decrease the patient's ability to perform physical activity.

Osteoarthritis

Patients with osteoarthritis have markedly reduced maximal aerobic capacities and muscle strength. It is estimated that untrained osteoarthritic patients have a

CASE STUDY 2

Case Study 2 was designed to evaluate the effectiveness of a muscle strengthening and endurance training program for on a 65-year-old severely deconditioned woman with osteoarthritis.

Before initiation of treatment, baseline data were obtained, including measures of muscle strength, joint active range of motion, joint circumference, Vo_2max during submaximal-intensity exercise, and functional activity level. The patient came to medical attention with unilateral knee pain and difficulty rising from a chair; she was unable to rise from the floor. It was thought that muscle weakness in relation to body weight limited her functional status. The woman had been receiving nonsteroidal antiinflammatory drug (NSAID) therapy (ibuprofen 800 mg three times daily) for 8 weeks before initiation of physical therapy. Ibuprofen at this dosage controlled pain and inflammation. The patient's ibuprofen dosage remained the same during the course of the investigation.

The supervised physical therapy program was 6 weeks in duration (three times per week) and consisted of the following:

1. Endurance component: Cycle ergometry at an intensity of 65% of Vo_2max, progressed every 2 weeks; initially duration was 10 minutes, and final duration was 45 minutes
2. Strength components: First, initial maximal concentric isokinetic exercise at moderate speed and moderate resistance (120 degrees per sec) and final eccentric isokinetic exercise at low speed and high resistance (60 degrees per sec) for four sets of 20 knee joint flexion and extension repetitions and, second, initial one-quarter squats from standing position, ending with three-quarter squats from standing position for four sets of 20
3. Antiinflammation component: Ice massage and pulsed ultrasound (20% ratio) administered to both knee joints

Results

The patient had a reduction in body weight of 8 kg (initial weight, 106 kg). Initially the patient had 70% of normal age-matched strength in her affected leg and 100% in the stronger leg. At the end of the study, muscle strength in her weaker leg had increased to 100% of age- and weight-matched normal strength and in her stronger leg the muscle strength was 120% of normal. Initially the patient had a Vo_2max of 15.8 ml/kg per minute. Her Vo_2max and ventilatory threshold both increased by 40% (up to 22.2 ml/kg per minute). In addition, her joint active range of motion in the affected knee (15 to 75 degrees initially, with bony block at the end of flexion range) increased slightly (ending at 5 to 75 degrees). The swelling markedly decreased in the affected knee joint.

deficit of 20% to 30% in aerobic capacity and a similar decline in muscle strength of both upper and lower extremities. Only one third of the deficit in Vo_2max can be explained by decreased cardiac function.[62] Therefore most researchers have concluded that these patients have detrained skeletal muscle, and it appears that type 2 muscle fibers are most severely affected.[69] However, patients with osteoarthritis can be trained to improve muscle strength[15,49] and aerobic capacity.[63]

Recommendations for types of exercise training for patients with osteoarthritis are similar to those for patients with rheumatoid arthritis, except that patients with osteoarthritis are encouraged to participate more in isotonic strengthening programs. Health and medical professionals treat osteoarthritis more aggressively than rheumatoid arthritis, since osteoarthritis has a slower disease course and the inflammatory component is nearly absent. In addition, the medications that patients with osteoarthritis generally take are not myopathic. Recently, nonsteroidal antiinflammatory drugs (NSAIDs) were the drugs of choice for reducing pain and inflammation in these patients. However, current data suggest that when the inflammatory process is not active, analgesics that are not antiinflammatory agents appear to be as effective as NSAIDs in combating joint pain.

Renal Failure

Patients with chronic renal failure have markedly reduced maximal aerobic capacity and muscle strength. It is estimated that untrained patients with end-stage renal failure have a deficit in aerobic capacity of 40% to 50%[96] and a similar decline in muscle strength of both upper and lower extremities. Many studies have indicated that there are high incidences of muscle atrophy and malnutrition in patients with chronic renal failure. In addition, there appears to be an impaired nutritive skeletal muscle blood flow in these patients during exercise of submaximal and maximal intensity.[8] Therefore most researchers have concluded that these patients have detrained skeletal muscle, and it appears that type 2b mus-

cle fibers are most severely affected.[8] Whether patients with chronic renal failure can be trained to improve muscle strength and aerobic capacity without prior correction of the inherent anemia or skeletal muscle blood flow, or both, is not known.[8,59]

Recommendations of types of exercise training for patients with end-stage renal failure, therefore, are not nearly as available as for patients with rheumatoid arthritis and osteoarthritis. Investigators who have evaluated exercise tolerance and limitations to exercise assert that the limiting factors must be addressed before a regimented strengthening or endurance program is initiated. These factors are limited blood flow to skeletal muscle, anemia, and in many cases poor nutritional status. Bradley et al.[8] recommended the use of vasodilators to increase blood flow. Metra et al.[59] recommended the use of human erythropoietin to improve anemia. Monteon et al.[65] did not observe abnormal metabolism of skeletal muscle but did note that these patients have muscle wasting resulting primarily from reduced energy intake that in some cases leads to malnutrition. If nutritional status, skeletal muscle blood flow, and hemoglobin concentration can be normalized, these patients may be trainable. Once an exercise program is initiated, it is imperative that higher energy levels be consumed.

Patients with chronic renal failure do tolerate cycling and treadmill exercise, but to a much lower level than normal. Zanconato et al.[96] found that children with end-stage renal failure were able to tolerate a maximal work load on cycle ergometer of only 25% (30 watts) of that for age-matched normal children (115 watts). Maximal heart rate was also significantly different: the end-stage renal patients attained maximal heart rates of 183 beats per minute, whereas normal heart rates were 202 beats per minute. Therapists must be aware that in these patients much lower work loads are required, to stimulate high heart rates. Training levels should be near the ventilatory anaerobic threshold, which is usually attained at 40% to 60% of maximal work load. Even at these extremely low work loads initial endurance is poor when duration of exercise is less than 5 to 10 minutes.

Muscle strengthening exercise, as well as cycling and treadmill exercise, should be part of the therapeutic intervention. Once again, however, the therapist should approach the training in a conservative manner initially, using the patient's body or body segment as the resistive force. The types of exercises may imitate activities of daily living that are difficult for the patient to perform. The clinical sign for appropriate repetitions and load is a sense of muscle fatigue related to lactic acid accumulation when the patient performs concentric activities. *When exercises such as repetitive squatting are intended to control the body weight, eccentric muscle control is required. The patient has a sense of fatigue but not the burning sensation associated with concentric muscle action. The sense of fatigue is that there is a loss of muscle control, and muscle quivering may occur. Rest between exercise bouts usually allows for full recovery.*

Chronic Fatigue Syndrome

Chronic fatigue syndrome appears to occur after certain viral infections (coxsackie virus and herpes virus). Clinical findings of weakness, lethargy, and fatigue during and after exercise activity have been reported. Patients complain for many months or years of flulike symptoms for which no definite cause can be found.

Patients with chronic fatigue syndrome have somewhat reduced maximal aerobic capacity; however, upper-extremity isometric muscle strength does not appear to be affected. It is estimated that when compared to normal individuals, untrained patients with chronic fatigue syndrome have a deficit in aerobic capacity of less than 20%[81] and have no decline in muscle strength of the upper extremities.[55] These patients appear to have a reduced cardiac function (maximal heart rate response) of 5% to 25%, depending on the mode of exercise testing.[64,81] In addition, Montague et al.[64] suspected decreased function of skeletal muscle metabolism that may result in an abnormally high level of acidosis during exercise of moderate to high intensity. Perceived effort during work does not appear to be abnormal for isolated isometric upper-extremity exercise tasks.[55] Yet, during whole-body dynamic ex-

ercising tasks, these patients perceive the work to be much harder than do normal individuals and consequently perform at a lower level.[64,81] Skeletal and cardiac muscles of these patients appear to be normal at rest but do not respond normally during exercise of moderate to high intensity. Although a lower heart rate response for maximal exercise occurs, heart rate response at any given submaximal work load is unclear. Montague et al.[64] found a slow acceleration of heart rate response and fatigue of exercising muscles long before peak heart rate occurred. The researchers observed that this response was compatible with data obtained in the study of patients with latent viruses.[64] Montague et al.[64] hypothesized that these effects on the cardiac system might be attributed to a blunting of the autonomic control of pacemaker cells. Riley et al[81] did not find a lowered chronotropic effect during exercise of submaximal intensity. They found that heart rate response was more accelerated than normal, which is similar to expected findings in individuals who are highly detrained. Regardless of the cardiac response, performance outcome appears to match the profile of detrained, sedentary normal individuals. However, individuals with chronic fatigue syndrome describe severe fatigue during and after moderate- and high-intensity activity.

No studies have been reported on the trainability of muscle strength, aerobic capacity, or perception of fatigue in patients with chronic fatigue syndrome. Investigators who have evaluated exercise tolerance and limitations to exercise have noted either a sluggish or an accelerated cardiac response, lowered maximal heart rates, and early perceived fatigue of skeletal muscle.

Patients with chronic fatigue syndrome are able to perform cycling and treadmill exercise. *It is imperative that therapists be aware that heart rate response may not be an accurate indicator of work load. Therefore it is highly recommended that perception of muscle fatigue and ventilatory response be used as a determinant in selecting an initial training work load.* For a training effect to occur, a proper intensity and appropriate duration and frequency of exercise must be assigned. The initial intensity selected may be conservative, since it appears that per-

CASE STUDY 3

Case Study 3 was designed to evaluate the effectiveness of an endurance training program for a 25-year-old woman with diagnosed chronic fatigue syndrome. She was a physical therapy student and was enrolled in a decelerated academic and clinical program. The endurance training program was begun 15 months after initial symptoms became evident.

Before initiation of treatment, baseline data were obtained during submaximal-intensity exercise, including estimates of Vo_2max and perceived effort during a three-stage cycle ergometer exercise test.

The supervised exercise program was 10 weeks in duration (three times per week) and consisted of an endurance component. The mode was cycle ergometry at an intensity of 65% of Vo_2max (70 watts), which corresponded to increased ventilation. This intensity was progressed every 2 weeks by determining the work load that increased ventilation and corresponded to an increased perceived level of muscular exertion. The initial duration of exercise was 20 minutes, and final duration was 45 minutes.

Initially the woman had an estimated Vo_2max of 30.8 ml/kg per minute. During the initial three-stage submaximal-intensity exercise evaluation, her heart rate response during stage 1 (150 kg-m [25 watts]) was 110 beats per minute and the Borg perceived exertion rating was 13, that is, somewhat hard. Her heart rate and perceived exertion responses during stage 2 (300 kg-m-[50 watts]) were 128 beats per minute and 15, that is, hard, respectively. The woman's heart rate response during stage 3 (450 kg-m [75 watts]) was 148 beats per minute, and rating of perceived exertion was 17, that is, very hard. The woman's initial Vo_2max was similar to reported values in the literature, and her subjective perception of the work as compared to heart rate response was higher than that normally expected for an individual of the same age group and fitness level.

Results

After the 10-week training program that consisted of cycle ergometry exercise her estimated Vo_2max increased by 26% (up to 38.8 ml/kg per minute). During the final three-stage submaximal-intensity exercise evaluation, her heart rate response during stage 1 (150 kg-m [25 watts]) was 96 beats per minute and the Borg perceived exertion rating was 11, that is, fairly light. Her heart rate and perceived exertion responses during stage 2 (300 kg-m [50 watts]) were 115 beats per minute and 12, that is, between fairly light and somewhat hard, respectively. The woman's heart rate response during stage 3 (450 kg-m [75 watts]) was 134 beats per minute, and the Borg rating of perceived exertion was 15, that is, hard. The woman's rating of perceived exertion as compared to heart rate response was still higher than that expected for the normal population but was not nearly as exaggerated as the rating obtained before training. Subjectively the student did describe fewer symptoms of fatigue and lethargy after completion of the exercise training program. She felt strongly that exercise was helpful for her in maintaining her studies and other personal activities.

ceived effort does not always match physiologic stress in these patients. This might be of some concern to practicing therapists. However, once an exercise regimen is begun and adaptations occur, intensity can be increased and work load optimized, as long as the exercise is tolerable to the patient.

Muscle strengthening is not usually a part of the therapeutic intervention unless specific deficits are noted. If the patient is unable to perform specific tasks because of muscle weakness, the therapist might consider, as for patients with chronic renal failure, a conservative approach, initially using the patient's body or body segment as the resistive force.

Spinal Cord Injury

Patients who have had spinal cord injury resulting in paralysis of the upper or lower limbs, or both, depend almost exclusively on upper-body activity for functioning. In addition, upper-body activity is necessary for locomotion and fitness training. Clinical findings for these patients depend on the cord level of the injury but in most cases include muscle paralysis and weakness, decreased muscular and cardiovascular endurance, and decreased ability to perform activities of daily living. In addition, medical problems include increased incidences of skin lesions and pulmonary dysfunction related directly to being wheelchair bound.[58]

Patients with spinal cord injury have a reduced maximum aerobic capacity, which, as mentioned earlier, is strongly correlated with level and completeness of cord lesion. Several factors are responsible for the decreased aerobic capacity, including decreased cardiac ability (innervation affected), decreased active muscle mass (paralyzed muscles), and decondition atrophy of the nonparalyzed skeletal and cardiac muscles.[43] Muscle strength is also affected, again depending on completeness and level of cord injury.[29] In addition, deconditioning of nonparalyzed skeletal muscle resulting in atrophy does occur in these patients.[18,20] It is estimated that untrained patients with spinal cord injury have a deficit in aerobic capacity of greater than 70% (quadriplegia) and 45% (paraplegia) as compared to normal aerobic capacity[11,26,42,51] and a decline of approximately 25% in muscle strength and power of nonparalyzed upper extremities (paraplegia).[33] Patients with spinal cord injury above the first thoracic (T-1) level have reduced cardiac function, since lesions above the T-1 level interrupt all sympathetic nerves that innervate the heart. As a result cardioacceleration (heart rate) and force of contraction (stroke volume) are less than appropriate for the metabolic need during exercise.

The ability to thermoregulate is impaired in patients with spinal cord injury.[23] The higher and more complete the lesion is, the greater the degree of thermoregulatory dysfunction is. Therefore when a patient with a spinal cord injury is exposed to a hot environment during exercise, core and skin temperatures increase at an abnormally high rate. These increases are due to decreased venous return of blood from lower extremities coupled with loss of vasomotor and sudomotor control over areas of insensate skin. The result is a decrease in cardiac output.[87]

As mentioned earlier, cardiac response is not normal in patients with quadriplegia (injured at cord level T-1 and above). Maximal heart rates range from 100 to 125 beats per minute during wheelchair ergometry and arm-cranking exercises.[11,42,51] Heart rate response is normal for patients with paraplegia who have lesions at low and moderate cord levels. Maximal heart rates during wheelchair ergometry and arm-cranking exercise ranged from 160 to 190 beats per minute.[32,42] However, cardiac output and stroke volume may be reduced by as much as 10% to 25% in patients with paraplegia, primarily because of blood pooling in the lower limbs that results from inactivity of the venous "muscle pump."[41]

Few studies have reported on the trainability of muscle strength and aerobic capacity in patients with spinal cord injury. Wheelchair-bound athletes have been evaluated and have much greater upper-body strength and power than normal.[18,33] Aerobic capacity can also be much higher than normal. Measurements of Vo_2max are greater than 50 ml/kg per minute in some competitively elite individuals with paraplegia.[26,32] Aerobic capacity in the sedentary wheelchair-bound patient is trainable. DiCarlo[22] demonstrated an improvement in aerobic capacity of greater than 90% in patients with quadriplegia who performed arm-cranking exercise. Earlier studies demonstrated the trainability of aerobic capacity in patients with paraplegia but improvements were not as dramatic.[22] Nilsson, Staff, and Pruett[67] found an improvement of approximately 20% in the aerobic capacity of patients with long-term paraplegia after the patients participated in an arm-cranking exercise program. Hooker and Wells[44] found similar improvements (12%) in a mixed group of patients with quadriplegia and paraplegia, but the results were not significant.

Other modes of aerobic training have been tried for patients with spinal cord injury. Cooney and Walker[16] evaluated the effect of low-resistance hydraulic arm exercise on oxygen consumption in

CASE STUDY 4

Case Study 4 was designed to evaluate the effectiveness of a muscle strengthening, endurance, and gait training program for a 52-year-old man with diagnosed lumbar spinal stenosis that resulted in lower-limb paralysis. The patient had progressive sensory and motor dysfunction for 3 months before loss of bowel and bladder control and lower-limb paralysis. The patient underwent several laminectomies at various levels and was referred for outpatient physical therapy 6 weeks after the surgical intervention.

Before initiation of treatment, baseline data were obtained for muscle strength of the trunk and all lower-extremity muscles bilaterally, and an estimate of Vo_2max at submaximal exercise intensity was performed by using a modified cycle ergometer as an arm-crank ergometer. In addition, transfers, bed mobility, sitting and standing balance, and gait were assessed.

The supervised physical therapy program was 16 weeks in duration (two 1-hour sessions per day, 5 days per week [10 total hours per week]) and consisted of muscle strengthening, endurance, and functional activity components. Initially the strengthening protocol incorporated concentric contractions against gravity or with gravity eliminated (depending on strength of muscle), eccentric contractions, and functional electrical stimulation (FES) for muscles with grades of 0, trace, and poor. As the patient's strength progressed, closed-chained concentric and eccentric contractions in functional patterns were used. Initially the mode used for endurance training was a wheelchair and an arm-crank ergometer. As the patient's lower-extremity muscle strength improved, cycle ergometry and gait exercise were used for cardiovascular endurance training. Functional activities were used for strength and endurance training. These included bed mobility activities, sitting balance, transfer from wheelchair to mat table and back, wheelchair activities, sit-to-stand and back-to-sit transfers, quadruped balance, standing balance, and gait exercise (parallel bars, walker, and crutches).

Initially the man had the following manual muscle strength ratings for the right leg and hip:

Gluteus maximus: Poor minus
Gluteus medius: Poor minus
Iliopsoas: Poor
Adductors: Poor plus
Quadriceps: Poor minus
Hamstrings: Poor minus
Gastrocnemius: Poor minus
Anterior tibialis: 0

Initial strength ratings for the left leg and hip were the following:

Gluteus maximus: Poor
Gluteus medius: Poor
Iliopsoas: Poor plus
Adductors: Poor plus
Quadriceps: Poor plus
Hamstrings: Poor
Gastrocnemius: Poor plus
Anterior tibialis: Poor plus

The estimated Vo_2max obtained during arm-crank ergometry was 15.8 ml/kg per minute. Blood pressure and heart rate responses were normal during the submaximal-intensity exercise evaluation. The man's initial Vo_2max was similar to reported values for patients with paraplegia who had low fitness levels. Initially the man was independent in bed mobility, wheelchair activities, and wheelchair-to-mat-and-back transfers. He had moderate sitting balance, required moderate assistance from one individual to go from sit to stand and back, was unable to attain standing balance, required moderate assistance from one individual for gait exercise in parallel bars, and was unable to perform gait exercise with a walker.

CASE STUDY 4 — cont'd

Results

After the 16-week training program his muscle strength improved for both lower extremities, aerobic capacity increased, and his level of functional activity improved. The patient's final strength ratings for the right leg and hip were the following:

Gluteus maximus: Fair
Gluteus medius: Poor plus
Iliopsoas: Fair
Adductors: Fair
Quadriceps: Fair
Hamstrings: Fair
Gastrocnemius: Fair
Anterior Tibialis: Poor

Final ratings for the left leg and hip strength were the following:

Gluteus maximus: Good minus
Gluteus medius: Fair
Iliopsoas: Good
Adductors: Good
Quadriceps: Good
Hamstrings: Good minus
Gastrocnemius: Good
Anterior tibialis: Good

His estimated Vo_2max, which was obtained during cycle ergometry, increased by 60% (up to 25.3 ml/kg per minute). At the end of the physical therapy program he was independent in going from sit to stand and back, had normal sitting balance and moderate standing balance, and was independent with a walker and crutches. Subjectively the patient described having much greater endurance, strength, and independence. The patient was initially somewhat depressed and did not believe he would be able to stand and walk. After the 16-week program he was quite "upbeat" about his accomplishments.

patients with quadriplegia. Improvements were in excess of 40% after 12 weeks of training. Other, predominantly upper-body exercise such as swimming has been used in training for patients with paraplegia, but few data exist that document the effectiveness of this training mode.[71]

As described earlier, cardiovascular response is less than optimal in patients with quadriplegia and paraplegia. The use of functional electrical stimulation (FES) of the lower extremities independently or as an adjunct to arm-crank ergometry training has been proposed to improve aerobic capacity and reduce cardiac strain.[80] The use of FES of the lower extremities in conjunction with arm-cranking exercise can increase cardiac output by 20% to 30% at near-maximal levels of exercise intensity.[19] When the use of arm-cranking exercise alone is compared with the use of the hybrid exercise of arm cranking and FES, however, Vo_2max is not altered.[19] Training that incorporates nonvolitional contractions of the lower extremities in pedaling a cycle ergometer can result in an increase in aerobic capacity.[78] However, this type of training does not enhance upper-extremity aerobic or work capacity.[78] Improvements or advantages gained during FES of the paralyzed lower extremities do not appear to carry over during bouts of combination arm and leg activity for oxygen consumption or during regular training for upper-extremity maximal aerobic capacity. Nonetheless, FES may enhance the life-style and independence of many patients with quadriplegia or paraplegia by means of multiple-channeled, computer-controlled gait and cycling systems. Investigations and implementation of these relatively new FES systems are progressing.[74,75]

Patients with spinal cord injuries are able to perform arm cranking, wheelchair exercise, FES cycling, and FES lower-extremity exercise. However, it is imperative that therapists be aware that in patients with quadriplegia heart rate response is not an accurate indicator of work load. In addition, during assessment of aerobic capacity in patients with quadriplegia it is important to increase work load at increments of 4 to 6 watts for each stage of arm-crank exercise. If the work load increment is increased by more than 8 to 10 watts, an accurate estimation of Vo_2max is not obtained.[51] Since heart rate response is abnormal in patients with quadriplegia, it is recommended that perception of muscle fatigue be used in selecting an initial training work load. In addition, the therapist must be cognizant of the exercise environment, since the ability to regulate temperature is impaired in patients with quadriplegia and in many patients with paraplegia. The exercise environment should be controlled, or clothing modified. One recommendation for clothing is to use a microclimate cooling vest to facilitate torso heat loss.[95]

The initial exercise intensity selected for untrained patients with spinal cord injury should be conservative, since cardiovascular response and thermoregulatory control may not match levels of physiologic stress in these patients. Once an exercise regimen is begun and adaptations occur, intensity can be increased and work load optimized, as long as exercise is tolerable to the patient.

The therapist must consider orthopedic injuries resulting from overuse of the shoulder, elbow, and wrist joints. These are fairly common in wheelchair-bound athletes and in individuals with spinal cord injury who are initiating exercise programs. Alternating training modes and, perhaps,

incorporating activities with limited joint stress, such as swimming, are recommended. Frequency and duration must be monitored so that when it is time for progression of exercise, the total exercise time does not increase by more than 20%.

Specific muscle strengthening, along with training for activities of daily living (for example, wheelchair transfers, bed mobility, dressing, and grooming), is an integral part of the therapeutic intervention. In general, muscle strengthening should be no different for nonparalyzed muscles than for normal muscles. However, after the trauma of a spinal cord injury the individual is almost always placed on a regimen of bed rest for a lengthy period until the spine can be stabilized. During this period of immobilization nonparalyzed muscles become weak. Therefore to prevent muscle damage and excessive soreness, initial training must be somewhat conservative. After a few training bouts muscle strengthening of the nonparalyzed muscles can be more aggressive.

Incomplete spinal cord injuries may result in muscles with excessive spasticity and flaccid (denervated) muscle. The muscles that have partial innervation can be trained by means of volitional contractions, but electrical stimulation has also been used. Electrical stimulation has been shown to improve muscle strength and reduce tone in patients with exaggerated extensor tone.[3] Muscle strength and hypertrophy can also be increased in flaccid or paralyzed muscles by the use of electrical stimulation and resistance training.[3,78] Muscle strengthening of uninvolved and involved musculature should eventually be oriented toward functional task performance. The ultimate goal of the patient is to be able to manipulate his or her body independently without excessive fatigue and with a reduced possibility of injury.

Mental Retardation

Individuals with mental retardation have a higher-than-normal incidence of obesity, an elevated mortality rate, and lower-than-normal levels of cardiovascular fitness. Reported clinical findings include muscle weakness, poor coordination, abnormal muscle tone (hypotonia and hypertonia),

CASE STUDY 5

Case Study 5 was designed to evaluate the effectiveness of a general fitness program for a 4-year-old girl with diagnosed Williams syndrome. Williams syndrome is a rare condition that occurs in approximately 1:50,000 live births.[79] Williams syndrome is characterized by the following signs and symptoms:

Cardiovascular disorders

Growth and developmental delays

Mild mental retardation in many cases

Poor visuospatial and motor skill development

Abnormal muscle tone and muscle weakness

"Elfin" facial features

Unusual, expressive vocabulary

The diagnosis was made when the girl was 8 months old, and an early-childhood intervention program was initiated at that time. Muscle strength and endurance were not the main focus of the intervention program, although the patient had hypotonia and muscle weakness. The initial focus was on fine and gross motor skills, visuospatial processing, and speech. Intervention was continued through special education in the school system when the child reached 3 years of age.

Before initiation of treatment, baseline data were obtained, including measures of muscle strength and descriptive evaluation of functional activities. The patient came to medical attention with decreased muscle strength in the trunk and upper and lower extremities, poor dynamic standing balance, and abnormal gait. It was thought that the decreased muscle strength paired with poor balance made it extremely difficult for this patient to play independently on age-appropriate toys such as slides and tricycles, thereby limiting her functional status. The girl had been receiving synthroid therapy (0.0375 mg per day) from the age of 8 months, after mild hypothyroidism had been diagnosed. Synthroid therapy, however, does not negatively affect muscle or connective tissue. The patient was also on regimens of various stool softeners for constipation from the age of 4 months, but it was thought that her decreased abdominal strength may also have affected her ability to evacuate fecal material. Drug therapy was not manipulated during the period of this case study.

The supervised training program was 16 weeks in duration (three times per week) and consisted of the following:

1. Pool therapy: Kicking, jumping from poolside, and practicing freestyle swimming stroke for 30   minutes

2. Therapeutic exercise: Climbing up and down the slide, playing on swings, and hanging on rings (total time of 30 minutes)

Results

After the training program the patient was able to perform playground activities of sliding and swinging independently. Her abdominal muscle strength improved, and she was able to perform 10 independent sit-ups, whereas before the training she had needed minimal assistance to perform a single sit-up repetition. After treatment the patient was able to attempt jumping and required minimal assistance to leave the ground, whereas before treatment the patient had been unable to jump and would not attempt a vertical jump maneuver.

poor endurance, and lethargy and fatigue during and after exercise activity. Psychologic and sociologic research investigations have documented high incidences of learning disabilities and disruptive behavior in these individuals.

Individuals with genetic conditions that are associated with mental retardation, such as Down's syndrome, commonly have a high incidence of heart and blood vessel abnormalities.[17] In addition, maximal heart rate response is slightly lower (by 5% to 10%) for these patients than for age-matched individuals in good health.[28,52] Therefore many patients with mental retardation have reduced maximal aerobic capacity. The percentage of decrease in oxygen consumption varies with the severity of the cardiac abnormalities, but oxygen consumption has been estimated to be approximately 25% less than that in sedentary age-matched normal individuals.[28,77] In addition to cardiac abnormalities, the propensity to be quite sedentary exists for these patients.[76] Findings of increased cardiac abnormalities coupled with inactive life-styles and poor diet have led to concern about the health of aging persons who are mentally retarded. The mortality rate for persons with mental retardation between the fifth and seventh decades of life is two to four times that for normal individuals.[13]

In addition to decreased cardiac function, muscle strength and endurance appear to be impaired. However, only limited data are available concerning evaluation of muscle strength in individuals with mental retardation. Jansma[45] reported that muscle strength can be impaired by as much as 50% in individuals with severe mental retardation. Hypotonia (low muscle tone) is common in patients with conditions such as Down's syndrome, which might explain some of the inherent muscle weakness in these individuals.[66] Muscle weakness appears to be greatest in the trunk and proximal limb musculature. In addition, many individuals with mental retardation have balance and visuospatial difficulties, which might explain the poor motor coordination observed in these individuals.[93]

Few studies have reported on the trainability of aerobic capacity in patients with mental retarda-

tion, and none was found that reported on muscle strength or motor coordination. Investigators who have evaluated exercise tolerance have noted lowered maximal heart rates and have had difficulty obtaining valid results from field-type aerobic fitness tests such as tests of walking or running distance.[27]

Patients with mental retardation are able to perform a variety of exercises and activities, including sports, stationary cycling, and treadmill exercise. It is imperative that therapists be aware that maximal heart rate response is lower than normal in these patients. Therefore, to select an appropriate intensity of exercise, the target heart rate response must reflect this lowered maximal response. Heart rate monitors (watch type) have been successfully used in a minimally supervised training program. The patients were capable of maintaining appropriate heart rates while exercising on a stationary cycle.[77] As with any group of patients, it is critical that exercise intensity be increased on a regular basis (every 2 to 6 weeks) and that appropriate duration (20 to 40 minutes) and frequency (3 or 4 times each week) of exercise be obtained.

Muscle strengthening should be a part of the therapeutic intervention. As mentioned earlier, weakness of the trunk and proximal limb musculature appears to be prevalent in patients with mental retardation.[66] Although the results of trunk muscle weakness are not well documented, it may lead to disfiguring and functionally impairing conditions such as scoliosis.[39] *Exercise that incorporates trunk stability in both static and dynamic functions should be included as a daily activity. Such exercise might include sports and recreational activities (such as swimming and hippotherapy–horseback riding) or specific muscle strengthening exercises that make use of the patient's body or body segment as the resistive force.*

SUMMARY

Limited published data exist concerning the responses of patients with severe deconditioning to exercise and exercise training. It does appear that many of these patients can improve muscle strength and endurance through exercise training.

Specific concerns and precautions for each patient group have been discussed, and strategies for cardiovascular and muscle strengthening for each patient group were described in the text and case studies.

REFERENCES

1. Armstrong R: Mechanisms of exercise-induced delayed-onset muscular soreness, *Med Sci Sports Exerc* 16:529, 1984.
2. Armstrong R: Muscle damage and endurance events, *Sports Med* 3:370, 1986.
3. Bajd T et al: Use of functional electrical stimulation in the rehabilitation of patients with incomplete spinal cord injuries, *J Biomed Eng* 11:95, 1989.
4. Belanger AY, McComas AJ: Neuromuscular function in limb girdle dystrophy, *J Neurol Neurosurg Psychiatry* 48:1253, 1985.
5. Bernstein LP, Antel JP: Motor neuron disease: decremental responses to repetitive nerve stimulation, *Neurology* 31:202, 1981.
6. Bobowick AR, Brody JA: Epidemiology of motor-neuron disease, *New Engl J Med* 288:1047, 1973.
7. Bohannon RW: Results of resistance exercise on patient with amyotrophic lateral sclerosis, *Phys Ther* 63:965, 1983.
8. Bradley JR et al: Impaired nutritive skeletal muscle blood flow in patients with chronic renal failure, *Clin Sci* 79:239, 1990.
9. Brain WR, Croft P, Wilkinson M: The course and outcome of motor neuron disease. In Norris FH, Kurland LT, editors: *Motor neuron diseases: research on amyotrophic lateral sclerosis and related disorders,* New York, 1969, Grune & Stratton.
10. Brooke MH: *A clinician's view of neuromuscular diseases,* Baltimore, 1977, Williams & Wilkins.
11. Burkett LN et al: Exercise capacity of untrained spinal cord–injured individuals and the relationship of peak oxygen uptake to level of injury, *Paraplegia* 28:512, 1990.
12. Carroll JE et al: Bicycle ergometry and gas exchange measurements in neuromuscular diseases, *Arch Neurol* 36:457, 1979.
13. Carter G, Jancar J: Mortality in the mentally handicapped: a 50-year survey at the State Park Group of Hospitals (1930-1980), *J Ment Defic Res* 2:143, 1983.
14. Castles JJ: Glucocorticoids. In McCarty DJ, editor: *Arthritis and allied conditions,* ed 10, Philadelphia, 1985, Lea & Febiger.
15. Chamberlain MA, Care G, Harfield B: Physiotherapy in osteoarthritis of the knees, *Intern Rehabil Med* 4:101, 1982.
16. Cooney MM, Walker JB: Hydraulic resistance exercise benefits cardiovascular fitness of spinal cord–injured, *Med Sci Sports Exerc* 18:522, 1986.

17. Cullum L, Liebman J: The association of congenital heart disease with Down's syndrome (mongolism), *Am J Cardiol* 24:354, 1969.
18. Davis GM et al: Cardiorespiratory fitness and muscular strength of wheelchair users, *Can Med Assoc J* 125:1317, 1981.
19. Davis GM et al: Cardiovascular responses to arm cranking and FNS-induced leg exercise in paraplegics, *J Appl Physiol* 69:671, 1990.
20. Dearwater S et al: Assessment of physical activity in inactive populations, *Med Sci Sports Exerc* 17:67, 1979.
21. Denys EH, Norris FH: Amyotrophic lateral sclerosis: impairment of neuromuscular transmission, *Arch Neurol* 36:202, 1979.
22. DiCarlo SE: Effect of arm ergometry training on wheelchair propulsion endurance of individuals with quadriplegia, *Phys Ther* 68:40, 1988.
23. Downey JA: The spinal patient and thermoregulation, *Thermal Physiol* 9:225, 1984.
24. Edstrom L, Grimby L: Effect of exercise on the motor unit, *Muscle Nerve* 9:104, 1986.
25. Ekblom B et al: Effect of short-term physical training on patients with rheumatoid arthritis, *Scand J Rheumatol* 4:80, 1975.
26. Eriksson P, Lofstrom L, Ekblom B: Aerobic power during maximal exercise in untrained and well-trained persons with quadriplegia and paraplegia, *Scand J Rehabil Med* 20:141, 1988.
27. Fernhall B, Tymeson GT, Webster GE: Cardiovascular fitness of mentally retarded individuals, *Adapt Phys Activity Q* 5:12, 1988.
28. Fernhall B et al: Maximal exercise testing of mentally retarded adolescents and adults: reliability study, *Arch Phys Med Rehabil* 71:1065, 1990.
29. Figoni SF: Spinal cord injury and maximal aerobic power, *Am Corr Ther J* 38:44, 1984.
30. Florence JM, Hagberg JM: Effect of training on the exercise responses of neuromuscular disease patients, *Med Sci Sports Exerc* 16:460, 1984.
31. Fowler WM, Taylor M: Rehabilitation management of muscular dystrophy and related disorders: the role of exercise, *Arch Phys Med Rehabil* 63:319, 1982.
32. Gass GC et al: Rectal and rectal vs. esophageal temperatures in paraplegic men during prolonged exercise, *J Appl Physiol* 64:2265, 1988.
33. Glaser RM: Arm exercise training for wheelchair users, *Med Sci Sports Exerc* 21:S149, 1989.
34. Haller RG, Lewis SF: Pathophysiology of exercise performance in muscle disease, *Med Sci Sports Exerc* 16:456, 1984.
35. Haller RG et al: Hyperkinetic circulation during exercise in neuromuscular disease, *Neurology* 33:1283, 1983.
36. Hanson PA, Rowland LP: Mobius syndrome and facioscapulohumeral muscular dystrophy, *Arch Neurol* 24:31, 1971.

37. Hanyu N et al: Degeneration and regeneration of ventral root motor fibres in amyotrophic lateral sclerosis: morphometric studies of cervical ventral roots, *J Neurol Sci* 55:99, 1982.

38. Harkom TM et al: Therapeutic value of graded aerobic exercise training in rheumatoid arthritis, *Arthritis Rheum* 28:32, 1985.

39. Harris SR, Tada TL: Genetic disorders in children. In Umphred DA, editor: *Neurological rehabilitation,* ed 2, St Louis, 1990, Mosby.

40. Hasson SM et al: Exercise training and dexamethasone iontophoresis in rheumatoid arthritis, *Physiother Can* 43:11, 1991.

41. Hjeltnes N: Oxygen uptake and cardiac output in graded arm exercise in paraplegics with low-level spinal lesions, *Scand J Rehabil Med* 9:107, 1977.

42. Hjeltnes N: Cardiorespiratory capacity in tetra and paraplegia shortly after injury, *Scand J Rehabil Med* 18:65, 1986.

43. Hjeltnes N, Vokac Z: Circulatory strain in everyday life of paraplegics, *Scand J Rehabil Med* 11:67, 1979.

44. Hooker SP, Wells CL: Effects of low- and moderate-intensity training in spinal cord–injured persons, *Med Sci Sports Exerc* 21:18, 1989.

45. Jansma P: A fitness assessment system for individuals with severe mental retardation, *Adapt Phys Activity Q* 5:223, 1988.

46. Johnson EW, Braddom R: Over-work weakness in facioscapulohumeral muscular dystrophy, *Arch Phys Med Rehabil* 52:333, 1971.

47. Kott E et al: Cell-mediated immunity to polio and HLA antigens in amyotrophic lateral sclerosis, *Neurology* 29:1040, 1979.

48. Kottke FJ: The effects of limitation of activity upon the human body, *JAMA* 196:117, 1966.

49. Kreindler H, Lewis CB, Rush S: Effects of three exercise protocols on strength of persons with osteoarthritis of the knee, *Top Geriatr Rehabil* 4:32, 1989.

50. Kuhn E et al: Early myocardial disease and cramping myalgia in Becker-type muscular dystrophy: a kindred, *Neurology* 29:1144, 1979.

51. Lasko-McCarthey, Davis JA: Effect of work rate increment on peak oxygen uptake during wheelchair ergometry in men with quadriplegia, *Eur J Appl Physiol* 63:349, 1991.

52. Lavay B, Reid G, Cressler-Chaviz M: Measuring the cardiovascular endurance of persons with mental retardation: a critical review, *Exerc Sport Sci Rev* 18:263, 1990.

53. Lee P, Kennedy AC, Anderson J: Benefits of hospitalization in rheumatoid arthritis, *Q J Med* 43:205, 1974.

54. Lewis SF, Haller RG: Skeletal muscle disorders and associated factors that limit exercise performance, *Exerc Sports Sci Rev* 17:67, 1989.

55. Lloyd AR, Gandevia SC, Hales JP: Muscle performance, voluntary activation, twitch properties and perceived effort in normal subjects and patients with the chronic fatigue syndrome, *Brain* 114:85, 1991.

56. Lyngberg K, Danneskiold-Samsoe B, Halskov O: The effect of physical training on patients with rheumatoid arthritis: changes in disease activity, muscle strength and aerobic capacity: a clinically controlled minimized crossover study, *J Clin Exp Rheumatol* 6:253, 1988.

57. Machover S, Sapecky AJ: Effect of isometric exercise on the quadriceps muscle in patients with rheumatoid arthritis, *Arch Phys Med* 47:737, 1966.

58. Mansel JK, Norman JR: Respiratory complications and management of spinal cord injuries, *Chest* 97:1446, 1990.

59. Metra M et al: Improvement in exercise capacity after correction of anemia in patients with end-stage renal failure, *Am J Cardiol* 68:1060, 1991.

60. Miller JR, Guntaka RV, Myers JC: Amyotrophic lateral sclerosis: search for polio-virus by nucleic acid hybridization, *Neurology* 30:884, 1980.

61. Milner-Brown HS, Miller RG: Muscle strengthening through high-resistance weight training in patients with neuromuscular disorders, *Arch Phys Med Rehabil* 69:14, 1988.

62. Minor MA et al: Exercise tolerance and disease-related measures in patients with rheumatoid arthritis and osteoarthritis, *J Rheumatol* 15:905, 1988.

63. Minor MA et al: Efficacy of physical conditioning exercise in patients with rheumatoid arthritis and osteoarthritis, *Arthritis Rheum* 32:1396, 1989.

64. Montague TJ et al: Cardiac function at rest and with exercise in the chronic fatigue syndrome, *Chest* 95:779, 1989.

65. Monteon FJ et al: Energy expenditure in patients with chronic renal failure, *Kidney Int* 30:741, 1986.

66. Morris AF, Vaughn SE, Vaccaro P: Measurement of neuromuscular tone and strength in Down syndrome children, *J Ment Defic Res* 26:41, 1982.

67. Nilsson S, Staff PH, Pruett EDR: Physical work capacity and the effect of training on subjects with long standing paraplegia, *Scand J Rehabil Med* 7:51, 1975.

68. Nordemar R: Physical training in rheumatoid arthritis: a controlled long-term study, *Scand J Rheumatol* 10:23, 1981.

69. Nordemar R et al: Changes in muscle fibre size and physical performance in patients with rheumatoid arthritis after 7 months of physical training, *Scand J Rheumatol* 5:233, 1976.

70. Nordemar R et al: Physical training in rheumatoid arthritis: a controlled long-term study. I. *Scand J Rheumatol* 10:17, 1981.

71. Ornstein LJ, Skrinar GS, Garrett GG: Physiological effects of swimming training in physically disabled individuals, *Med Sci Sports Exerc* 15:110, 1983.

72. Partridge RH, Duthie JR: Controlled trial of the effect of complete immobilization of the joints in rheumatoid arthritis, *Ann Rheum Dis* 22:91, 1963.

73. Perlman S et al: Dance-based aerobic exercise for rheumatoid arthritis, *Arthritis Care Res* 3:29, 1990.

74. Petrofsky JS, Phillips CA, Hendershot D: The cardiorespiratory stresses which occur during dynamic exercise in paraplegics and quadriplegics, *J Neuro Ortho Surg* 6:252, 1985.

75. Petrofsky JS et al: Bicycle ergometer for paralyzed muscle, *J Clin Eng* 9:13, 1984.
76. Pitetti KH, Campbell KD: Mentally retarded individuals: a population at risk? *Med Sci Sports Exerc* 23:586, 1991.
77. Pitetti KH, Tan DM: Effects of a minimally supervised exercise program for mentally retarded adults, *Med Sci Sports Exerc* 23:594, 1991.
78. Pollack SF et al: Aerobic training effects of electrically induced lower-extremity exercises in spinal cord–injured people, *Arch Phys Med Rehabil* 70:214, 1989.
79. Preus M: The Williams syndrome: objective definition and diagnosis, *Clin Genet* 25:422, 1984.
80. Ragnarsson KT: Physiologic effects of functional electrical stimulation–induced exercises in spinal cord–injured individuals, *Clin Orthop Res* 233:53, 1988.
81. Riley MS et al: Aerobic work capacity in patients with chronic fatigue syndrome, *Br Med J* 301:953, 1990.
82. Russell WR, William FM: Recovery of muscular strength after poliomyelitis, *Lancet* 1:330, 1954.
83. Saltin B, Rowell LB: Functional adaptations to physical activity and inactivity, *Fed Proc* 39:1506, 1980.
84. Saltin B et al: Response to exercise after bed rest and after training, *Circ* 38(suppl)7:37, 1968.
85. Sanjak M, Reddan W, Brooks BR: Role of muscular exercise in amyotrophic lateral sclerosis, *Neurol Clin* 5:251, 1987.
86. Sanjak M et al: Physiologic and metabolic responses to progressive and prolonged exercise in amyotrophic lateral sclerosis, *Neurology* 37:1217, 1987.
87. Sawka MN, Latzka WA, Pandolf KB: Temperature regulation during upper-body exercise: able-bodied and spinal cord–injured, *Med Sci Sports Exerc* 21:S132, 1989.
88. Sharfstein SS, Sack DS, Fauci AS: Relationship between alternate day corticosteroid therapy and behavioral abnormalities, *JAMA* 248:2987, 1982.
89. Siegel IM: The management of muscular dystrophy: a clinical review, *Muscle Nerve* 1:453, 1978.
90. Smith PEM et al: Practical problems in the respiratory care of patients with muscular dystrophy, *New Engl J Med* 316:1197, 1987.
91. Smith RD, Palley HF: Rest therapy for rheumatoid arthritis, *Mayo Clin Proc* 53:141, 1978.
92. Sockolov R et al: Exercise performance in 6- to 11-year-old boys with Duchenne muscular dystrophy, *Arch Phys Med Rehabil* 58:195, 1977.
93. Trauner DA, Bellugi U, Chase C: Neurologic features of Williams and Downs syndromes, *Pediatr Neurol* 5:166, 1989.
94. Vignos PJ: Physical models of rehabilitation in neuromuscular disease, *Muscle Nerve* 6:323, 1983.
95. Young AJ et al: Cooling different body surfaces during upper- and lower-body exercise, *J Appl Physiol* 63:1218, 1987.
96. Zanconato S et al: Exercise tolerance in end-stage renal disease, *Child Nephrol Urol* 10:26, 1990.

STUDY QUESTIONS

■ What are the benefits of exercise training for patients with progressive degenerative motor neuron and neuromuscular diseases?

■ Describe what factors the clinician must be aware of that negatively impact muscle hypertrophy and the effect of these factors on the rehabilitation process.

■ Describe exercise tolerance and response to exercise training in patients with rheumatoid arthritis and osteoarthritis.

■ Describe exercise tolerance and response to exercise training in patients with chronic renal failure and chronic fatigue syndrome.

■ What are the benefits of exercise training for patients with spinal cord injuries, and what are potential complications?

■ What are the benefits of exercise training for patients with mental retardation?

CHAPTER 10

EVALUATION OF POSTURAL STABILITY, MOVEMENT, AND CONTROL
Exercise Tolerance and Training for Patients with Neurologic Dysfunction and Balance Disorders

Lewis Nashner

Maintaining postural stability is a complex process involving the coordinated actions of biomechanical, sensory, motor, and central nervous system components. A relatively simple biomechanical definition for postural stability can be formulated in terms of the position of the body center of gravity relative to the base of support. The body movements used to maintain postural stability, however, are complex because of the number of joint systems and muscles involved. Sensing the position of the body relative to gravity and the base of support is also complex and involves combinations of visual, vestibular, and somatosensory inputs. Central adaptive processes are required to modify the sensory and motor components so that stability can be maintained under a wide variety of task conditions.

The major emphases of this chapter are the following: (1) to define the biomechanics of postural stability and movement, (2) to describe the physiology and methods for assessment of postural movement control, (3) to describe the physiology and methods for assessment of sensory postural control, (4) to describe the diagnostic and training applications of computerized dynamic posturography, and (5) to describe additional applications in disability rating and occupational risk assessment.

BIOMECHANICS OF POSTURAL STABILITY

Definition of Postural Stability

To maintain stability with the feet in place, the body's center of gravity (COG) must be positioned vertically over the base of support.[48,60,78] When this condition is met, a person can both resist the destabilizing influence of gravity and actively move the COG. If the COG is positioned outside the perimeter of the base of support, the person has exceeded the in-place limits of stability. At this point, to prevent a fall, a rapid step or stumble to reestablish the base of support beneath the COG or additional external support is required.

A person's postural stability is best described in terms of angular displacement of the COG from the gravitational vertical. COG sway is then defined as the angle formed by the intersection of a first line from the center of the base of support

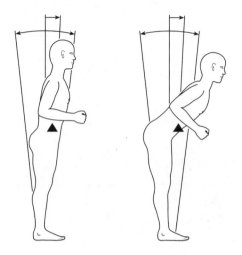

Fig. 10-1 Center of gravity (COG) sway angle in relation to the limits of sway (LOS) cone. The figure on the left is moving about the ankles; the figure on the right is moving about the hips. Center of gravity sway angles of the two figures are the same. Triangles show the body COG positions.

through the COG and a second line extending vertically from the center of support (Fig. 10-1). This definition of stability pertains whether the person moves about the ankles or the hips or about both joints and also takes height into account.[87] Thus a given sway angle indicates a comparable state of postural stability for all body movement patterns and heights. This definition of stability is further discussed in the section on limits of stability.

Base of Support

The base of support for standing on a flat, firm surface is defined as the area contained within the perimeter of contact between the surface and the two feet. The base of support area is nearly square when the feet are placed comfortably apart during quiet standing. Similarly a diagonal stance produces a parallelogram-shaped base of support that extends forward on one side and backward on the other, and a tandem stance or position creates a long but narrow base of support.

When the support surface area is smaller than the feet or when surface irregularities limit the con-

tact between the feet and the surface, the base of support is reduced. Standing sideways on a narrow beam, for example, provides a base with a normal width but short length. Thus the person's limits of stability are effectively reduced in the anterio-posterior (AP) dimension but not in the lateral dimension.

Limits of Stability

The limits of stability (LOS) measure is a two-dimensional quantity defining the largest possible COG sway angle as a function of sway direction from the center position.[60,72] The LOS depends on the placement of the feet and the base of support. In normal adults standing on a flat, firm surface with feet spaced comfortably apart, the LOS perimeter can best be described as an ellipse Fig. 10-1; see Fig. 10-3). The AP dimension of this ellipse is approximately 12.5 degrees from the most backward point to the most forward point on the perimeter.[87] Although height of the COG above the surface and foot length affect the AP limits of stability, these two features covary, resulting in approximately the same AP limits for persons of various heights.[41]

The lateral LOS depends on the person's height relative to the spacing between the feet. When the feet of a person 180 cm (70 inches) tall are placed 10 cm (4 inches) apart, for example, the lateral dimension of the LOS ellipse is approximately 16 degrees from the farthest point on the left to the farthest point on the right on the perimeter. To produce a 16-degree ellipse, a wider spacing between the feet is required for taller individuals, whereas shorter people can place their feet closer together.

The biomechanical properties that determine the LOS are similar for standing in place, walking, and sitting without trunk support (Fig. 10-2). During in-place standing the COG moves randomly within an LOS perimeter determined by the base of support and the placement of the feet. During walking the COG progresses forward through the LOS in a smooth rhythmic movement.[81,85] At heel strike an LOS is established with the COG positioned at the posterior perimeter. As the step progresses, the COG moves forward within the LOS. As the COG

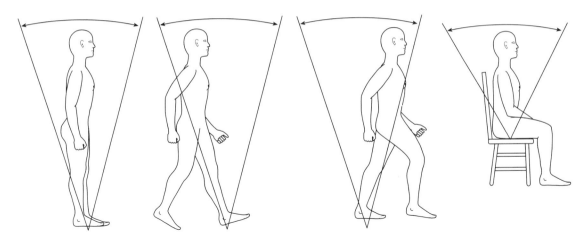

Fig. 10-2   Boundaries of limits of sway during standing, walking, and sitting.

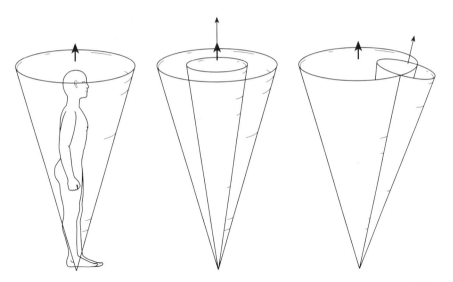

Fig. 10-3   Relationships of the LOS, the sway envelope, and the COG alignment. *Middle,* The COG alignment (*fine arrows*) centered within the LOS (*heavy arrows*). *Right,* The COG aligned forward relative to the center.

approaches the anterior perimeter of the LOS, the next step establishes a new LOS and the rhythmic process is repeated. When a person is sitting without trunk support the height of the COG above the support surface is lower and the base area is larger. Therefore the LOS perimeter is larger when a person is seated than during quiet standing.

Limits of Sway

It is impossible to maintain a motionless COG because in-place standing is an inherently unstable task requiring periodic corrections to overcome the destabilizing influence of gravity.[9,26,31,99] Thus a person attempting to maintain balance sways spontaneously back and forth and from side to side.

The limits of sway measure is a two-dimensional quantity defining the largest spontaneous COG sway angle as a function of the sway direction (Fig. 10-3). A person's limits of spontaneous sway vary with the sensory conditions and the configuration of the base of support, But unless the person loses balance, the limits of sway are always well within the LOS.

Center of Gravity Alignment

A point at the center of the area contained within the limits of sway perimeter defines the COG alignment (Fig. 10-3). This definition of COG alignment is based on the assumption that a person is attempting to maintain a COG position that is at the center of the limits of sway perimeter. When a normal person is asked to stand erect, COG alignment is placed accurately above the center of the base of support.

Understanding the concepts of limits of sway and COG alignment is important because each affects a person's balance differently. When the COG is aligned over the center of the base of support, the limits of sway can be as large as the LOS before balance is lost. A person whose COG alignment is offset forward, backward, or to one side of the center of support is not as stable as a person whose COG alignment is centered, even when the limits of sway are similar in the two. The person with the offset COG alignment is less stable because smaller sway angles in the direction of the offset move the COG beyond the LOS perimeter.

Limits of Stability and Sway Frequency

The actual LOS depends on the COG sway frequency as well as on placement of the feet and size of the base of support.[91] When COG sway is slow, gravity is the only significant destabilizing force that must be overcome and the COG can be moved within the full range of the LOS. For the average adult, COG movements within the full range of the LOS are possible when sway oscillations (front to back or side to side and then back again) take 2 or 3 seconds or longer. In contrast, when the COG moves rapidly, the momentum of the body acts as an additional destabilizing force. When a sway os-

cillation is completed in 1 second or less, the LOS contracts to approximately 3 degrees.

Understanding the impact of COG sway frequency is important in assessing a person's balance. Since higher frequencies reduce the effective LOS, a person using fast sway movements is closer to exceeding the LOS than is an individual swaying slowly through a comparable arc.

Summary

A human subject standing in an erect posture with the feet in place is inherently unstable because the COG of the body is located a significant distance above a relatively small base of support. These biomechanics are used (1) to define the postural stability in terms of the angular position of the COG relative to the center of support and (2) to define the LOS in terms of the COG position relative to the perimeter of the area of support. Postural stability at a given time is the angular distance between the current COG position and the LOS. Both the static alignment of the body and the dynamic sway affect the postural stability.

BIOMECHANICS OF POSTURAL MOVEMENT
Anatomy of Movement About a Single Joint

A detailed description of the large number of muscles controlling ankle, knee, and hip joint motions is beyond the scope of this chapter. Instead, this section focuses on the key muscle groups involved in balance and on the general physiologic principles governing coordination of these muscles during the production of postural movements.

Motions about a given joint are controlled by the combined actions of at least one pair of muscles working in opposition. All leg and lower trunk joints have multiple pairs of opposing muscles. Furthermore, many leg muscles act about two neighboring joints. At the ankle joint the gastrocnemius and tibialis anterior are the major extensor (plantar flexor) and flexor (dorsiflexor) muscles, respectively. The quadriceps is the major knee extensor; the hamstrings and gastrocnemius muscles are both knee flexors. The hamstrings and lower back muscles are hip extensors, whereas hip flex-

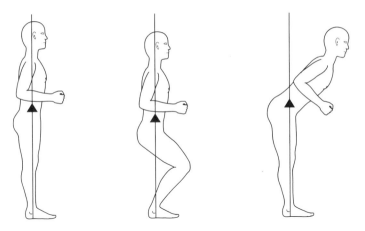

Fig. 10-4   Stable postures.

ion is controlled by quadriceps and abdominal muscles.

An isolated muscle acts like a spring, tending to resist attempts to stretch the muscle beyond a resting length.[52] The degree of the muscle's resistance to stretch is referred to as muscle stiffness. Both the resting length of the muscle and the muscle stiffness vary depending on how strongly the muscle is being activated. An inactive muscle has an extended rest length and offers little resistance to stretching. The rest length of a highly active muscle is shorter, and the muscle vigorously resists stretching.

When the forces exerted by pairs of opposing muscle are combined about a joint, the effect is to resist rotation of the joint relative to a resting position. The degree to which the joint resists rotation is referred to as the joint stiffness. The resting position and the stiffness of the joint are each independently altered by changing the activation levels of one or both muscles. Joint resting position and joint stiffness, however, are by themselves an inadequate basis for controlling postural movements because the stiffness properties of muscle are highly nonlinear. Although resistance to a small displacement from the resting position is strong, the resistance breaks down over larger displacements unless the activation level is increased.[61]

During erect standing with the arms at the side or folded at the waist, the COG is located in the area of the lower abdomen, and the exact position at a given moment depends on the relative positions of the ankle, knee, and hip joints.[72] Because there are three principal joint systems—ankles, knees, and hips—between the base of support and the COG during standing, a wide variety of postures can be assumed with the COG over the center of the base of support[79] (Fig. 10-4). For similar reasons a wide variety of active ankle, knee, and hip movement patterns can be used to produce similar shifts in COG position. This diversity of postures and balance movement patterns can be observed in individuals performing highly trained dance and martial arts routines.

Multijoint Postural Movement

The major joint and muscle systems controlling the COG during standing are illustrated in Fig. 10-5. Postural movements involve the coordinated actions of the ankle, knee and hip joints and, frequently, also the neck. The motions about each of these joints, however, are not determined simply by the muscles acting directly about the joint; leg and trunk muscles also exert indirect forces on neighboring joints through the inertial interaction forces among body segments.[80,87] For example, when the ankle muscles contract to extend the

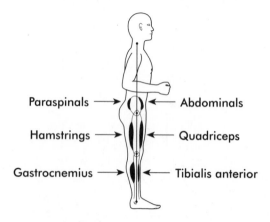

Paraspinals →   ← **Abdominals**

Hamstrings →   ← **Quadriceps**

Gastrocnemius →   ← **Tibialis anterior**

Fig. 10-5 Functional anatomy of the major joint and muscle systems controlling the body COG during standing.

lower leg segments backward, the hips flex unless thigh and lower trunk muscles are activated to stabilize these joints. The hips flex in the absence of additional stabilizing forces because the inertia of the trunk tends to make its movements lag behind those of the legs.

Because of the indirect inertial effects of muscular forces, the function of leg and trunk muscles during posture control can differ quite dramatically from their traditional anatomic classification, as summarized in Table 10-1. When a person is standing on a rigid surface, contraction of the tibialis anterior (anatomically classified as an ankle dorsiflexor) also causes knee flexion, although there is no anatomic insertion of this muscle at the knee. As dorsiflexion of the ankle moves the lower leg forward, inertia causes the thigh to lag behind and

the knee flexes as a result. Although the gastrocnemius is anatomically classified as an ankle extensor and knee flexor, its functional effect on the knee during standing is extension rather than flexion. The knee extends because of inertial interactions similar to those previously mentioned.

Contractions of thigh and lower trunk muscles exert similar indirect effects on the knee and ankle joints. The quadriceps muscle not only is a hip flexor and knee extensor by direct action but also is an ankle extensor by indirect action. The hamstrings muscle, in addition to having direct knee flexor and hip extensor functions, is an indirect ankle flexor.

One common example of an abnormal movement pattern is the destabilization of a proximal knee or hip joint during postural movement. This problem is often called proximal joint instability. Although it is tempting to attribute an unstable knee or hip joint to weakness or inactivity in the muscles acting directly about these joints, the instability can also be caused by the indirect effects of delayed ankle muscle activation.[89]

Coordination of Postural Movements into Strategies

When a person's postural stability is disrupted by an external perturbation, one or a combination of three different strategies is typically used to coordinate movement of the COG back to a balanced position. When the perturbation displaces the COG beyond the LOS perimeter, a step or stumbling reaction is the only movement strategy effective in preventing a fall. When the COG remains within the LOS, two different strategies or combi-

Table 10-1 Functional anatomy of muscles involved in balance movements

Joint	Extension		Flexion	
	Anatomic	**Functional**	**Anatomic**	**Functional**
Hip	Paraspinal, hamstrings	Paraspinal, quadriceps	Abdominal, quadriceps	Abdominal, hamstrings
Knee	Quadriceps	Quadriceps, gastrocnemius	Hamstrings, gastrocnemius	Hamstrings, tibialis
Ankle	Gastrocnemius	Gastrocnemius	Tibialis	Tibialis

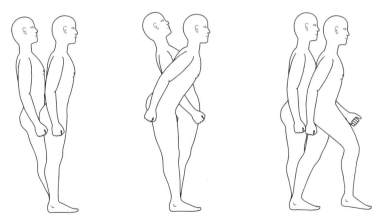

Fig. 10-6   Functional properties of the ankle and hip and stepping strategies for moving the COG relative to the base of support.

nations thereof can be used to move the COG while maintaining the initial placement of the feet on the support surface.

The ankle strategy shifts the COG while maintaining the placement of the feet by rotating the body as an approximately rigid mass about the ankle joints (Fig. 10-6). This rotation is accomplished by contracting the ankle joint muscles and exerting torque about the ankle joints. At the same time, contractions of thigh and lower trunk muscles are required to resist the destabilization of these proximal joints.

Movements organized into the hip strategy are centered about the hip joints with smaller opposing ankle joint rotations (Fig. 10-6). The COG shifts in the opposite direction from the hip because the inertia of the trunk moving in one direction generates an opposite horizontal (shear) reaction force against the support surface.[55,87] The tendency toward destabilization of the knee joints is resisted by coordination of the muscular actions about the ankle, knee, and hip joints.

Appropriate Use of Postural Movement Strategies

The relative effectiveness of ankle, hip, and stepping strategies in repositioning the COG over the base of support depends on the configuration of

the base of support, the COG alignment in relation to the LOS, and the speed of the postural movement.[55,71,87] For example, the ankle strategy is most effective in executing relatively slow COG movements when the base of support is firm and the COG is well within the LOS perimeter. The ankle strategy is also effective in maintaining a static posture when the COG is offset from the center.

The amplitude and speed of ankle movements are biomechanically limited by the torque that can be exerted about the ankles before the feet lift off from the support surface.[91] The reader can experience this biomechanical constraint by increasing the amplitude and frequency of sway about the ankles until the feet begin to lift off from the floor. The strengths of the ankle joint muscles are not the limiting factors. Gastrocnemius strength is determined by the force requirements for running and jumping and therefore far exceeds the requirements for executing ankle movements. The maximal force capabilities of the anterior tibialis muscles, in contrast, are more closely matched to the requirements for balance. Thus reductions in ankle muscle strength impair a person's use of ankle movements more than the use of hip movements in recovering from backward COG displacements.

Hip movements rely on horizontal shear forces rather than ankle torques to shift the COG and are therefore not limited by constraints on ability to exert torque about the ankles. Thus hip movements are effective when the COG is positioned near the LOS perimeter and when the LOS boundaries are contracted by a narrowed base of support. The reader can experience the conditions requiring the use of hip movements by attempting to shift posture while standing on tiptoe or with the feet placed laterally heel to toe.

Hip movements have biomechanical limitations inasmuch as they cannot produce large shifts in COG position. In addition, because hip movements rely on inertial reaction forces, they cannot be used to effectively maintain balance when the COG is offset from the center.

When the COG is displaced beyond the LOS, a step or stumble is the only effective strategy for preventing a fall. Stepping and stumbling are subject to fewer biomechanical limitations than are ankle and hip movements, but the former are inefficient, disruptive, and usually inappropriate when simpler ankle or hip movements are effective.

Summary

Corrective postural movements move the COG relative to the base of support. Because there are three major joint systems between the base of support and the body COG, different movement patterns or strategies can be used to move the COG. Each movement strategy operates within a specific set of biomechanical constraints and is therefore useful for maintaining postural stability under particular task conditions. The ankle strategy moves the COG slowly to positions well within the limits of stability and is most effective when the person is standing on a firm base of support. The hip strategy, in contrast, is most effective for performing small, rapid shifts in COG position when the base of support is narrow or when the COG is near the limits of stability.

PHYSIOLOGY OF POSTURAL MOVEMENT CONTROL
Reflex Movements

The influences of stretch reflex and automatic and volitional movement systems on standing bal-

ance are reviewed in Table 10-2. Among the three systems of movement control, the stretch reflex system is the earliest mechanism for increasing the activation level of the muscles of a joint after an externally imposed rotation of the joint. This response component is initiated by inputs from muscle spindles, tiny stretch sensitive receptors embedded within the muscle. Output fibers from the muscle spindles enter the spinal cord and, via single synapses within the cord, activate muscle fibers within the same muscle from which the spindle inputs originated.[61]

Current theory suggests that the myotatic stretch reflexes improve the nonlinear stiffness properties of muscle in controlling the effects of external disturbances during movement control.[61] Thus during large joint displacements reflexes rapidly increase activation of the stretching muscles and decrease activation of the shortening antagonists, thereby preventing the breakdown of joint stiffness.

Stretch reflexes, however, play almost no direct role in controlling a person's coordinated active postural movements in response to external balance perturbations,[42,47] since the combined effects of the muscle stiffness properties and the stretch reflexes are still insufficient to maintain standing balance. First, the level of ankle joint stiffness resulting from these two mechanisms does not fully counteract the large destabilizing forces of gravity and external perturbations during sway.[42,76] Second, because rotations of the support surface can elicit stretch reflexes inappropriate for balance control, other response mechanisms not dependent on local stretch inputs are required to maintain balance when the support surface is irregular or unstable.[76]

Automatic Postural Movements

Automatic postural movements are the earliest functionally effective responses helping to maintain stability when a standing individual's balance is perturbed.[76,77,90] Automatic postural movements resemble reflex responses in some respects and voluntary movements in others. Like reflexes, automatic movements are triggered by external stimuli, occur at fixed latencies, and are relatively

Table 10-2 Properties of the three movement systems

Property	Reflex	Automatic	Voluntary
Mediating pathways	Spinal cord	Brain stem, subcortical	Brain stem, cortical
Mode of activation	External stimulus	External stimulus	Self-generated or stimulus
Response properties	Localized to point of stimulus, highly stereotyped	Coordinated among leg and trunk muscles, stereotypic but adaptable	Unlimited variety
Role in posture control	Regulate muscle forces	Coordinate movements across joints	Generate purposeful behaviors
Onset time	Fixed at 35 to 40 msec	Fixed at 85 to 95 msec	Varies with difficulty, 150 + msec

stereotypic. Like voluntary postural movements, automatic responses involve the coordinated actions of many leg and trunk muscles, and the amplitudes and patterns of automatic responses adapt to the task conditions. Although the pathways mediating automatic postural movements have not been fully elucidated, the 85- to 95-msec latencies of electromyograph (EMG) responses are sufficient to include significant brain stem and subcortical involvement.[43,70,73]

Local somatosensory input from the feet and ankle joints is by itself sufficient to trigger an automatic postural movement.[56] The direction of the automatic movement is also determined by the triggering somatosensory stimulus.[55,77,90] A backward movement is triggered by forward displacement of the body COG, such as when the support surface moves backward or when the person pulls backward on a rigid object. A forward movement follows a backward COG displacement caused by forward movement of the surface or pushes against a rigid object.

Although the amplitude of the automatic movement is related to the intensity of the triggering somatosensory stimulus,[28a] visual input, vestibular input, and the past experiences of the individual also influence the response amplitude.[76,82] The pattern of movement response among leg and lower trunk muscles, in contrast, is determined not by the triggering stimulus but by the configuration of the support surface and the prior experience of the individual.

When an automatic postural movement is initiated by an external stimulus, the onset of muscular EMG activity occurs within 85 to 95 msec, and the resulting patterns of activation among leg and lower trunk muscles are directionally specific and relatively stereotypic (Fig. 10-7). The onset of active movement force is delayed an additional 20 to 40 msec because there is a delay between electrical activation and force generation in a muscle.[6]

Ankle movements are generated by EMG responses that begin at 85 to 95 msec in the directionally appropriate ankle joint muscles.[55,77,90] The gastrocnemius muscles are activated for backward postural movements, whereas anterior tibialis contractions produce forward movements. Electromyograph activity then radiates in sequence to the thigh and to the lower trunk muscles on the same dorsal or ventral aspect of the body. Activation of the thigh and lower trunk muscles stabilizes the knees and hips, allowing the body to move as a unit about the ankles. Thigh and trunk muscle EMG onsets occur, on average, 10 to 30 msec later than do those of the ankle. Prior activation of the ankle muscles provides proximal muscles with a stable movement base.

Hip movements are generated by activation of the directionally appropriate thigh and lower trunk muscles at 80- 90-msec latencies.[55] Quadriceps and abdominal muscles are activated to flex the hips and move the COG backward. The knee remains relatively stable because the quadriceps and

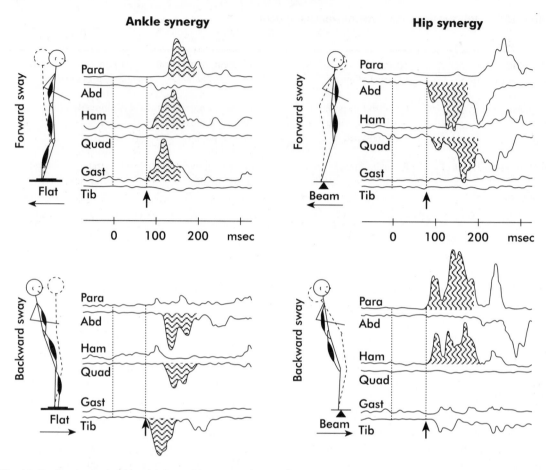

Fig. 10-7 Patterns of ankle, thigh, and lower trunk muscle EMG responses during executions of movements, organized into ankle and hip strategies. Muscle patterns for paraspinal, abdominal, hamstring, quadriceps, gastrocnemius, and anterior tibial muscles are shown. Electromyographic signals have been full-wave rectified and low-pass filtered. Traces are averages of five trials. Traces of antagonist muscles acting about the same joint are grouped. The trace of the functional extensor muscle is displaced upward by increased activation. The functional flexor trace is displaced downward during activation. (From Horak FB, Nasher LM: *J Neurophysiol* 55:1369, 1986.)

abdominal muscles have opposite functional effects about this joint. Paraspinal muscle and hamstrings activations extend the hips and move the COG backward. Opposing functional effects of these two muscles also stabilize the knees. During movements in both directions the ankle muscles are relatively inactive.

The strategy selected for responding to an external perturbation is set in advance, depending on the person's immediate past experience, not on a conscious decision made at the time of response.[55,71] When a person is well practiced at standing on a particular support surface, a relatively pure example of the appropriate movement strategy described in the preceding sections is observed. In contrast, a more complex movement combining the two pure strategies is observed during the initial practice trials that follow a change in support surface conditions. After 10 or 15 practice trials on the new surface, however, the less appropriate component is progressively reduced and reliance on the well-practiced pure strategy increases. Movement strategies are not voluntarily changed by instruction alone, even if a person is familiar with the pattern and motivated to quickly change it.

Voluntary Postural Movements

Voluntary postural movements can occur in the presence or absence of external stimuli. The variety of possible movement patterns under voluntary control is almost limitless. Unlike the highly repeatable latencies of reflex and automatic responses, voluntary response latencies vary with the complexity of the task and the person's attention to it, ranging from a minimum of 150 msec to much longer times.[84]

A person's voluntary actions either directly alter the posture or involve the arms, trunk, and head in ways that have an indirect effect. Examples of voluntary changes in posture include shifting weight from one side to the other or changing the placement of the feet on the surface. Actions having the largest indirect effect on posture are those exerting force against external objects. When a freely standing person pulls open a heavy door, for example, the force on the door is offset by an equal and opposite force on the body COG. Voluntary actions not involving external objects, for example, raising an arm from the side to a forward pointing position, have relatively little impact on a person's postural stability.

Research has shown that voluntary actions with the potential for disturbing postural stability are actively delayed so that an associated postural response can establish a stable base of support. For example, when a freely standing person performs a voluntary action involving external forces, an automatic postural movement is initiated in leg muscles in advance of the activation of the arm muscles.[10,23,84] The coordination of voluntary and postural components depends on the requirements for postural stability. When the need for active stabilization is removed by providing trunk support during the standing arm pull, the stabilizing postural responses in the leg muscles are abolished and voluntary activations of arm muscles are initiated more quickly.

Summary

Three movement systems with unique characteristics control the motor actions of the body. Reflex movements are extremely rapid, but their effectiveness in posture control is severely limited because reflexes are localized to the source of the stimulus and are relatively fixed, regardless of the task conditions. Automatic postural movements are more rapid than voluntary responses but are slightly slower than reflexes. They are well suited to providing the first line of defense in posture control because they are rapid, coordinated, and highly adaptable to the task conditions. Voluntary movements are the most versatile and varied of the three systems. They are poorly suited for posture control because they are substantially slower when the task conditions are complex and they require continuous mental effort.

METHODS FOR CLINICAL ASSESSMENT OF POSTURAL MOVEMENT CONTROL
Assessing Integrity of Sensory and Motor Pathways

Posture evoked response test. The posture evoked response test (PER) is used to analyze the peripheral nerve, spinal cord, brain stem, and subcortical pathways mediating postural movements. In PER testing, responses are elicited by rapidly rotating the support surface on which the patient is standing about the ankle joint axis. When rotational velocities are 50 degrees per second or faster, the posture control system receives a highly saturating stretch stimulus at the ankle joints while the body COG remains initially stationary over the base of support[30,75] (Fig. 10-8). The addition of random time intervals between

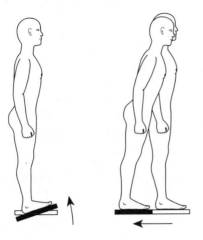

Fig. 10-8 Support surface rotation and horizontal translation methods for eliciting automatic postural responses.

rotations minimizes the patient's ability to anticipate stimuli.

Normal posture evoked response test results. Posture evoked responses are measured by recording surface EMG signals simultaneously from the gastrocnemius and tibialis anterior muscles of the two legs. Results of toes-up rotations for a typical individual with normal health are shown in Fig. 10-9. Toes-up rotations of the support surface elicit short latency (SL) responses in the gastrocnemius muscles of both legs. Average SL responses are 35 to 37 msec with less than 2 msec of variation among normal individuals.[8,35,62,75] Short latency responses are attributed to the monosynaptic stretch reflex system involving the sensory and motor peripheral nerves and first-order synapses in the spinal cord.[25,75] Medium latency (ML) responses are identifiable in the gastrocnemius muscles of some normal individuals at average latencies of 75 to 80 msec, with individual variations of less than 5 msec.[2,7,21,25] These ML responses are attributed to polysynaptic segmental reflex mechanisms.[39,40] Because the directions of ankle joint rotation and induced body sway are opposite when the surface is rotated, muscle forces generated by the SL and ML responses tend to destabilize rather than stabilize the posture.[76]

Well-defined long latency (LL) responses to toes-up surface rotations are recorded in the tibialis anterior muscles of both legs in all normal individuals.[3,34] Average LL responses are 120 msec, with individual variations of less than 10 msec.[8,35,62,75] In contrast to the SL and ML components, LL responses are mediated by requirements for postural stability rather than by the local stretch inputs.[29,75,76] These LL responses are the person's main line of defense against many types of unexpected postural disturbances.[55,83,90] Long latency responses are thought to involve the ascending sensory and descending motor pathways of the spinal cord and the brain stem and subcortical motor control centers. Although LL responses are longer than the SL and ML responses, they are still too short to be initiated under voluntary control.[84]

Because stretch reflexes are relatively inactive in the flexor leg muscles of humans, SL responses are typically not observed in tibialis anterior muscles after toes-down rotations of the support surface. The ML and LL responses in the tibialis anterior and gastrocnemius muscles, respectively, are similar to those reported for toes-up rotations.

Assessing the Coordination of Automatic Postural Responses

Automatic postural response test. When the support surface is unexpectedly translated forward or backward, the body initially remains stationary and becomes offset relative to the base of support[77,90] (Fig. 10-8). This type of perturbation elicits an automatic postural response that can be analyzed for a range of velocities and directions by the use of forward and backward translations varying in magnitude (threshold, intermediate, and saturating) and timing (random intervals between stimuli).

In the standard protocol used in the EquiTest (R) (NeuroCom, Inc., Portland, Oregon) the support surface translates at a constant velocity during a fixed interval of time. The exact velocities and

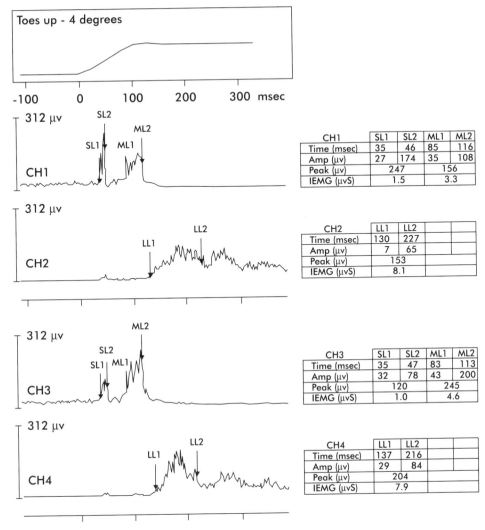

Fig. 10-9 Summary of a typical posture evoked response (PER) test result. *CH1*, Left gastrocnemius; *CH2*, left tibialis anterior; *CH3*, right gastrocnemius; *CH4*, right tibialis anterior. See text for descriptions of LL, ML, and SL components.

amplitudes of translations are adjusted in accordance with the height of the individual patient, to achieve a predetermined velocity and amplitude of body sway.[28a] The slowest translation is scaled to rotate the body about the ankle joints at 2.8 degrees per second for a total distance of 0.7 degrees. This scale approximately represents the threshold displacement required to elicit an automatic postural response. A higher velocity translation rotates the body about the ankle joints at 6 degrees per second for a total distance of 1.8 degrees. The highest velocity translation rotates the body at 8 degrees per second for a total distance of 3.2 degrees. This stimulus produces an approximately maximal amplitude automatic response in normal individuals.[54] Displacement velocities used in the physiologic range for the automatic response test are much slower than the rapid rotational velocities used to produce responses in the PER test.

The coordination of lower leg, thigh, and lower trunk muscles is analyzed by imposing a sequence of identical forward or backward translations while recording the surface EMG activities of the gastrocnemius, anterior tibialis, hamstrings, quadriceps, paraspinal, and abdominal muscles of both legs.[55,77] Each raw EMG signal is full-wave rectified and low-pass filtered to provide a quantitative measure of the muscle activation level. The results are then averaged over a sequence of identical forward or backward translation trials relative to the onset times of the individual stimuli. Fig. 10-7 shows normal EMG patterns.

Normal automatic postural responses. As the body is displaced forward (or backward) relative to the base of support, the initial resistance to the sway is due to the inherent stiffness of the ankle joints. This small resistance is insufficient to stabilize the COG sway.[47,76] Because velocities of support surface translation rotate the body about the ankle joints at rates falling within the physiologic range of postural sway (0 to 8 degrees per second), the SL and ML responses are either too weak or too inhibited during standing to have a significant impact on the active force response.[42,47]

When individuals are adapted to using the ankle strategy by standing on a flat, firm support surface, activations of leg and lower trunk muscles return the body to the stable, centered position by rotating the body as a coordinated unit about the ankle joints. Activations begin in the stretching ankle joint muscles at 85- to 95-msec latencies.[55,77,90] These activations exert torque about the ankle joints, which greatly enhances the resistance to sway rotation about the ankles. Contractile activity then radiates proximally to the thigh and to lower trunk muscles on the same dorsal or ventral aspect of the legs after additional delays of 10 to 30 msec. These proximal muscle activations help stabilize the knee and hip joints so that the body moves as a coordinated unit about the ankle joints.

When the ankle strategy is used to compensate a sway perturbation, backward displacements of the surface result in the activation of gastrocnemius, hamstrings, and paraspinal muscles in distal to proximal sequence. In response to forward support surface displacements, anterior tibialis, quadriceps, and lower abdominal muscles are activated in sequence.

The strengths of the ankle joint torques generated by the automatic responses are coordinated in relation to the velocity of the support surface translations to return the body to the stable, centered position with minimal undershoot or overshoot. The ankle torque exerted by each leg is recorded by means of a separate force plate. Ankle torque increases abruptly 20 to 40 msec after onset of the EMG responses in ankle joint muscles.[76,77,90] Ankle torques are equal in the two legs and, as shown in Fig. 10-10, the total torque generated by the two closely approximates that necessary to return the body to the original centered position.

Summary

For purposes of assessment, postural responses can be elicited by a variety of support surface displacements. The resulting motor outputs are measured by means of surface EMG recordings of leg muscles, by analysis of the forces exerted by the feet against the support surface, and by analysis of the resulting body motions. Because automatic responses are relatively stereotypic among normal individuals, patient results can be compared to those of age-matched normal individuals, to identify components of abnormal motor control.

Rapid ankle joint rotation provides a supersaturating stimulus to the posture control system and therefore is an ideal stimulus for assessing the integrity of the sensory and motor pathways mediating the SL, ML, and LL response components. Surface EMG recordings of the resulting muscle activations provide the most accurate measure of response onsets. A relatively slower translation of the support surface provides a physiologic stimulus that is useful in assessing the coordination and adaptation characteristics of automatic postural responses. Response coordination is quantified by the analysis of the surface reaction forces or the muscle EMG recordings, or both.

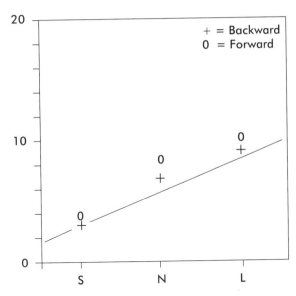

Fig. 10-10 Strengths of normal active force responses (+ and *0*) as compared with the strengths required to recenter the COG over the base of support (*heavy line*) as a function of support surface translation size. Strengths are shown in units of angular momentum per unit of body mass. *S, M,* and *L* are small, medium, and large translations.

PHYSIOLOGY OF SENSORY POSTURAL CONTROL
Senses Involved in Postural Control

Sensing the position of the COG relative to gravity and the base of support requires a combination of visual, vestibular, and somatosensory (tactile, deep pressure, joint receptor, and muscle proprioceptor) inputs. Use of the three balance senses is reviewed in Table 10-3. Three senses are required because no single sense directly measures COG position. Vision measures the orientation of the eyes and head in relation to surrounding objects. Somatosensory inputs provide information on the orientation of the body parts relative to one another and to the support surface. The vestibular system does not provide orientation information in relation to external objects. Rather, it measures gravitational, linear, and angular accelerations of the head in relation to inertial space.

No single combination of the three senses provides accurate COG information under all conditions, since one or more of the senses may provide information that is misleading or inaccurate for purposes of balance control. For example, when a person stands next to a large bus that suddenly

Table 10-3 Use of the senses for balance

Sense	Reference	Conditions favoring use	Conditions disrupting use
Somatosensory	Support surface	Fixed support surface	Irregular or moving support
Visual	Surrounding objects	Fixed visible surrounds, irregular or moving support	Moving surrounds, darkness
Vestibular	Gravity, inertial space	Irregular or moving support, moving surrounds, darkness	Unusual motion environments

begins to move forward, momentary disorientation or unsteadiness may result. A fraction of a second is required for the brain to determine whether the resulting visual stimulus indicates backward sway of the person or forward movement of the bus. If a downwardly tilted support surface is encountered, the brain must determine whether the surface is tilted downward or the surface is level and the body is tilted back. During situations of sensory conflict the brain must quickly select the sensory inputs providing accurate orientation information and ignore the misleading ones. The process of selecting and combining appropriate sensory information is called sensory organization.

Somatosensory Control

Somatosensory input derived from the contact forces and motions between the feet and the support surface is the dominant sensory input to balance under normal (fixed) support surface conditions. [4,28,33,38,49] When a person stands on a firm, level surface, the extent of COG sway is small relative to the LOS. Closing the eyes to eliminate vision causes little if any functionally significant increase in COG sway. Even a well-compensated patient with a bilateral vestibular loss sways well within the LOS with the eyes closed. [11,12,83,105]

Visual Control

Vision plays a significant role in balance, especially when the support surface is unstable. [9,36,68,95,96] For example, when toes-up and toes-down tilting of the surface in direct relation to the AP sway disrupts somatosensory input useful for balance, COG sway is significantly less with eyes open than with eyes closed. [11,12,83] The stabilizing effect of vision is also illustrated by comparing eyes-open and eyes-closed sway while a person stands on a compliant foam rubber pad. Vision also influences COG alignment. For example, when a person is exposed to a constant linear or rotational movement of the visual field, the alignment of the COG over the base of support shifts in the direction of the visual field motion. [22,69]

Vestibular Control

When functionally useful somatosensory and visual inputs are available, vestibular inputs play a minor role in controlling COG position, [19,83,105] since the somatosensory and visual inputs are more sensitive to body sway than is the vestibular system. [91] The primary role of vestibular input under these conditions is most probably to allow independent, precise control of head and eye positions. Precise head and eye control is critical in the execution of many complex motor activities such as running and kicking or catching a moving ball.

Vestibular input is critical for balance when both the somatosensory and visual inputs are misleading or unavailable. [2,18,45] The patient with a profound bilateral vestibular loss, for example, is unsteady when standing in darkness on a compliant or irregular surface. Because vestibular input is seldom misleading (except in cases of disease and in unusual motion environments), it is critical to balance when conflicting visual and somatosensory information requires a person to identify and quickly ignore misleading input. [11,12] Patients with peripheral vestibular deficits frequently complain of dizziness and unsteadiness during exposure to conflicting visual and support surface stimuli.

Exposure to a specific gravity of 0 or to a simulation of zero gravity is thought to cause changes in the way the brain interprets orientation input from the vestibular system. The utricular otoliths normally sense both the linear acceleration of the head and the tilt angle of the head with respect to gravity. Under zero-gravity conditions the brain must adapt to an absence of the tilt angle component of the otolith input. The adaptive changes in interpretation of the vestibular input after such exposure may be viewed as a temporary, environmentally induced disorder. [93,114] These maladaptive changes, for example, in astronauts, are most potent immediately after return to normal terrestrial conditions and are most pronounced when the returning astronauts are exposed to conflicting visual conditions. [93]

Summary

Three senses—somatothesis, vision, and vestibular—provide redundant information relative to an individual's state of erect postural stability. Under normal conditions somatosensory and visual inputs are the most sensitive. Both of these senses, however, may provide functionally inappropriate information relative to postural stability under some task conditions. Although the vestibular input is perhaps the least sensitive, it is the least impaired by the external conditions. Normal individuals maintain stability under a wide variety of conditions by quickly suppressing the influence of the sense(s) providing inaccurate information. In patients with sensory deficits, postural stability can be impaired by the loss of critical sensory information and by the inability to select the functionally appropriate sense(s) under conflict conditions.

SENSORY ORGANIZATION TESTING
Sensory Conditions

The six conditions of the sensory organization testing (SOT) protocol are designed to assess the patient's ability to effectively use visual, vestibular, and somatosensory inputs to maintain postural stability and to select the input(s) providing the most functionally appropriate orientation information under a variety of conditions. Sensory organization is evaluated by selectively disrupting somatosensory or visual information, or both, regarding body COG orientation in relation to the gravitational vertical and then measuring the patient's ability to maintain balance.

Somatosensory or visual information is disrupted by a method commonly termed "sway referencing." This method involves the tilting of the support surface or the visual surround, or both, about an axis colinear with the ankle joints, to directly follow the patient's COG sway in the AP direction.[83] Under sway-referenced conditions the orientation of the support surface or the visual surround, or both, remains constant in relation to the COG sway angle. Although the somatosensory and visual systems continue to provide information during sway-referenced conditions, these inputs

contain no functionally useful information relating the orientation of the body COG to the gravitational vertical.

Information from a sense subjected to sway referencing suggests that the orientation of the body COG relative to gravity is not changing, when in fact it is. Normally individuals ignore a sway-referenced sensory input that is functionally inaccurate and maintain balance by using other sensory inputs. In addition to sway referencing, eyes-closed conditions are used to further isolate the somatosensory and vestibular systems. There is no noninvasive way to selectively disrupt vestibular orientation information.

Protocol

The SOT exposes the patient to the six sensory conditions illustrated in Fig. 10-11. The six conditions consist of all combinations of normal (fixed), eyes-closed, and sway-referenced visual and support surface sensory conditions.[14,83] The six conditions are presented beginning with the simplest, eyes open on a fixed support surface, and ending with the most challenging, in which the support surface and the visual surround are both sway referenced.

During sensory conditions 1 and 2, the support surface and visual surround are fixed, and the patient stands with eyes open and eyes closed, respectively. These trials provide baseline measures of the patient's postural stability. During sensory condition 3, the surface remains fixed while the patient stands with eyes open in a sway-referenced visual surround. In the last three test conditions, the support surface is sway referenced while the patient stands with eyes open and the visual surround fixed (condition 4), with eyes closed (condition 5), and with eyes open and the visual surround sway referenced (condition 6).

The complete protocol consists of 18 20-second trials, three consecutive trials for each of the six sensory conditions. During each trial the patient is instructed to ignore any surface or visual surround motion and remain upright and as steady as possible. The use of three trials for

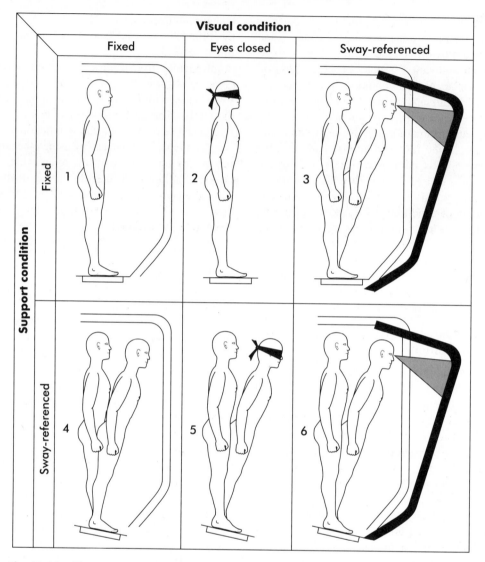

Fig. 10-11   The six sensory organization test (SOT) conditions.

each sensory condition improves the reliability of the resulting measures. The repeated measures also provide an opportunity to determine whether the patient's performance improves under a given condition with practice.

Quantifying Results

Equilibrium scores.   During each trial the COG sway angle is calculated in real time based on the biomechanical relations among the position of the center of vertical force (COF) exerted by the feet against the support surface, the position of the COG, and the limits of stability.[65,98] When the frequency of COG sway is below 0.5 Hz, the COG is located vertically above the COF. As COG sway frequency increases, movements of the COG lag behind the COF and decrease in relative size.[91,98]   A   real-time, multiple-pole digital filter is used to approximate these amplitude and frequency relations among the COF and COG motions.

A separate measure of stability, called the equilibrium score, is calculated for each trial. The equilibrium score is a nondimensional percentage that compares the patient's peak amplitude of AP sway with the theoretic AP limits of stability (LOS). The patient's theoretic LOS is the maximal forward and backward COG sway angles that can be achieved by a normal individual of similar height and weight. Equilibrium scores near 100% indicate little sway; scores approaching 0% indicate that sway is nearing the LOS. Trials in which the patient exceeds the LOS and loses balance are arbitrarily assigned equilibrium scores of 0%.

Center of gravity alignment. Separate AP and lateral alignment scores are calculated for each SOT trial by averaging the AP and lateral positions of the COG sway angle during the 20-second test interval. These calculations are based on the assumption that the patient's spontaneous COG swaying during the course of the trial occurs symmetrically at about the point of COG alignment.

Ankle versus hip movements. When ankle movements are used to control sway, the associated low-frequency motions of the COG generate relatively little horizontal shear force against the support surface. Higher-frequency hip and upper-body movements, in contrast, generate small but rapid shifts in COG position and much larger horizontal shear forces.[55,87] Based on this biomechanical principle, the relative amounts of ankle and hip movement are determined by comparing the peak-to-peak amplitude of the horizontal shear force to a theoretic normal limit for a person of similar weight. Although this method provides an accurate measure of the extent of hip and upper-body movement activity, this score does not measure the time-dependent trajectory of the actual body motion.

Summary of test results. The graphic summary of typical SOT results is shown in Fig. 10-12. The first plot, Fig. 10-12, *A*, summarizes the equilibrium scores obtained from a maximum of three trials under each of the six sensory conditions. Each equilibrium score is presented as a bar.

All areas of the plot in which equilibrium scores fall below the fifth percentile relative to results for the age-matched normal sample are indicated by stippling. The second plot, Fig. 10-12, *B*, summarizes the sensory ratios, movement patterns, and COG alignment.

Normal Test Results

Equilibrium scores. Table 10-4 summarizes the ranges of equilibrium and composite scores for a sample of 194 normal individuals. Equilibrium scores for sensory conditions 3 through 6 are based on the average of scores for the three trials. Equilibrium scores of 0 are substituted for trials in which individuals lost balance. Sizable studies of the normal population have found similar normal SOT results.[63,97]

The equilibrium scores of normal individuals of all ages are the highest for the first three sensory conditions because somatosensory inputs dominate balance when the support surface is fixed, regardless of the status of visual and vestibular inputs. Although equilibrium scores decrease when the functionally useful somatosensory input is disrupted (sway-referenced support surface) during conditions 4 through 6, normal individuals continue to maintain balance well within the LOS. The scores for sensory condition 4 are the highest of these three conditions because normal visual inputs are available. The lowest equilibrium scores occur during conditions 5 and 6, when both somatosensory and visual inputs are disrupted and individuals must rely on vestibular inputs alone to maintain balance.

Center of gravity alignment. Normal individuals align the COG very near the center of the base of support during all six sensory conditions. Although sway amplitudes increase significantly during conditions 5 and 6, the average COG positions remain very nearly centered.

Strategy analysis. The individual's movement strategy during each SOT trial is analyzed by plotting the resulting movement strategy score against the corresponding equilibrium score (Fig. 10-12). Points falling in the upper left quadrant of the strategy plot indicate trials in which the COG sway excursions are small but the amplitude of hip

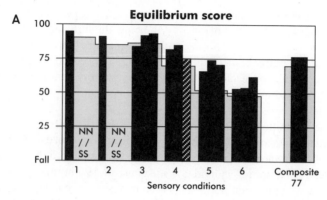

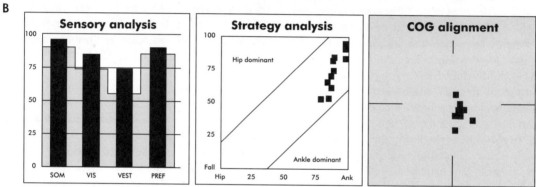

Fig. 10-12 Graphic summary of SOT results for a typical individual in normal condition. **A,** Equilibrium scores for the six sensory conditions (up to three trials per condition) and the composite equilibrium score. **B,** The four sensory analysis ratios, the analysis of movement patterns versus equilibrium scores, and the COG alignment. Shaded areas show scores falling below normal, based on the normal population study.

Table 10-4 Ranges of sensory organization test scores as a function of age for 194 normal adults

	Population equilibrium scores (means [fifth percentiles])		
Condition	20 to 59 years of age (N = 112)	60 to 69 years of age (N = 54)	70 to 79 years of age (N = 28)
1	94 (90)	94 (90)	89 (70)
2	92 (85)	91 (86)	86 (63)
3 (average)	91 (86)	89 (80)	88 (82)
4 (average)	82 (70)	85 (77)	78 (69)
5 (average)	69 (52)	65 (51)	61 (45)
6 (average)	67 (48)	65 (49)	53 (27)
Composite	798 (704)	776 (676)	729 (638)

and upper-body movements is large. Therefore this region of the plot is labeled "hip dominant." Points in the lower right quadrant indicate trials in which COG sway excursions are large, but the movements are primarily about the ankle joints. Therefore this region is labeled "ankle dominant." Points falling along an upper right to lower left diagonal indicate trials in which the amplitude of hip and upper-body movements increase in proportion to the amplitude of the COG sway.

In the strategy analysis plots of the normal population, points corresponding to individual trials fall along a diagonal. This result occurs because individuals normally use ankle movements when the COG is well within the LOS (high equilibrium scores) and increase their use of hip movements as the COG approaches the LOS (low equilibrium scores). When points in the strategy analysis plot fall along a nearly vertical line, the patient is abnormally dependent on ankle movements. Points along a horizontal line indicate that the patient is abnormally dependent on hip movements.

Summary

A patient's ability to effectively use each of the three sensory inputs to posture control and to select the functionally appropriate sense(s) under a variety of conditions is assessed by systematically exposing the patient to six sensory conditions. Ability to maintain postural stability under each sensory condition is assessed by determining the distance between the COG and the LOS during sway. The patient's postural stability relative to normal is determined by comparing stability scores based on weighted averages of the six sensory conditions. In patients with reduced stability the specific dysfunctional sense or senses are then determined by the pattern of normal versus abnormal equilibrium scores obtained during the six conditions.

Strategy analysis assesses a patient's ability to make effective use of ankle and hip movement strategies over a range of sway amplitudes. Normal individuals use primarily ankle movements when sway is small and use progressively more hip

movements as the sway amplitude approaches the stability limits. The COG alignment score assesses the patient's ability to maintain the body sway when centered over the base of support.

DIAGNOSTIC APPLICATIONS FOR COMPUTERIZED DYNAMIC POSTUROGRAPHY
Patient Selection

Some components of computerized dynamic posturography (CDP) results correlate with specific types of disease and therefore are applicable during the diagnostic process. Other components of the CDP results identify the patient's adaptive strategies for coping with the balance disorder. These results are most useful in designing a course of treatment and monitoring the outcome. Still other CDP components correlate with the patient's functional capabilities in daily life. These later results are applicable to the objective assessment of the patient's disability. In all instances, however, the clinical value of the posture evoked response, motor coordination, and sensory organization test results is maximized in combination with the patient's history and the results of other clinical tests.

The clinical applicability of CDP assessment varies with the chief complaints of the individual patient and the clinical goals of the physician or therapist. In the diagnostic process CDP has the most clinical value for patients with symptoms of unsteadiness, disorientation, or vertigo, or a combination of these, in whom the history and physical examination do not suggest an obvious localized cause. In such cases the underlying disease process is unknown, and the initial clinical goal is to identify the process. Symptoms in such patients include the following:

Dysequilibrium of unknown origin

History of falls

Vertigo or dizziness that does not respond to the usual medications

Persistent disequilibrium with normal vestibular function test results and rotational-chair results

Gait or postural disorders when the neurologic examination results either are within normal

Table 10-5 Patterns of posture evoked response test results and their clinical significance

Probable disease or disorder	Responses		
	Short latency	Medium latency	Long latency
Normal peripheral nerve, spinal, brain stem, and subcortical pathways	Normal	Normal	Normal
Brain stem or subcortical deficit, or both	Normal	Normal or prolonged	Prolonged
Peripheral nerve deficit, possible brain stem or subcortical involvement, or both	Prolonged	Prolonged	Prolonged

limits or reveal only soft signs that do not account for the symptoms

Persistent symptoms after aminoglycoside therapy, chemotherapy, or inner-ear surgery

Progressive rigidity or spasticity

Interpretation of Posture Evoked Response Test Results

Analysis of the EMG latencies of the three response components provides information that can assist in localizing disease within the sensory and motor pathways of the spinal cord, brain stem, and subcortical areas involved in maintaining postural stability. Localization is possible because the three EMG components assessed by the PER test are mediated at different levels of the central nervous system.[25] Additional localizing information is provided by the distribution of normal and abnormal latencies between the two legs and movement directions.

Table 10-5 presents the typical patterns of normal and abnormal results for a single leg and movement direction and the probable CNS lesion sites associated with each pattern. Delay of all three response components strongly suggests peripheral nerve disease, although a combination of peripheral nerve disease and central nervous system (CNS) disease cannot be ruled out on the basis of the absolute latencies alone.[25] Because the peripheral nerve sensory and motor pathways are common to three response components, it is physiologically impossible for only the SL response to be delayed.

The distribution of prolonged latencies between the two legs provides additional information relative to the location of a lesion because the efferent spinal and brain stem pathways mediating long-loop responses are anatomically distinct for the two legs and movement directions. Bilateral and bidirectional prolongations of latencies are most likely the result of global CNS deficits such as polyneuropathy, neurotoxic exposure, and multiple sclerosis. Unilateral prolongations are indicative of localized CNS lesions, which may be peripheral (for example, peripheral nerve injury) or central (for example, brain stem stroke). Unidirectional prolongations of latencies are most likely caused by CNS deficits localized to efferent branches of the brain stem, spinal cord, and peripheral nerve circuits, although this has not been verified by clinical trials. The muscle proprioceptor inputs responsible for triggering automatic responses are bidirectionally sensitive, and delay or disruption of sensory input limited to one direction of movement is unlikely.

Prolonged latencies are evidence for abnormality in any one or a combination of components that make up the long-loop automatic system and therefore are strong indications for nonvestibular, spinal cord, brain stem, or subcortical involvement.[7,66,107] Delay of the ML and LL of only the LL component is suggestive of a spinal cord or brain stem lesion, or both.[29,32,62] Delays limited to the ML or LL component, or both, have been reported in patients with multiple sclerosis,[32] posterior column lesions,[29] and Huntington's disease.[107] Additional research suggests that PER test and electroencephalogram (EEG) scalp recordings can be combined to further isolate delays in the third component to the afferent (sensory) or the efferent (motor) branches of the long-loop system.[1]

Peripheral neuropathy,[66] multiple sclerosis,[94] neurotoxic exposure,[7] and age-related disorders[113] are commonly associated with bidirectional and bilateral prolonged latencies. Localized brain stem lesions such as those associated with stroke[81a] and cerebral palsy[89] commonly cause unilateral latency abnormalities, whereas global brain stem disorders result in bilaterally prolonged latencies.[107] Prolonged latencies associated with orthopedic injuries also have been reported, but these have not been formally verified by clinical trials. In contrast, prolonged latencies are not commonly associated with cerebellar deficits and Parkinson's disease,[8,25,53,57] although the cerebellum and basal ganglia influence other characteristics of the automatic responses.

Interpretation of Abnormal Automatic Postural Responses

Abnormalities in the magnitudes of automatic responses occur in patterns similar to those described for the latencies. Bilateral and bidirectional magnitude abnormalities are likely to be caused by adaptive deficits in the neural modulation of automatic responses. For example, large bilateral magnitude elevations are observed in patients with cerebellar deficits.[53] Less dramatic bilateral elevations are seen in patients with profound bilateral vestibular losses who (presumably) become increasingly responsive to the alternative somatosensory input.[53]

Unilateral reductions in magnitude are likely to occur in the presence of localized neural or musculoskeletal lesions. For example, patients with hemiplegia caused by brain stem stroke show not only increased latency responses but also reduced magnitudes on the affected side.[81a]

Interpretation of Sensory Organization Test Results

Normal versus abnormal results. A person's overall level of performance on the SOT is best characterized by the composite equilibrium score, which is the average of the following 14

equilibrium scores: the condition 1 average score, the condition 2 average score, and the three scores from each trial of the conditions 3 through 6. The resulting composite score is a weighted average that emphasizes the equilibrium scores for conditions 3 through 6. This weighting is used because sensory balance deficits are more readily reflected during testing of the more difficult sensory conditions.

Physiologic inconsistency. In one form of inconsistent pattern a patient with an abnormal composite score obtains equilibrium scores for the more difficult sensory conditions, 4, 5, and 6, that are equal to or better than those obtained for the easier conditions, 1, 2, and 3.[50] In the typical inconsistent pattern (Fig. 10-13) the equilibrium scores for sensory conditions 5 and 6 are both within the normal range, whereas scores for the easier conditions, 1, 2, and 3, and the composite score are abnormal. In any of the previously described instances the SOT is internally inconsistent, and the patient's sensory organization should be considered normal.

A second form of inconsistency occurs when a poor SOT result is seen in a patient whose balance and locomotor capabilities are not obviously impaired in daily life. Specifically, substantially abnormal scores for conditions 1 and 2 are physiologically inconsistent when observed in a patient who does not have ataxia and ambulates without the use of balance aids. The preceding types of results are judged inconsistent because research has shown a strong correlation between SOT findings and other clinical measures of balance system disability.[64]

For example, physiologically inconsistent results of the previously described types occur when the patient exhibits a regular but well-controlled sway oscillation that does not increase as the task becomes more difficult or when the patient simply exaggerates sway during the easier conditions. An inconsistent SOT pattern in the absence of any other findings is interpreted as positive evidence that the patient is exaggerating symptoms of postural instability.

Vestibular dysfunction. When a patient's composite equilibrium score is in the abnormal

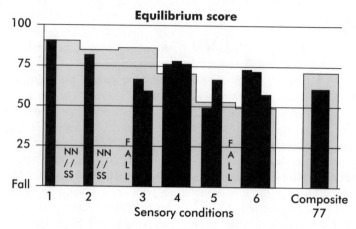

Fig. 10-13 Example of a physiologically inconsistent SOT result. Because the sensory analysis is invalid in these cases, only the equilibrium score is shown.

range and no evidence of inconsistency exists, the ratio scores determined by sensory organization analysis are examined, to identify the dysfunctional sense(s). A sense is said to be dysfunctional when the patient either cannot or does not effectively use information from the sense to maintain balance. A dysfunctional sense may be caused by loss of the peripheral input, disruption of CNS pathways processing the input, adaptive suppression of the input, or a combination of these factors.

A patient's ability to make effective use of the vestibular input is reflected by the ratio between the equilibrium scores for sensory conditions 5 and 1. Condition 5 provides the most definitive assessment of the vestibular input because useful somatosensory inputs are disrupted by sway referencing and vision is removed by eye closure. The patient with vestibular dysfunction experiences instability when both the support surface and visual inputs are reduced by conditions such as darkness in conjunction with an irregular or compliant support surface.

Vestibular dysfunction patterns similar to that shown in Fig. 10-14 are seen in virtually all patients with bilateral peripheral vestibular deficits. These patients perform relatively normally during sensory conditions 1 through 4, but free-falling

occurs repeatedly during sensory conditions 5 and 6.[13,56,74,83,105] Similarly, patients with uncompensated unilateral peripheral lesions perform abnormally during sensory condition 5 only or during conditions 5 and 6.* In these patients free-falling may occur, or they may either fall after attempts to regain balance or remain standing but score well below normal limits.

Because the SOT tests the patient's ability to effectively use sensory inputs but does not test the peripheral senses themselves, the vestibular dysfunction pattern does not distinguish between peripheral and CNS vestibular lesions.[50] Similar vestibular dysfunction patterns are seen in patients with peripheral vestibular lesions and in patients with CNS lesions affecting central pathways of the vestibular system, for example, patients with cerebellar ataxia.[89] For similar reasons the SOT does not detect well-compensated unilateral vestibular lesions. Patients who compensate after unilateral injuries typically return to normal SOT performance within 2 to 4 weeks of the initial insult.[17,44,46]

Vision preference. A patient's ability to suppress input from the visual system when it is available but functionally inaccurate is reflected by the

---

*References 5, 17, 20, 24, 27, 44, 46, 58, and 110.

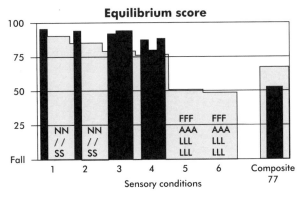

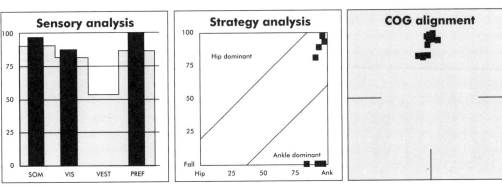

Fig. 10-14 Sensory organization test results for a patient with vestibular dysfunction.

ratio comparing the sum of equilibrium scores for conditions 3 and 6 with the sum of those for conditions 2 and 5. When functionally inaccurate (sway-referenced) visual inputs are presented, the normal individual ignores the visual input and performs as if the eyes were closed. In contrast, the patient who balances normally in the absence of vision but who prefers the conflicting visual input is less stable during sway-referenced visual conditions 3 and 6 than during the comparable eyes-closed conditions 2 and 5. An example of a vision preference pattern is shown in Fig. 10-15. Patients with an abnormal vision preference experience unsteadiness and disorientation in environments containing many moving visual stimuli.

An abnormal preference for vision, either alone or in combination with vestibular dysfunction, is most frequently observed in patients with posttrau-matic vertigo and unsteadiness.[11] Some elderly patients with unsteadiness also demonstrate an abnormal preference for vision, especially during their first few exposures to conditions 3 and 6.[113] Although the pathologic basis for vision preference is unknown, the previously described origins suggest that the deficit is more likely to occur in the CNS processing of vestibular and visual information.

Somatosensory dysfunction. The use of the somatosensory input is reflected by the ratio between the eyes-open and eyes-closed equilibrium scores obtained during conditions 1 and 2. This ratio is equivalent to the classic "Romberg quotient" and is interpreted in the same manner.[96] In normal individuals who are standing on a fixed, regular support surface the somatosensory input dominates the control of balance under both eyes-open and eyes-closed conditions. Hence, in a

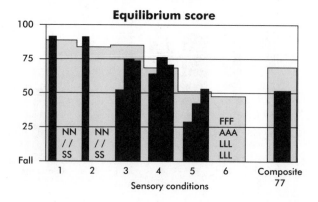

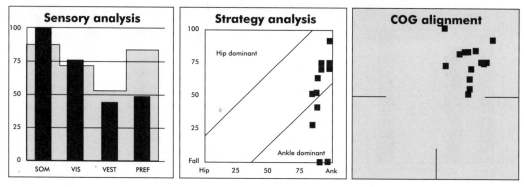

Fig. 10-15 Sensory organization test results for a patient with an abnormal preference for vision.

normal individual sway decreases little if at all when the eyes are closed.[15,16]

The patient who relies on the visual rather than somatosensory input to maintain balance during fixed surface conditions shows significantly increased sway with eye closure (Fig. 10-16). Sway increases with eye closure, even if the vestibular input is functioning normally, because the vestibular input is not as sensitive in controlling sway as the somatosensory or visual inputs are. The patient who depends on vision is expected to show ataxia and instability during normal ambulation because use of vision can be difficult when the patient is moving.

Vision dysfunction. The ability to make effective use of the visual input to maintain balance is reflected by the ratio between the equilibrium scores for sensory conditions 4 and 1. This ratio extends the concept of the Romberg quotient to the visual system, which is isolated by means of a sway-referenced support surface (condition 4) to remove the useful somatosensory input. If the patient cannot or does not make effective use of vision in the absence of useful somatosensory inputs, sway increases abnormally during condition 4 (Fig. 10-17). Patients with visual dysfunction ambulate normally on a fixed, level support surface. The patient with vision dysfunction, however, is destabilized by compliant, irregular, or moving support surfaces.

A patient in whom two of the three senses are dysfunctional exhibits what is generally called multisensory pattern.[50,88] The patient with multi-

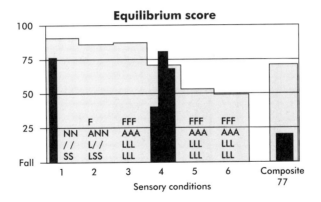

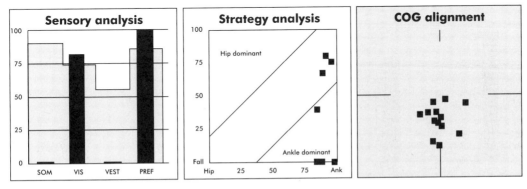

Fig. 10-16   Sensory organization text results for a patient with vestibular and somatosensory dysfunction.

sensory pattern depends on a single sense for balance. When both visual and vestibular inputs are dysfunctional, for example, the patient depends at all times on the somatosensory input for balance. This patient is unsteady whenever the support surface is irregular, compliant, or moving. The patient with dysfunctional somatosensory and vestibular inputs depends at all times on vision for balance and is unsteady whenever the visual surround is obscured or in motion.

Clinical research has shown that multisensory patterns occur principally in patients with CNS lesions extending beyond the peripheral or CNS vestibular system. In support of this conclusion, many patients with multisensory SOT patterns also demonstrate prolonged latencies, another CDP finding consistent with CNS disease.[107,111]

Interpretation of Strategy Analysis and Center of Gravity Alignment Results

Inappropriate use of ankle and hip movements can be caused by many different types of disorders. Weakness of the ankle joint muscles, for example, limits the torsional forces that can be exerted about the ankles and forces the patient to rely on hip movements. Ankle muscle weakness is more likely to affect the anterior tibialis (dorsiflexor) and the associated forward body movements. Because the strengths of the gastrocnemius and soleus muscles (ankle plantar flexors) are determined by requirements for running and jumping, their strengths are normally many times greater than the strengths of the muscles required for balance.

Loss of ankle joint mobility forces a patient to rely more heavily on hip joint movements, whereas

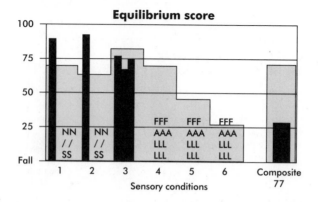

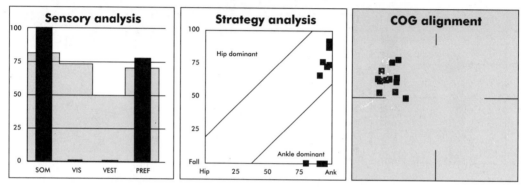

Fig. 10-17 Sensory organization test results for a patient with vestibular and vision dysfunction.

loss of hip joint mobility leads to an increased reliance on ankle movements. The patient who has pain with movement about the ankles or hips may also alter the movement strategy to minimize movements about the affected joints. Research suggests that patients who have lost sensations in the feet and ankle joints modify their patterns to rely more heavily on hip movements.[56]

Many disorders can result in lateral shifts in COG alignment. Examples include pain with weight bearing, limb weakness resulting from musculoskeletal injury, unilateral neurologic deficits affecting limb sensations and motor responses, and central vestibular system disease disrupting the sense of position relative to vertical.[102] Posturography information alone may not differentiate among the other possible causes of an asymmetry

in weight bearing. When localized brain stem disease such as stroke causes a lateral shift in COG alignment, prolonged response latencies, reduced response magnitudes, or both latency and magnitude abnormalities are likely to occur in one of the two legs. In cases of localized brain stem disease, however, the resulting latency and magnitude abnormalities may occur in either leg relative to the lateral shift in COG alignment.

Summary

Dynamic posturography provides objective measures of the major sensory and motor components of balance. Some of the measures provide diagnostic information relative to the sensory and motor systems. Other measures provide information relative to the patient's functional status within a variety of tasks. These latter measures are useful for establishing goals for treatment and monitoring the results. Because posturography incorporates a number of independent measures of posture control, it is possible to identify inconsistencies among the independent test results. This information can be useful in identifying nonphysiologic causes such as anxiety and deliberate exaggeration of symptoms.

BALANCE TRAINING APPLICATIONS OF COMPUTERIZED DYNAMIC POSTUROGRAPHY
Patients Likely to Benefit from Balance Training

Training focused on improving dysfunctional components of balance can have a positive impact on the overall performance capabilities of patients with dizziness or unsteadiness, or both. Patients likely to benefit from balance training are identified by the history, diagnosis, psychologic profile, and other life-style factors. A thorough description of the positive indications for balance training have not been fully articulated because CDP is a relatively new approach. The evidence, however, suggests that elderly persons with balance problems,[100] patients with vestibular deficit and symptoms of dizziness and unsteadiness,[51,103,104,106] and those with brain injuries resulting from trauma and stroke[102] are among the appropriate candidates for balance training.

Problems in patients who are likely to benefit from the use of CDP in treatment design and monitoring include the following:

Balance dysfunction resulting from head trauma
Stroke-related balance and mobility problems
Developmental disorders such as cerebral palsy and certain learning disorders involving balance and motor coordination
Age-related balance problems in an otherwise normal individual
Balance dysfunction resulting from vestibular disease

Setting Goals for Balance Training

Once the decision to use balance training has been made, additional information is needed to identify which of the patient's functions can be improved by training and which are best managed by modifying the patient's life-style and expectations. Such information is necessary because preliminary clinical research indicates that balance training focused on the specific functional problems of the patient is more effective than generalized conditioning.[21,51,100,101,103] For example, a normally sighted person making ineffective use of vision or having an abnormal preference for vision under conflict conditions can be trained to make more effective use of vision. In contrast, a patient with profound bilateral loss of vestibular dysfunction cannot regain the vestibular balance capability and must be counseled to avoid environments with inadequate lighting and unstable surfaces.

Directing Treatment Toward the Patient's Functional Problems

Understanding the patient's primary functional problems and the higher-level adaptive strategies used to cope with these problems is critical to designing an optimal treatment approach, whether the treatment includes surgery, drugs, physical therapy, or a combination of approaches. This understanding is critical because adaptation and motor learning are the primary means by which a patient optimizes performance in the presence of both temporary and irreversible changes in the nervous system. Of course, other factors extending beyond the scope of this chapter must also be considered before undertaking treatment. These include the probable course of the disease process, the presence of other exacerbating conditions, and the patient's life-style and treatment expectations.

The purpose of some CDP tests is to provide objective, quantitative information relative to the patient's functional problems and higher-level adaptive strategies. The process predicting the outcome of a treatment approach is usually complex because balance capabilities are influenced by the interactions of multiple components and adaptive strategies and because the correlations between any known disease or disorder and the nature and extent of the individual's functional balance disability are frequently weak. In some cases consideration of all the factors can lead to an adequate understanding of the patient's problem in advance of treatment. In other cases the patient's underlying disease or disorder is never well understood. In either case a treatment aimed at reducing symptoms and improving performance must be undertaken, if possible.[22,51,100,101,103]

Functional Problems Treated by Postural Stability Training

Vestibular dysfunction. Patients with abnormal vestibular SOT patterns may be improved by training, depending on the underlying diagnosis.[51,104,106] In patients with profound bilateral loss of vestibular function training cannot be used to restore postural stability in the absence of useful visual and somatosensory inputs. In contrast, training can be a primary mode of treatment in patients with vestibular dysfunction patterns caused by incomplete compensation for partial peripheral CNS vestibular lesions, or both. Training is also a useful adjunct when drugs or surgery are also used to treat the latter conditions.

Multisensory disorders with and without prolonged latencies. Vestibular and vision dysfunction, vestibular and somatosensory dysfunction, and either of these patterns combined with prolonged latencies are all indicative of additional CNS disease, which may or may not be documented by other clinical tests.[110] Although clinical studies substantiating the experiences of these patients are incomplete, anecdotal evidence suggests that the prognosis for improvement with training may be more limited when the latencies are also prolonged.

Exaggerated symptoms of postural unsteadiness. Inconsistent results in the absence of other clinical findings suggest that the patient's postural stability is physiologically normal but impaired either by intense anxiety or by deliberate exaggeration of the symptoms. In the presence of other clinical findings an inconsistent SOT pattern suggests that the patient's stability problems are aggravated by anxiety or exaggeration. A diagnosis of exaggerated

symptoms is further substantiated in patients who refuse to cooperate with training. If the patient improves with training, deliberate exaggeration may be ruled out, although the actual cause might never be determined.

Vision preference. In the patient with an abnormal preference for vision, none of the three senses are dysfunctional. The three sensory ratios are within the normal range, indicating normal performance during sensory conditions 2, 4, and 5. Rather, the patient has an adaptive problem in determining when to ignore the visual information. Scores are below the normal range during sensory condition 6 or conditions 3 and 6. Thus when visual information is functionally useful (for example, in a fixed and visible surround), the patient makes effective use of vision and stands normally, even when somatosensory inputs are disrupted. However, the patient uses the visual input when it provides erroneous information.

Inappropriate movement strategies. A normal individual moves primarily about the ankles when sway amplitudes are well within the LOS and increases the use of hip movement when sway approaches the LOS. Postural movements are ineffective in the patient who uses ankle strategy movements to control sway displacements of large amplitude. The patient who depends on ankle movements falls prematurely when sway amplitudes are large. The patient using hip movements to control sway of small amplitude is inefficient and expends a needlessly high level of energy to maintain a centered COG position.

Ineffective use of movement strategies may be caused by an abnormal adaptation or by an inability to produce one of the two movement patterns. For example, inappropriate use of hip movements during sway of small amplitude might be an abnormal adaptation caused by anxiety or by misperception of the LOS. In these cases training aimed at teaching the appropriate conditions for using ankle movements can have a positive impact. In contrast, weakness of ankle joint muscles, loss of ankle sensation, reduced mobility about the ankles, or combinations of these factors prevent the patient from generating effective ankle movements and are contraindications for movement strategy training unless the underlying physiologic factors also are addressed.

Inappropriate use of ankle movements during sway of large amplitude might be an abnormal adaptation used by a dizzy patient to minimize head movements and associated stimulation of the vestibular system. When inappropriate use of ankle movement is an abnormal adaptation, training is likely to have a positive effect. Contraindications to teaching appropriate use of hip movements might include weakness or loss of mobility about the hip joints. There is also clinical evidence suggesting that patients with profound bilateral loss of peripheral vestibular function cannot effectively coordinate hip movements and that training in these cases is ineffective.[105]

Abnormal center of gravity alignment. A normal individual maintains the COG very nearly centered over the base of support. Although sway increases significantly during difficult sensory conditions, normal individuals continue to maintain the COG alignment near the center. The patient whose COG is maintained forward, backward, or to one side of the center of the base of support cannot tolerate larger COG displacements in the direction of the misalignment without loss of postural stability. A misaligned COG increases the risk for falls, especially when displacement is in the backward direction.

Like inappropriate movement strategies, abnormal COG alignment can be the result either of an abnormal adaptation or of underlying musculoskeletal deficits. Examples of disorders inhibiting normal COG alignment include muscular weakness or contractures and orthopedic disorders. In the absence of musculoskeletal deficits that prevent normal COG alignment, biofeedback therapy in which the patient's COG position is displayed relative to the LOS can be successful in teaching patients to monitor the COG position.[46]

Abnormal response magnitudes. Abnormally weak automatic responses can be caused by neuromuscular deficits, by CNS deficits affecting the input drive to the postural muscles, or by adaptive abnormalities. When response weakness is unilateral, the cause is likely to be neuromuscular. When adaptive abnormalities are involved, the automatic responses are more frequently bilaterally reduced or increased. Central adaptive abnormalities such as those caused by cerebellar deficits are always the cause when the automatic responses are abnormally strong.[53] The effects of training on automatic response strengths are unknown.

Summary

Training focused on the primary functional problems and secondary adaptive strategies of the individual can have a positive effect on postural stability in a variety of patients. The most effective training program, however, incorporates all the information from the patient's history, physical examination, and clinical test results. Dynamic posturography is particularly useful in identifying adaptive strategies related to use of sensory inputs, movement patterns, COG alignment, and response strengths.

COMPUTERIZED DYNAMIC POSTUROGRAPHY APPLICATIONS IN DISABILITY AND RISK ASSESSMENT
Elderly Persons

Although many factors contribute to loss of mobility in elderly persons, impaired postural stability is an important component.[92,112] In addition, fall-related injury is a major cause of morbidity in this age group. Because of the prevalence of stability and mobility disorders that have a major negative impact on the quality of life and independence of elderly persons,[108] fall risk assessment and intervention are appropriate for these patients.

Although aging can affect a wide range of factors that contribute to abnormal postural stability, including the biomechanical, musculoskeletal, and sensorimotor systems, recent evidence suggests that the ability to quickly adapt to unexpected conditions and challenges provides a sensitive indication of the risk of impending falls in normal elderly individuals.[58,67,97,113] Results from recent clinical studies suggest that certain elements of CDP can be appropriate objective tools for assessing the potential impact of impaired postural stability on safe mobility in elderly individuals. Recent study results further indicate that training can substantially improve balance function, even in elderly persons of advanced age.[67]

Occupations Requiring Exceptional Balance Skills

Assessment of postural stability can be a major challenge in persons with such occupations as commercial and military flying, which require exceptional spatial orientation and coordination skills. Given the time and expense of training pilots, methods are being sought to more quickly identify those unlikely to qualify for the work. Similarly, when a qualified pilot develops a medical problem involving the balance system, accurate information is needed to determine whether or when the individual should return to work.

No standards have been established for occupational assessment of postural stability. However, recent investigations indicate that the stressful and life-like balance function tests (particularly those requiring persons to perform in a variety of tasks and environments) do provide an accurate, objective measure of the individual's overall performance capabilities. For example, a recent retrospective study of the Royal Danish Air Force concluded that the vestibular autorotation test is more sensitive than the traditional caloric test in setting minimal vestibular function test standards for high-performance pilots.[109] Similarly, the SOT protocol of CDP consistently shows the inability of astronauts to suppress inappropriate visual cues to balance during the early phases of readaptation after prolonged exposure to zero-gravity and zero-gravity simulator conditions.[93] In addition, the results of the SOT component correlates well with the dizziness handicap inventory test results in patients with documented balance disorders.[64]

Medical-Legal Cases Involving Balance Disorders

Medical-legal cases involving complaints of unsteadiness or dizziness, or both, can be difficult to settle equitably because there are no well-established correlations between the traditional hard clinical signs of disease and the actual extent of a patient's symptoms and functional impairment. Although suspicion that the patient is exaggerating symptoms for secondary gain is raised by negative results on the classic clinical tests, these tests provide only indirect circumstantial evidence. That is, they are not based on the patient's functional capabilities in an interactive test situation. Thus the information gained from CDP can be of significant assistance in two ways. First, CDP test protocols provide an objective assessment of the patient's balance function that can be related to his or her capabilities in daily life. Second, when CDP results are physiologically inconsistent, they can provide positive evidence for exaggeration of symptoms.

CONCLUSION

Postural stability is a major requirement for many activities of daily living and is therefore receiving increased attention from medical practitioners. A systematic model of the biomechanical and physiologic mechanisms underlying normal postural stability has evolved over the past 20 years, although our knowledge is still incomplete. The systematic model of postural functions is allowing researchers and clinicians to divide the process into its component parts and to understand the interactions among the components under a variety of task conditions.

The systematic model of postural stability has guided the development of new methods for assessment, medical treatment, and training of abnormal postural functions. In the area of training the systematic model and improved assessment methods are allowing clinicians to design more effective treatments focused on the patient's specific abnormal functions and to objectively monitor the outcomes of these treatments. At the same time, the aging population, new laws granting additional rights to disabled workers, and increased concern for occupational liability are shifting the clinical focus toward prevention and quality-of-life issues. Assessment and training applications of dynamic posturography will continue to play an important role in these areas.

REFERENCES

1. Ackermann H, Diener HC, Dichgans J: Mechanically evoked cerebral potentials and long-latency muscle responses in the evaluation of afferent and efferent long-loop pathways in humans, *Neurosci Lett* 66:233, 1986.
2. Allum JHJ, Honegger F, Pfaltz CR: The role of stretch and vestibulospinal reflexes in the generation of human equilibrating reactions. In Allum, JHJ, Hulliger M, editors: *Progress in brain research,* vol 80, New York, 1989, Elsevier.
3. Allum JHJ, Keshner EA: Vestibular and proprioceptive control of sway stabilization. In Bles W, Brandt Th, editors: *Disorders of posture and gait,* New York, 1986, Elsevier.
4. Aggashyan RV et al: Changes in spectral and correlation characteristics of human stabilograms at muscle afferentation disturbance, *Agressologie* 14:5, 1973.
5. Asai M et al: Clinical evaluation of the EquiTest system in peripheral vestibular patients. In Brandt Th et al, editors: *Disorders of posture and gait,* New York, 1990, Georg Thieme Verlag.
6. Bawa P, Stein RB: Frequency response of human soleus muscle, *J Neurophysiol* 39:788, 1976.
7. Beckley DJ et al: *Dynamic posturography in the assessment of cisplatyn neurotoxicity* (abstract), Annual meeting, American Academy of Neurology, Boston, April 1991.
8. Beckley DJ et al: Electrophysiological correlates of postural instability in Parkinson's disease, *Electroenceph Clin Neurophysiol* 81:263, 1991.
9. Begbie JV: Some problems of postural sway. In deReuck AVS, Knight J, editors: *CIBA Foundation symposium on myotatic, kinesthetic and vestibular mechanisms,* London, 1967, Churchill-Livingstone.
10. Belen'kii VY, Gurfinkel VS, Pal'tsev YI: On the elements of voluntary movement control, *Biophysics* 12:135, 1967.
11. Black FO, Nashner LM: Vestibulospinal control differs in patients with reduced versus distorted vestibular function, *Acta Otolaryngol* 406:110, 1984.
12. Black FO, Nashner LM: Postural control in four classes of vestibular abnormalities. In Igarashi M., Black FO, editors: *Vestibular and visual control of posture and locomotor equilibrium,* Basel, 1985, Karger.
13. Black FO, Wall C III, Nashner LM: Effect of visual and support surface references upon postural control in vestibular deficit subjects, *Acta Otolaryngol Scand* 95:199, 1983.
14. Black FO, Wall C III, O'Leary DP: Computerized screening of the human vestibulospinal system, *Ann Otol Rhinol Laryngol* 87:853, 1978.
15. Black FO et al: Normal subject postural sway during the Romberg test, *Am J Otolaryngol* 3:309, 1982.
16. Black FO et al: Abnormal postural control associated with peripheral vestibular disorders. In Pompeiano O, Allum JHJ, editors: *Progress in brain research,* vol 76, New York, 1988, Elsevier.
17. Black FO et al: Effects of unilateral loss of vestibular function on the vestibuloocular reflex and posture control, *Ann Otol Rhinol Laryngol* 98:884, 1989.
18. Bles W, de Jong JMBV: Unilateral and bilateral loss of vestibular function. In Bles W, Brandt Th, editors: *Disorders of posture and gait,* New York, 1986, Elsevier.
19. Bles W, de Jong JMBV, de Wit G: Somatosensory compensation for loss of labyrinthine function, *Acta Otolaryngol* 97:213, 1984.
20. Bowman CA, Mangham CA: Clinical use of moving platform posturography, *Sem Hearing* 10:161, 1989.
21. Brandt Th, Daroff RB: Physical therapy for benign paroxysmal positional vertigo, *Arch Otolaryngol* 106:484, 1980.
22. Brandt Th, Paulus W, Straube A: Vision and posture. In Bles W, Brandt Th, editors: *Disorders of posture and gait,* New York, 1986, Elsevier.
23. Cordo PJ, Nashner LM: Properties of postural adjustments associated with rapid arm movements, *J Neurophysiol* 47:287, 1982.
24. Cyr DG, Moore GF, Moller CG: Clinical application of computerized dynamic posturography, *Entechnology* 9:36, 1989.
25. Dichgans J, Diener HC: Clinical evidence for functional compartmentalization of the cerebellum. In Bloedel JR, Dichgans J, Precht W, editors: *Cerebellar functions,* New York, 1985, Springer-Verlag.
26. Dichgans J, Diener HC: Different forms of postural ataxia in patients with cerebellar diseases. In Bles W, Brandt Th, editors: *Disorders of posture and gait,* New York, 1986, Elsevier.
27. Dichgans J, Diener HC. The contribution of vestibulospinal mechanisms to the maintenance of human upright posture, *Acta Otolaryngol Scand* (in press).
28. Diener HC, Dichgans J: On the role of vestibular, visual, and somatosensory information for dynamic postural control in humans. In Pompeiano O, Allum JHJ, editors: *Progress in brain research,* vol 76, New York, 1988, Elsevier.
28a. Diener HC, Horak FB, Nashner LM: Influence of stimulus parameters on human postural responses, *J Neurophysiol* 59:1888,
29. Diener HC et al: Characteristic alterations of long-loop "reflexes" in patients with Friedrich's disease and late atrophy of the cerebellar anterior lobe, *J Neurol Neurosurg Psychiatr* 47:679, 1984.
30. Diener HC et al: Early stabilization of human posture after sudden disturbance: influence of rate and amplitude of displacement, *Exp Brain Res* 56:126, 1984.
31. Diener HC et al: Quantification of postural sway in normals and patients with cerebellar diseases, *Electroencephalogr Clin Neurophysiol* 57:134, 1984.
32. Diener HC et al: The significance of delayed long-loop responses to ankle displacement for the diagnosis of multiple sclerosis, *Electroencephalogr Clin Neurophysiol* 57:336, 1984.

33. Diener HC et al: The significance of proprioception on postural stabilization as assessed by ischemia, *Exp Brain Res* 296:103, 1984.

34. Diener HC et al: Long loop reflexes in a standing subject and their use for clinical diagnosis. In Igarashi M, Black FO, editors: *Vestibular and visual control on posture and locomotor equilibrium,* Basel, 1985. Karger.

35. Diener HC et al: Medium- and long-latency responses to displacements of the ankle joint in patients with spinal and central lesions, *Electroencephalogr Clin Neurophysiol* 60:407, 1985.

36. Diener HC et al: Role of visual and static vestibular influences on dynamic posture control, *Human Neurobiol* 5:105, 1986.

37. Reference deleted in proofs.

38. Dietz V, Horstmann GA, Berger W: Significance of proprioceptive mechanisms in the regulation of stance. In Allum JHJ, Hulliger M, editors: *Progress in brain research,* vol 80, New York, 1989, Elsevier.

39. Dietz V, Quintern J, Berger W: Corrective reactions to stumbling in man: functional significance of spinal and transcortical reflexes, *Neurosci Lett* 44:131, 1984.

40. Dietz V et al: Cerebral potentials and leg muscle EMG responses associated with stance perturbation, *Exp Brain Res* 57:348, 1985.

41. Duncan PW et al: Functional reach: a new clinical measure of balance, *J Gerontol* 45:M192, 1990.

42. El'ner AM, Popov KE, Gurfinkel VS: Changes in stretch reflex system concerned with the control of postural activity of human muscle, Agressologie 13:19, 1972.

43. Evarts EV, Tanjii J: Gating of motor cortex reflexes by prior instruction, *Brain Res* 71:479, 1974.

44. Fetter M, Diener HC, Dichgans J: Recovery of postural control after an acute unilateral vestibular lesion in humans, *J Vest Res* 1:373, 1991.

45. Fregly AR: Vestibular ataxia and its measurement in man. In Kornhuber HH, editor: *Handbook of sensory physiology,* vol 6, no 2, Berlin 1974, Springer-Verlag.

46. Goebel JA, Paige GD: Dynamic posturography and caloric test results in patients with and without vertigo. *Otolaryngol Head Neck Surg* 100:553, 1989.

47. Gurfinkel VS, Lipshits MI, Popov KY: Is the stretch reflex the main mechanism in the system of regulation of the vertical posture of man? *Biophysics* 19:744, 1974.

48. Gurfinkel VS, Osevets M: Dynamics of the vertical posture in man, *Biophysics* 17:496, 1972.

49. Gurfinkel VS et al: The state of the stretch reflex during quiet standing in man, In Homma H, editor: *Progress in brain research,* vol 44, New York, 1976, Elsevier.

50. Hamid MA, Hughs GB, Kinny SE: Specificity and sensitivity of dynamic posturography: a retrospective analysis, *Acta Otolaryngol suppl* 481:596, 1991.

51. Herdman SJ: Management of balance disorders in vestibular deficiency, *Rehab Management* 4:68, 1991.

52. Hill AV: The mechanics of active muscle, *Proc R Soc Lond* 141B:104, 1953.

53. Horak FB: Comparison of cerebellar and vestibular loss on scaling of postural responses. In Brandt Th et al, editors: *Disorders of posture and gait,* New York, 1990, Georg Thieme Verlag.

54. Horak FB, Diener HC, Nashner LM: Influence of central set on human postural responses, *J Neurophysiol* 62:841, 1989.

55. Horak FB, Nashner LM: Central programming of postural movements: adaptation to altered support surface configurations, *J Neurophysiol* 55:1369, 1986.

56. Horak FB, Nashner LM, Diener HC: Postural strategies associated with somatosensory and vestibular loss, *Exp Brain Res* 82:167, 1990.

57. Horak FB, Nutt JG, Nashner LM: Postural inflexibility in Parkinsonian subjects, *J Neurol Sci* 111:46, 1992.

58. Horak FB, Shupert CL, Mirka A: Components of postural dyscontrol in the elderly: a review, *Neurobiol Aging* 10:727, 1989.

59. Horak FB et al: Vestibular function and motor proficiency of children with impaired hearing or with learning disability and motor impairment. *Dev Med Child Neurol* 30:64, 1988.

60. Koozekanni SH et al: On the role of dynamic models in quantitative posturography, *IEEE Trans Biomed Engl* 27:605, 1980.

61. Houk JC: Regulation of stiffness by skeletomotor reflexes, *Ann Rev Physiol* 41:99, 1979.

62. Huttunen J, Homberg V: EMG responses in leg muscles to postural perturbations in Huntington's disease, *J Neurol Neurosurg Psychiatr* 53:55, 1990.

63. Jackson RT, Epstein CM: Effect of head extension on equilibrium in normal subjects, *Ann Otol Rhinol Laryngol* 100:63, 1991.

64. Jacobson GP et al: Balance function test correlates of the dizziness handicap inventory, *J Am Acad Audiol* 2:253, 1991.

65. Koles ZJ, Casttelein RD: The relationship between body sway and foot pressure in normal man, *J Medical Eng Technol* 4:279, 1980.

66. Ledin T et al: Dynamic posturography in assessment of polyneuropathic disease, *J Vest Res* 1:123, 1991.

67. Ledin T et al: Kronhed AC, Moller C, Moller M, Odkvist LM, Effects of balance training in elderly evaluated by clinical tests and dynamic posturography, *J Vest Res* 1:129, 1991.

68. Lee DN, Lishman JR: Visual proprioceptive control of stance, *J Hum Move Stud* 1:87, 1975.

69. Lestienne F, Soechting J, Berthoz A: Postural readjustments induced by linear motion of visual scenes, *Exp Brain Res* 28:363, 1977.

70. Marsden DC, Merton PA, Morton HB: Latency measurements compatible with a cortical pathway for the stretch reflex in man, *J Physiol (Lond)* 230:58, 1973.

71. McCollum G, Horak FB, Nashner LM: Parsimony in neural calculations for postural movements. In Bloedel J, Dichgans J, Precht W, editors: *Cerebellar functions,* Berlin, 1984, Springer-Verlag.

72. McCollum G, Leen TK: Form and exploration of mechanical stability limits in erect stance, *J Motor Behav* 21:225, 1989.

73. Melvill Jones G, Watt DGD: Observations on the control of stepping and hopping movements in man, *J Physiol (Lond)* 219:709, 1971.

74. Mirka A, Black FO: Clinical application of dynamic posturography for evaluating sensory integration and vestibular dysfunction. In Arenberg IK, Smith DB, editors: *Neurologic clinics: diagnostic neurotology,* Philadelphia, 1990, WB Saunders.

75. Nardone A et al: Responses of leg muscles in humans displaced while standing, *Brain* 113:65, 1990.

76. Nashner LM: Adapting reflexes controlling the human posture, *Exp Brain Res* 26:59, 1976.

77. Nashner LM: Fixed patterns of rapid postural responses among leg muscles during stance, *Exp Brain Res* 150:403, 1977.

78. Nashner LM: Analysis of stance posture in humans. In Towe AL, Luschei ES, editors: *Handbook of behavioral neurobiology,* vol 5, New York, 1981, Plenum.

79. Nashner LM: Strategies for organization of human posture. In Igarashi M, Black FO, editors: *Vestibular and visual control of posture and locomotor equilibrium,* Basel, 1985, Karger.

80. Nashner LM: A functional approach to understanding spasticity. In Struppler A, Weindl A, editors: *Electromyography and evoked potentials,* Berlin, 1985, Springer-Verlag.

81. Nashner LM: The organization of human postural movements during standing and walking. In Grillner S et al, editors: *Neurobiology of posture and locomotion,* London, 1986, Macmillan.

81a. Nashner LM: Computerized dynamic posturography. In Jacobson GP, Newman CW, editors: *Handbook of balance function testing,* St. Louis, 1992, Mosby.

82. Nashner LM, Berthoz A: Visual contribution to rapid motor responses during posture control, *Brain Res* 150:403, 1978.

83. Nashner LM, Black FO, Wall C: Adaptation to alteres support and visual conditions during stance: patients with vestibular deficits, *J Neuroscience* 2:536, 1982.

84. Nashner LM, Cordo PG: Relation of automatic postural responses and reaction-time voluntary movements of human leg muscles, *Exp Brain Res* 43:395, 1981.

85. Nashner LM, Forssberg H: Phase-dependent organization of postural adjustments associated with arm movements while walking, *J Neurophysiol* 55:538,

86. Reference deleted in proofs.

87. Nashner LM, McCollum G: The organization of human postural movements: a formal basis and experimental synthesis, *Behav Brain Sci* 8:135, 1985.

88. Nashner LM, Peters JF: Dynamic posturography in the diagnosis and management of dizziness and balance disorders. In Arenberg IK, Smith DB, editors: *Neurologic clinics: diagnostic neurotology,* Philadelphia, 1990, WB Saunders.

89. Nashner LM, Shumway-Cook A, Marin O: Stance posture control in selected groups of children with cerebral palsy: deficits in sensory organization and muscular coordination, *Exp Brain Res* 197:393, 1983.

90. Nashner LM, Woollacott M, Tuma G: Organization of rapid responses to postural and locomotor-like perturbations of standing man, *Exp Brain Res* 36:463, 1979.

91. Nashner LM et al: Organization of posture controls: an analysis of sensory and mechanical constraints. In Allum JHJ, Hulliger M, editors: *Progress in brain research,* vol 80, New York, 1989, Elsevier.

92. Overstall PW et al: Falls in the elderly related to postural imbalance, *Br Med J* 1:261, 1977.

93. Paloski WH et al: Vestibular ataxia following shuttle flights, *Am J Otol* 14:9, 1993.

94. Panzer VP et al: Functional evaluation of clinical status in multiple sclerosis, *Am Neurol Acad* (abstract) 1991.

95. Paulus WM, Straube A, Brandt Th: Visual stabilization of posture: physiological stimulus characteristics and clinical aspects, *Brain* 107:1143, 1984.

96. Paulus W, Straube A, Brandt Th: Visual postural performance after loss of somatosensory and vestibular function, *J Neurol Neurosurg Psychiatr* 50:1542, 1987.

97. Peterka RJ, Black FO: Age-related changes in human posture control: sensory organization tests, *J Vest Res* 1:73, 1991.

98. Riley P, Mann RW, Hodge A: Modelling of the biomechanics of posture and balance, *J Biomech* 23:503, 1990.

99. Scott DE, Dzendolet F: Quantification of sway in standing humans, *Aggressologie* 13:35, 1972.

100. Shepard NT: The clinical use of dynamic posturography in the elderly, *Ear Nose Throat J* 68:940, 1989.

101. Shepard NT, Telian SA: Balance disorders (the dizzy patient). In Jacobson GP, Northern, editors: *Diagnostic audiology,* Austin, Tex, 1991, Pro Ed.

102. Shumway-Cook A, Anson D, Haller S: Postural sway biofeedback: its effect on reestablishing stance stability in hemiplegic patients, *Arch Phys Med Rehab* 69:395, 1988.

103. Shumway-Cook A, Horak FB: Vestibular rehabilitation: an exercise approach to managing symptoms of vestibular dysfunction, *Sem Hearing* 10:196, 1989.

104. Shumway-Cook A, Horak FB: Vestibular rehabilitation: an exercise approach to managing symptoms of vestibular dysfunction, *Neurol Clin North Am* 8:44, 1990.

105. Shupert CL et al: Coordination of head and body in response to support surface translations in normals and patients with bilaterally reduced vestibular function. In Amblard B, Berthoz A, Clarac F, editors: *Posture and gait: development, adaptation and modulation,* New York, 1988, Elsevier.

106. Smith-Wheelock M, Shepard NT, Telian SA: Physical therapy program for vestibular rehabilitation, *Am J Otol* 12:218, 1991.

107. Tian J-R, Herdman SJ, Zee DS: Postural instability in Huntington's disease, *Soc Neurosci (abstract)* 15:691, 1989.

108. Tinetti M, Speechley M, Ginter SF: Risk factors for falls among elderly persons living in the community, *New Engl J Med* 319: 1701, 1988.

109. Vesterhauge S, Mansson A: The vestibular autorotation test (VAT): its application in Danish aviation medicine. In Haid CT, editor: *Vestibulare diagnosis and neurootosurgical management of the skull base,* Grateifing, 1991, Demeter Verlag.

110. Voorhees RL: The role of dynamic posturography in neurotologic diagnosis, *Laryngoscope* 99:995, 1989.

111. Voorhees RL: Dynamic posturography findings in central nervous system disorders, *Otolaryngol Head Neck Surg* 103:96, 1990.

112. Wolfson L et al: Stressing the postural response: a quantitative method for testing balance, *J Am Geriatr Soc* 34:845, 1986.

113. Wolfson L et al: A dynamic posturography study of balance in healthy elderly, *Neurology* 42:2069, 1992.

114. Young LR et al: Spatial orientation in weightlessness and readaptation to earth's gravity, *Science* 225:202, 1984.

STUDY QUESTIONS

■ How does an individual maintain a stable posture?

■ Define the terms "limits of stability" and "limits of sway."

■ How are postural movements controlled, and how are they assessed in the clinic?

■ What is the interaction of vision and vestibular and somatosensory input for controlling posture, and how is somatosensory and visual input tested in the clinic?

■ Describe patients who may benefit from balance exercise training and factors that must be considered in developing the exercise training program.

PART V

EXERCISE FOR CHILDREN, ADOLESCENTS, AND ELDERLY PERSONS

■ *KEEP IN MIND WHILE YOU READ . . . In Chapter 11 Roy Shephard describes the effect of exercise training and limitations of exercise for healthy and frail elderly persons. Recommendations for exercise prescription are given, along with hints for motivating these patients. In Chapter 12 Oded Bar-Or describes factors that limit exercise tolerance for adolescents and children. In addition, the effects of exercise training are described for adolescents and children with asthma, cerebral palsy, cystic fibrosis, diabetes, hypertension, muscular dystrophy, or obesity. Excellent recommendations for determining intensity and mode of exercise are given. Special populations like elderly persons and children with chronic disease are rarely discussed in the literature. However, these two world-renowned physicians bring to light their experience in working with these patients. ■*

CHAPTER 11

TRAINING CONSIDERATIONS FOR HEALTHY AND FRAIL ELDERLY PERSONS

Roy J. Shephard

KEY TERMS

- Aging
- Cardiorespiratory function
- Exercise prescription
- Fitness
- Safety

In this chapter exercise programs and training responses for healthy ("normal") and frail elderly individuals are discussed. It may be helpful initially to define the two categories of elderly patients and to examine the anticipated influence of aging on the cardiorespiratory and neuromuscular systems.

DEFINITION OF HEALTH AND FRAILTY IN ELDERLY PATIENTS
Threshold of Old Age

Because of considerations of safety and convenience, many training studies supposedly dealing with elderly individuals have been focused on persons in the latter half of their working careers, with participants ranging in age from 40 to 65 years. Most geriatricians would regard such individuals as late middle-aged rather than elderly.

Attainment of the age of retirement from work is one obvious milestone that indicates the formal transition of status from a worker to a senior citizen. This threshold is currently reached at an age of 65 years in both Canada and the United States, but it occurs a few years earlier in some European countries.[126] Certainly the marker is not firmly fixed. In North America "equal opportunity" and "human rights" legislation is now tending to push back the age of mandatory retirement. On the other hand, automation is leading to much redundancy of workers and unemployment among people who were previously regarded as late middle-aged; for them, the threshold is being moved downward.

Gradations of Physical Condition

Even if the threshold of old age could be agreed upon, elderly persons do not form a homogenous group. Most people show a substantial deterioration in physical condition between the ages of 65 and 85 years. Thus one simple method of classification is to categorize elderly persons on the basis of calendar age. For instance, we might recognize the "young old" (65 to 75 years of age), the "middle old" (75 to 85 years of age), and the "very old" (over 85 years of age).

However, such a categorization ignores the potential for substantial differences in physical condition in persons who share an identical calendar age.[26,60] Because of interindividual differences in training, health, and inheritance, age gives only a crude guide to function. Attempts have been made to develop scales of biologic age by using a variety of anthropometric, physiologic, and psychologic markers, but such initiatives have foundered because it has been far from clear how to combine data obtained from such disparate disciplines either with each other or with measures of chronic disease. Too often, calculations of biologic age have proved little more than a complicated way of determining a person's calendar age.[126]

Functional Categorization

Since neither calendar age nor biologic age is entirely satisfactory as a means of categorizing elderly persons, there seems much to commend a simple functional classification, particularly when the concern is to prescribe an appropriate training program.

The *"young old"* might be considered a group of persons who are freed from the responsibilities of child care and are often retired from work and yet can live independently, with little or no restriction of physical activity. The *"middle old"* face increasing physical disability as a result of chronic disease or aging, or both, and require an increasing amount of assistance with their daily activities, whereas the *"very old"* are those who have become almost totally dependent, requiring either extensive support from a devoted relative or nursing care within some type of institution.

Relative Numbers of "Normal" and Frail Elderly Persons

The Canada Health Survey[20] found that 26.5% of individuals over the age of 65 years were frail and had some major limitation of habitual physical activity and that 8.9% of senior citizens were "very old" and had a total inability to undertake major physical activities. On average, Canadian senior citizens currently live for 8 to 10 years in the "frail, middle-old" category and for a final year in the "very old," that is, totally dependent, category before dying.[127]

In the United States Lenfant and Wittenberg[81] noted that 80% of elderly persons had some type of chronic disability; arthritis (44%) and heart disease (27%) were the most common problems. The active life expectancy of a United States citizen at the age of 60 years was 60% of a remaining 16.5 years, but by 85 years of age the active expectancy had dropped to only 40% of a remaining 7.3 years.[69]

Nevertheless, the proportions of "normal" and "frail" elderly persons depend somewhat on where the old-age threshold is placed; if it is placed at 55 rather than 65 years of age, the total number of elderly persons in the community is almost doubled but most persons in the 55- to 65-year-old category who are added to the sample are classed as "normal elderly."

Impact of Chronic Disease

One important variable that often limits both the ability to exercise and the training response of elderly persons is the onset of chronic disease.[126,127] Nearly 85.6% of Canadians over the age of 65 years report chronic health problems,[20] and in the Canada Fitness Survey[21] a substantial proportion of elderly persons perceived "illness" as a major barrier to an increase in personal physical activity. Certainly many of the chronic diseases that afflict senior citizens call for an adaptation of the training regimen, but the diseases are often relative rather than absolute contraindications to participation in an exercise program.[127] Substantial gains in physical condition remain possible with an appropriate exercise prescription.

Distinctions among the effects of aging, physical inactivity, and disease are far from clear-cut. For example, it has generally been held that elderly persons have difficulty in sustaining cardiac stroke volume as maximum aerobic effort is approached. However, myocardial function is adversely affected by both a sedentary life-style and ischemic myocardial fibrosis. Further, acute ischemia can limit cardiac responses to a given bout of exercise. Weisfeldt, Gerstenblith, and Lakatta[157] thus have argued that if a person has a decline in stroke volume at high work rates, this reflects undiagnosed cardiac disease. In the view of these researchers, if silent myocardial ischemia can be excluded by rigorous electrocardiography, echocardiography, and other techniques, an elderly person can compensate for the inevitable decline in peak heart rate by the Frank-Starling mechanism, developing a sufficient increase in stroke volume to sustain the peak cardiac output observed in a younger person (Fig. 11-1). In the context of the classification used in this chapter, the study of Weisfeldt, Gerstenblith, and Lakatta[157] focused on normal elderly persons,

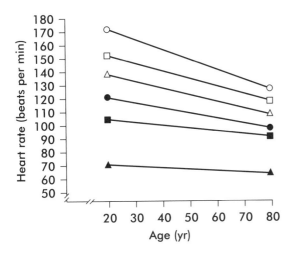

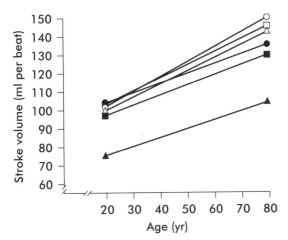

Fig. 11-1   Graphs demonstrating the possible compensation for a decline in maximal heart rate by an increase in peak stroke volume. Based on data from the Boston longitudinal study of aging for persons free of ischemic heart disease on stress electrocardiography and scintigraphy. Each line represents a progressively greater work rate. (From Andres R, Bierman EL, editors: *Principles of geriatric medicine*, New York, 1985, McGraw-Hill.)

whereas other investigators have been testing frail elderly persons.

As age advances, normal elderly persons constitute a diminishing fraction of the total population, and the dividing line between health and illness becomes progressively blurred. Although an extensive battery of clinical tests could be applied to establish "good health," interpretation of such investigations is hampered by the high proportion of "falsely positive" abnormal test results. Contrary to predictions from Bayes theorem,[50] the proportion of false-positive test results seems to rise with age. Thus I prefer the following simple, operational definition of "normal": the absence of any well-defined symptoms, gross medical condition, or use of medication that would restrict effective participation in a progressive conditioning program.

Influence of Age on Cardiorespiratory and Neuromuscular Function

General considerations. One common metaphor of aging has been "the downhill slope."[131,135] Whether in cardiorespiratory function, speed of neural responses, or muscular strength, performance deteriorates in a linear or even an accelerating fashion with advancing age.[135] However, it is less clear whether the decline of function is an inevitable consequence of aging or whether it reflects a combination of declining physical activity, social influences, and intercurrent disease.[18,71,111,112,128]

Some patients show a small, immediate increase in physical activity with the free time that becomes available at retirement,[126] but with the possible exceptions of walking and gardening,[96] the overall trend is for physical activity to progressively decline as a person becomes older (Fig. 11-2). On the other hand, Kasch and Kulberg,[67] Kasch, Wallace, and Van Camp,[68] and Åstrand[5] have suggested that when training is sustained or even increased, the downward slope in cardiorespiratory function can be checked for periods of 10 to 20 years.

Retirement often leads to a diminution of both responsibilities and social contacts. The community expects elderly persons to "slow down" and "enjoy a well-earned rest" in the comfort of their homes. This tendency toward social isolation, sometimes described as "disengagement," is exacerbated by such factors as increasing poverty, impairment of sight or hearing, and death of a spouse. Thus the slowing of reactions, impairment

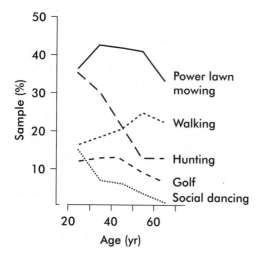

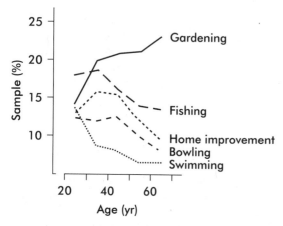

Fig. 11-2 Influence of age on patterns of physical activity for the community of Tecumseh, Michigan. With the exception of walking and gardening the percentage of the population pursuing various common types of physical activity declines with age. (From Montoye HJ: *Physical activity and health: an epidemiological study of an entire community,* Englewood Cliffs, NJ, 1975, Prentice Hall.)

of memory, and limitation of intelligence that have been described in some samples of elderly persons may reflect a lack of practice of the required skills rather than any inherent or unavoidable consequence of aging.

The proportion of the population that is affected by chronic disease increases progressively with age. Brown and Shephard[17] invited older female employees (from 40 to 70 years of age) of a department store to participate in a simple work site fitness test. Approximately 50% of the group reported some type of chronic disease, and in about 25% of the entire sample the condition was judged to have decreased the individual's cardiorespiratory fitness. The issue of myocardial ischemia and its potential impact on peak cardiac performance has already been raised. However, a condition as prevalent as varicose veins can also limit cardiac output by reducing the preloading of the heart, and osteoarthritis of the hip or instability of the knees can have a less direct effect on cardiorespiratory function by discouraging habitual activity. Any description of aging should ideally exclude cases of intercurrent disease, but there are at least two major practical difficulties. First, many of the pathologic processes such as ischemic limitation of myocardial function or destruction of pulmonary tissue in the chronic smoker remain ''silent'' until the process is far advanced. Second, in the very old the healthy make up only a small proportion of the total population, so it becomes arguable that certain forms of chronic disease are the anticipated ''norm'' for this age group.

Cardiorespiratory function

Lung volumes. Lung volumes such as vital capacity and forced expiratory volume decrease steadily as a person becomes older (Fig. 11-3). Unpleasant breathlessness (dyspnea) occurs when exercise demands a tidal volume that is more than 50% of vital capacity. For a young adult to reach the 50% limit a heavy intensity of exercise is required, but in elderly persons even moderate tasks may induce severe breathlessness. The situation is worsened if the lungs have been exposed to large amounts of cigarette smoke or certain industrial air contaminants and if weakened muscles cause a poor perfusion in the active limbs with a resultant lowering of ventilatory threshold.

Diffusing capacity. The maximal pulmonary diffusing capacity decreases with age, but since the peak pulmonary blood flow is also smaller in an older person, exercise does not normally induce any decrease in the oxygen saturation of arterial

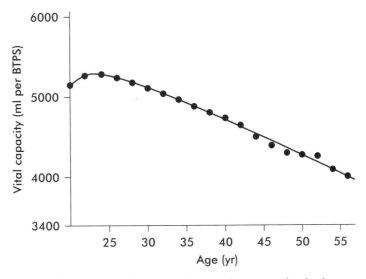

Fig. 11-3 Decrease in vital capacity (ml of air expired, measured at body temperature and pressure, saturated with water vapor [BTPS]) with aging. Mean curve based on work of Graimprey (Graimprey J: *Rev Med de Nancy* 79:648, 1954) and Needham, Rogan, and McDonald (Needham CD, Rogan MC, and McDonald I: *Thorax* 9:313, 1954). (From Shephard RJ: The physiological sequelae of segmental resection and other forms of thoracic treatment in flying personnel, *Royal Air Force Flying Personnel Research Committee* 1007, 1956.)

blood. The exception is in the patient who has a poor distribution of inspired gas because of chronic obstructive lung disease and chronic bronchitis (the "blue bloater").

Cardiac output. Because arterial oxygen saturation in the older person normally remains close to 100%, maximal cardiac output remains the main determinant of maximal oxygen intake and thus of cardiorespiratory performance.[119,126] Maximal cardiac output is the product of peak heart rate and stroke volume. The peak heart rate ($f_h$max) declines progressively with age. Some authors have assumed the formula of $f_h$max = 220 − age (years), although a wide interindividual variation exists[3] (Fig. 11-4); some 65-year-old patients can reach heart rates 40 beats per minute faster than the 155 beats per minute suggested by the standard formula. A high peak heart rate gives a wider-than-expected margin of cardiac function. Values lower than the anticipated maximum value may be encountered when exercise is halted by anginal pain (a "symptom-limited" test), when the cardiac

pacemaker fails to show a normal response to exercise (the sick sinus syndrome), when ischemia causes some form of heart block, or when the person stops exercising because of muscle weakness.

During exercise of submaximal intensity the cardiac stroke volume of a healthy elderly person is essentially the same as that in a young adult; values for men range from 110 to 135 ml (depending on habitual activity patterns), and values for women are approximately 20 to 25 ml lower. Niinimaa and Shephard[98] found that their patients (apparently healthy individuals in their final years of employment at a university) showed a decline in stroke volume as maximal effort was approached (Fig. 11-5). The authors reasoned that the aging myocardium had difficulty in sustaining cardiac ejection against the heavy afterload of vigorous exercise. Weisfeldt, Gerstenblith, and Lakatta[157] argued that such observations were a consequence of silent myocardial ischemia. If care was taken to exclude patients with a poor coronary blood flow by means of screening with a

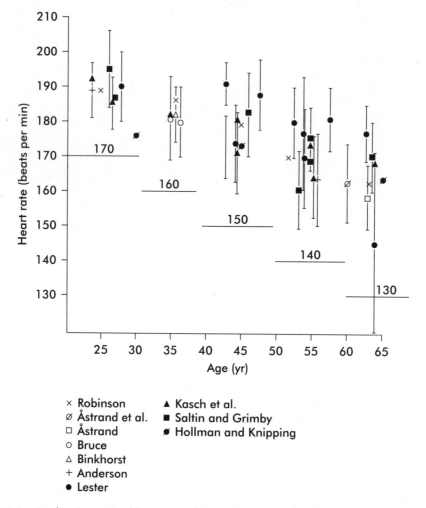

Fig. 11-4 Decline in maximal heart rate with age. Summary of various reported studies. See original monograph for details of references. (From Andersen KL et al: *Fundamentals of exercise testing,* Geneva, 1971, World Health Organization.)

combination of exercise electrocardiography and scintigraphy the healthy heart compensated for the decline in peak heart rate, invoking the Frank-Starling mechanism to develop a larger maximal stroke volume than that observed in a young adult. The main weaknesses in their study were that maximal oxygen intake was not measured and that, considering the reported peak heart rates, it seems unlikely that patients were stressed maximally. Thus it remains possible that Weisfeldt,

Gerstenblith, and Lakatta[157] might have observed a decrease in stroke volume if their tests had been pursued to higher intensities of effort. Moreover, there is worldwide agreement that maximal oxygen intake decreases with aging,[126] a finding that seems incompatible with a full compensation for the decrease in peak heart rate by increases in stroke volume.[128] The peak oxygen pulse rate, a simple surrogate measure of stroke volume, also shows a regular decrease with aging.[128] Thus,

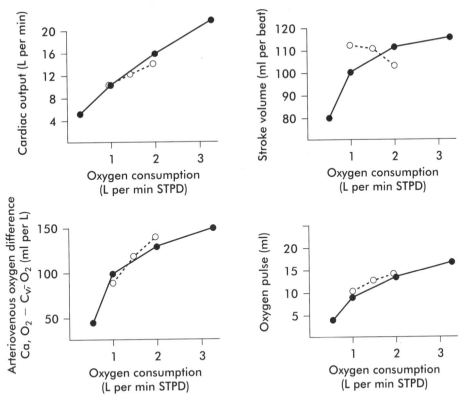

Fig. 11-5 Comparison of cardiovascular responses to exercise in young adults (average age 25 years) and elderly persons (average age 65 years). *STPD,* standard temperature and pressure, dry. (From Niinimaa V, Shephard RJ: *J Gerontol* 33:362, 1978.)

although the hypothesis of Weisfeldt, Gerstenblith, and Lakatta[157] is interesting, it would seem that at most it applies to persons in a small, rather specialized subsegment of the elderly population who have an unusually well-preserved coronary circulation.

The decrease in peak stroke volume more normally observed than the increase described in the previously cited study may reflect a combination of poor preloading (diminished venous tone, frank varicosities, a reduction in blood volume because of a low-salt diet, and a delayed relaxation of the ventricles[146]), a decrease in myocardial contractility (loss of sarcoplasm and fibrosis of the ventricular wall, reduced enzyme activities, and a decrease in the number and sensitivity of the catecholamine receptors[156]), and an increase of af-

terloading (a rise in systemic blood pressure and a loss of elasticity in the arterial wall[41,61]). Because of these many handicaps, it would be surprising if the peak stroke volume were not decreased rather than increased in elderly persons.

A variable that influences peak oxygen transport is the maximal arteriovenous oxygen difference. In a young adult, peak values typically range from 140 to 160 ml per L, but in elderly persons the maximum arteriovenous oxygen difference decreases to about 120 ml per L. The peak arteriovenous oxygen difference observed at any given age depends on the arterial oxygen saturation, the hemoglobin level, the completeness of oxygen extraction in the working muscles, and the distribution of blood flow between the working muscles and other tissues from which less oxygen is extracted. As previously noted, the arterial oxygen saturation remains close to 100% when older persons undertake maximal exercise. In the frail elderly person a poor diet, internal bleeding, or both may reduce the hemoglobin level and result in a corresponding decrease in potential arterial oxygen content, but healthy elderly persons usually are not anemic.[43] Some authors have argued that poor capillarization and reduced tissue enzyme activity reduce peripheral oxygen extraction in the working muscles of older persons, but that the margin of function in the young adult[116] is such that this change is unlikely to have a major impact on oxygen transport. A more important issue is the relative distribution of cardiac output in the muscles (where oxygen extraction is virtually complete), the viscera (where there is less oxygen extraction) and the skin (where little oxygen is extracted).[11,140] Since the peak cardiac output is lower in an elderly person despite essentially unchanged visceral oxygen needs, the muscles inevitably receive a smaller fraction of peak blood flow; this tendency is exacerbated when an increase in skin blood flow is required for heat dissipation in persons with obesity.[65]

Functional implications. Maximal oxygen intake is the prime determinant of endurance performance.[119] However, the use that is made of a given maximal oxygen transport depends on cardiac and respiratory oxygen usage, body mass, and mechanical efficiency. The onset of myocardial ischemia may also prevent an older person from realizing a true maximal oxygen transport during some types of exercise.

The chest muscles and the myocardium together consume approximately 5% of the observed maximal oxygen intake, even in a young person. In patients with advanced chronic obstructive lung disease, the energy cost of breathing can consume most of the available oxygen supply that is developed during vigorous exercise. Even in a healthy elderly person, stiffening of the rib cage causes some increase in respiratory work rates.

The energy cost of many tasks is almost directly proportional to body mass,[17,55] so a given absolute maximal oxygen intake (in liters per minute) allows a poorer performance if body fat accumulates with aging.

Movements become mechanically less efficient in an older person. This is partly an expression of nervousness and lack of recent practice, partly a result of tissue changes (collagen cross-linkages, deterioration of joint surfaces, and stiffening of articulations), and partly a consequence of changes in the central nervous system (poor coordination, poor postural control, tremor, and other extraneous movements). In healthy elderly persons the cumulative effect of these various factors is quite small; for example, we have noted an average net mechanical efficiency of 21.5% on the cycle ergometer, rather than the figure of 23% anticipated in a young adult.[126]

To a first approximation the cardiac work rate is proportional to the product of heart rate and systolic blood pressure. Any form of exercise thus increases cardiac oxygen consumption, sometimes four- or fivefold. If the coronary vessels are healthy, vasodilation allows a corresponding increase of myocardial blood flow, but in many older persons coronary vasodilation fails to meet the increased demand and effort may become limited by symptoms of angina. This is particularly likely when forms of exercise are attempted that induce a large rise in systemic blood pressure, such as sustained isometric contractions or endurance exercise using small muscle groups (for instance, arm work, with the hands raised above the head).

Neuromuscular function

Nervous system. Aging is associated with a progressive impairment of central nervous system function. Recent memory is poor, the special senses deteriorate, reflexes are slow, coordination is impaired, and extraneous movements develop.

The loss of memory has been attributed to cell death in the central nervous system, and this is certainly a factor in Alzheimer's disease, but in the healthy older person the problem seems related more to perceptual difficulties (weakness of vision or hearing), to lack of practice, and even to a lack of motivation to rehearse and store recent information. If there is an inherent functional problem, the limitation is probably in the ability to associate

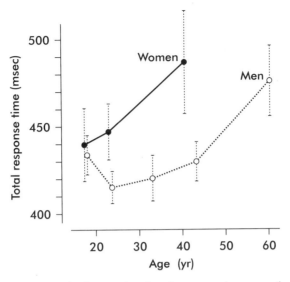

Fig. 11-6 Influence of age on brake reaction time for men and women of various ages. (From Wright GR, Shephard RJ: *Arch Environ Health* 33:141, 1978.)

ideas and thus to transfer information from the short-term to the long-term memory store.[126]

The loss of vision with aging is well documented. A progressive circumscription of the visual field leads to an eventual "tunnel vision" and a danger of collisions and accidents involving obstacles outside the central field of view. At the same time, there is a progressive loss of elasticity in the lens of the eye, so its focal length becomes almost fixed. Unless the patient is willing to wear contact lenses, the need for spectacles minimizes participation in many active sports. A yellowing of the lens and the development of opacities reduce the amount of light entering the eye, so there is difficulty in seeing objects when illumination is poor. In a proportion of the elderly population pathologic changes such as glaucoma and diabetic retinitis lead to total blindness.[126]

The deterioration in hearing initially affects the hearing of high-frequency sounds, which are important to the understanding of conversation. In a proportion of the elderly population, problems of decreased auditory acuity are compounded by tinnitus and a poor signal-to-noise ratio. Some compensation is possible by means of hearing aids, but the use of such equipment is not compatible with all types of sport. Deafness has an adverse effect on the social aspects of physical activity, which can be important in the motivation of an older participant. Failure to hear may also reduce performance in some sports and can increase the risk of accidents in pursuits as simple as walking.

Reflexes and movement times slow substantially with aging,[160] but the sex difference observed even in young adults suggests that factors other than the speed of neural conduction and synaptic transmission contribute to test scores (Fig. 11-6). Partly because of impaired vision and hearing, older persons tend to be more cautious in reacting to signals. They have more difficulty in distinguishing true signals from noise both at the receptor level and within the central nervous system[114]; thus they delay their responses.

Impaired coordination is reflected in the poor posture, increased sway, and low mechanical efficiency observed during the performance of many tasks. If balance is disturbed during a movement, it takes longer than normal for equilibrium to be reestablished.[101] The speed with which a coordinated task can be performed is also slower than normal. There is a tendency toward tremor when steady movements are required, which is particularly marked in patients with pathologic degenerations of the midbrain such as Parkinson's disease and Huntingdon's chorea.

Muscle function. A progressive loss of lean tissue is a marked feature of aging,[139,145] although often the decrease in lean tissue is masked by a parallel accumulation of body fat. The lean tissue mass value by 65 years of age is commonly 25% less than in the young adult, and there appears to be an accelerating loss of lean tissue thereafter.

Measurements of peak isometric force show a parallel decrease of strength in all the main muscle groups (Fig. 11-7). The peak force changes little between 25 and 40 years of age, but decline accelerates thereafter. There seems to be a selective loss of fast-twitch (type 2) fibers,[34] so the loss of function is greatest for rapid movements, whether these be tested by means of an isokinetic dynamometer or simple field tests.

Again, it is unclear to what degree the observed functional changes are an inevitable consequence of aging and to what degree they reflect a lack of training, an absence of recent practice, or a poor coordination of available motor units.[30,77]

Exercise Programming and Anticipated Training Responses in Healthy Elderly Persons

Preliminary screening

Need for assessment. At one time it was argued that for any person over the age of 35 or 40 years a stress electrocardiogram (ECG) was a necessary prelude to training.[28] This doctrine was always held more strongly in the United States than in Canada and other countries, but time and experience have led to a universal reconsideration of this view. Often, the results of screening tests were puzzling because of silent diseases or minor disorders[122,123] and the discovery of a seemingly dangerous condition led to an unnecessary prohibition of moderate training in a patient who until that time had been enjoying exercise. Screening is certainly desirable if a major training program is contemplated (for example, if the patient is preparing

seriously for some type of Masters' competition).[99] Changes in test score may also help personal motivation during training, and group scores can be used to assess the effectiveness of training programs. In frail elderly persons a stress test may further elucidate obscure symptoms, may help in diagnosis and prognosis, and may help determine the results of individual medical or surgical treatment, including rehabilitation. However, exercise testing is not needed when only a moderate increase in current daily exercise is contemplated. Indeed, because of the suggestion that an increase in physical activity is dangerous, insistence on rigorous laboratory testing may be counterproductive.

Many exercise programs for healthy elderly persons focus on endurance activities; thus the main objective of any exercise testing, as for those in younger age groups, remains the measurement or the estimation of maximal oxygen intake. Whether assessing the individual or the program, it is also helpful to have information on the electrocardiographic and blood pressure responses to a graded laboratory exercise test, together with data on muscle function, body composition, and flexibility.

Maximal oxygen intake. A determination of maximal oxygen intake may be helpful in setting a safe upper limit for the person who wishes to undertake a vigorous endurance exercise program. Normally an elderly person should hold sustained bouts of physical activity to an intensity below the ventilatory threshold[154]; this can be ensured by prescribing an activity that demands no more than 65% to 70% of maximal oxygen intake, but it can equally well be established by a progressive submaximal-intensity exercise test. The maximal oxygen intake also indicates the likely fatigue threshold for various durations of activity; for instance, fatigue is likely to develop if the average energy consumption exceeds 40% of maximal oxygen intake during an 8-hour period.[63,121]

Healthy elderly persons are well able to undertake standard laboratory tests of aerobic power: treadmill walking, cycle ergometry, and stair climbing. However, if a person has not undertaken vigorous exercise recently, both habituation and task learning are

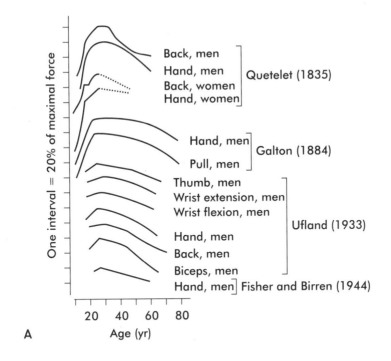

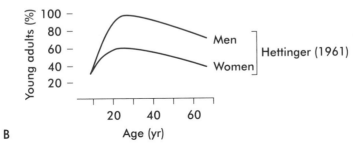

Fig. 11-7 **A** and **B**, Decrease in isometric force in various muscle groups with age. (**A** from Fisher MB, Birren JE: *J Appl Psychol* 31:490, 1947; **B** from Hettinger T: *Physiology of Strength,* Springfield, Ill, 1961, Charles C Thomas.)

slowed. An elderly person should thus be allowed more time than a young person to become familiar with both the laboratory and the test equipment that is to be used. As in a younger person, the most accurate method of determining maximal oxygen intake is to carry a progressive stress test through to voluntary exhaustion.[29,136,149] If a treadmill is used, the only changes of protocol necessary relative to a younger person are a longer period of "warm-up," smaller increments of speed or slope per test stage, and a lower peak rate of working. If a stepping bench is the chosen means of exercise, a step height of 35 to 40 cm rather than 45 cm may suffice to elicit maximum effort.

A traditional "plateau" of oxygen consumption can be demonstrated in as many as three quarters of the healthy elderly persons who undertake a maximal stress test on the treadmill[136]; however, because the peak oxygen intake is less than in a young adult, the usually accepted criterion of a plateau (<2 ml/kg per minute increment of oxygen consumption with an increment of power output[119]) also provides a less certain measure of maximal power. Moreover, the proportion of patients reaching such a plateau has been rather low in some studies,[149] although the peak oxygen intake for a given patient has nevertheless remained quite reproducible from one test day to another, showing a test-retest correlation as high as 0.90. Ancillary criteria demonstrating that a person has reached maximal effort (peak heart rate, blood lactate concentration, and respiratory gas exchange ratio[119]) all become more fallible in elderly persons, so if the patient fails to reach a plateau, the only option is to report the peak voluntary effort that is attained.

If maximal exercise tests are conducted on a cycle ergometer, peak performance may be halted by quadriceps weakness and fatigue rather than by the intended central circulatory limitation of oxygen transport.[126,127] Maximal cycle ergometer performance results tend to show a steeper age-related decline than do the corresponding treadmill or step-test data.[7]

Tests at submaximal exercise intensity. Because of fears about the safety of maximal-intensity tests, some authors have preferred to predict the maximal oxygen intake from data obtained during exercise of submaximal intensity. Such predictions (which are already imprecise in young adults) become progressively more unsatisfactory with aging, since the maximal heart rate (an essential element in the prediction) shows a large, variable decrease with aging[3] (Fig. 11-4). The coefficient of variation for heart rate predictions of maximal oxygen intake is 15% to 25% in 65-year-old persons, and there is sometimes a superimposed systematic error.[126,127] Such values

can possibly be used in population surveys, but they have little value when prescribing exercise for the individual. Attempts to estimate oxygen consumption from the rate of working (as in the usual Bruce protocol) make the test even more unsatisfactory. The elderly patient tends to walk in a mechanically inefficient manner, using short, tentative steps, and the energy cost of treadmill exercise is further modified relative to anticipated values because the patient usually clutches the handrail while walking. Likewise, an older person climbs stairs awkwardly, and the mechanical efficiency of cycle ergometry is less than the 23% anticipated in a young adult.[119,126]

Electrocardiographic evaluation. As patients become older, an ever-increasing proportion show exercise-induced abnormalities of ECG wave form and rhythm[96,137] (Fig. 11-8), including ST segmental depression and premature ventricular contractions. However, as in younger patients, questions remain about the reliability and the validity of such information in the diagnosis of myocardial ischemia[120] and the extent to which the exercise prescription should be modified if, indeed, true ischemia is present.

Because of an increased prevalence of patients with significant myocardial ischemia, it has been argued that the number of false-positive results should decrease in an elderly population. At first inspection Bayes' theorem[50] would certainly support such a hypothesis. However, the interpretation of the exercise record is complicated by a high incidence of resting ECG abnormalities, and a lack of overall physical condition may prevent the older person from reaching a diagnostically adequate level of cardiovascular stress. The number of erroneous interpretations may thus increase rather than decrease with aging.

An abnormal ECG is more likely to be a true, positive result if it is associated with other cardiovascular risk factors such as smoking, obesity, hypertension, or a poor lipid profile. False-positive test results can generally be clarified by means of further laboratory investigations (echocardiography, scintigraphy, and angiograms) but at a substantial cost to the insuring agency and at some risk to the patient.

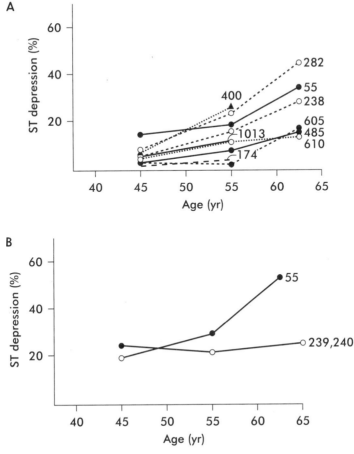

Fig. 11-8 Influence of age on the frequency of exercise-induced ECG abnormalities, **A**, in men and, **B**, in women. Dots and triangles refer to different studies. See Shephard RJ: *Physical activity and aging*, London, 1987, for details of references. (From Sidney KH, Shephard RJ: *Br Heart J* 39:1114, 1977.)

A proportion of patients with exercise-induced ECG changes undoubtedly have significant silent myocardial ischemia with implications of an adverse prognosis. This situation raises the following questions: (1) Is it safe for such individuals to undertake regular bouts of physical exercise? (2) Should continuous electrocardiographic monitoring be provided during training? (3) Can the intensity of exercise during which such abnormalities appear be used as a guide in exercise prescription?

Safety. The safety of appropriately prescribed exercise is increasingly recognized, even in pa-tients with established cardiovascular disease. A survey of 167 cardiac rehabilitation programs[150] provided data on 2,351,916 person-hours of pre-scribed exercise. There were 21 incidents of car-diac arrest and eight myocardial infarctions across the 167 programs, with incidence rates of 1 per 111,996 patient-hours of exercise for cardiac arrest, 1 per 293,990 patient-hours for myocardial infarction, and 1 per 783,972 patient-hours for a fatality. The risks were apparently similar for programs of large and small scale and were not influenced by the availability of continuous

Table 11-1   Risk of death during selected types of exercise relative to sedentary conditions for three age groups.

Type of exercise	Relative risk of death		
	20-39 yr	**40-49 yr**	**50-69 yr**
Nonstrenuous	2.5	3.6	2.5
Strenuous	10.0	13.1	5.3
Walking	0.0	0.2	0.5
Jogging	9.3	4.7	0.7
Nordic skiing	9.3	9.0	6.1

From Vuori I, Suurnakki L, Suurnakki T: *Med Sci Sports Exerc* 14:114, 1982.

electrocardiographic monitoring. In Toronto, 20 years' experience with some 5000 "postcoronary" patients has yielded similar statistics.[134] It seems unlikely that healthy elderly persons are at greater risk than patients who have recovered from a myocardial infarction, provided that the elderly persons undertake a similar pattern of moderate, progressive activity appropriate to their initial states of training. Indeed, Vuori, Suurnakki, and Suurnakki[153] have argued that because elderly persons are less likely to undertake vigorous pursuits for which they are ill prepared, the risk of death as a result of either "nonstrenuous" or "strenuous" exercise is relatively less in the 50- to 69-year-old category than in younger age groups (Table 11-1). Moreover, if account is taken not just of the period of physical activity but rather of the entire 24-hour day, the modestly active person has a better prognosis than does someone who remains sedentary.[141]

Continuous monitoring. Continuous ECG monitoring is costly and time-consuming and gives the patient a false impression that moderate-intensity exercise is a dangerous habit. Considering that such a regimen is, indeed, safe and that it is usually difficult to encourage an older person either to begin or to adhere to an exercise prescription, it seems counterproductive to insist on continuous electronic surveillance of training for the average healthy elderly person,[54] although such instrumentation may be warranted for certain candidates with high-risk ECG abnormalities.

Prescription ceiling. A better method of avoiding an exercise catastrophe than ECG monitoring is to set an appropriate ceiling to an exercise prescription and to insist that the patient not exceed this intensity. Some "type-A," time-conscious individuals are inclined to think that if benefit is obtained from 30 minutes of exercise at a heart rate of 130 beats per minute, much greater benefit will result from a similar period of activity at a heart rate of 160 beats per minute. Highly competitive, aggressive individuals are at particular risk for trying to beat the training response of a friend or defeat someone at a game of tennis, even though they are in poor physical condition. The ideal ceiling of exercise is a little below the ventilatory threshold, at an intensity of effort that results in some breathlessness but during which conversation is still possible. Downward adjustment of the prescription is recommended for activities that involve the use of relatively small muscles, an awkward posture, isometric straining, the prolonged support of body mass, or the use of the arms above the head. Caution is also needed when recent illnesses, intercurrent emotional stress, and adverse environmental conditions such as extremes of heat and cold are present.

Blood pressure monitoring. Normally exercise leads to a progressive rise in systolic blood pressure as the body attempts to sustain the perfusion of vigorously contracting muscles.[73,84,85,87,115] During isometric straining against a closed glottis, large increases in blood pressure can develop within a minute (see Chapter 6). A slower increase in systolic pressure occurs during 10 to 15 minutes of vigorous endurance activity. In some apparently healthy older persons the myocardium may be weakened by chronic fibrotic degeneration, or left ventricular contractility may be impaired by a silent myocardial ischemia; such persons not only have a decrease in stroke volume (as just described) but also find difficulty in sustaining the blood pressure at high work rates. Failure of the blood pressure to show the anticipated rise with a further increase in work rate is an ominous sign, warning the investigator that exercise should be halted immediately.[1]

Baroreceptor reflexes are less sensitive than normal in elderly persons,[110] and postural hypotension may thus develop after exercise, particularly if the patient has some initial tendency toward hypotension.[33,86] Common causes are lack of an adequate "warm-down" and standing in hot, humid shower areas.[120] Consciousness is usually regained quite quickly if the patient lies down, but there is a risk that a hypotensive incident may provoke a cardiac arrhythmia, and if consciousness is lost, the person can also be injured in falling.

Muscle function. Standard laboratory tests can be used to assess isometric, isokinetic, and isotonic muscle strength.[126,127] Observations have commonly been limited to measurements of peak isometric force made on a few key muscle groups,[126] although isokinetic data are now becoming available for older persons.[40,53] Hand-grip force is simple to determine and important to function, but it does not provide a good indication of a person's overall body strength. An adequate warm-up is important in preventing musculoskeletal injuries during testing, and prolonged straining against a closed glottis is also to be avoided because of the associated rise in systemic blood pressure. An elderly person may need longer periods of practice than young persons require to reach stable scores.

Under field conditions explosive strength could theoretically be evaluated by a standing broad jump or a jump-and-reach test, although lack of recent practice of gymnastic skills frequently leads to scores that are unrepresentatively low relative to actual strength.[38] A combination of muscle strength and endurance can also be assessed from such items as timed push-ups and sit-ups,[125] but such tests are hard on an aging vertebral column and may give rise to undesirably large elevations in systemic blood pressure. The observed scores for most strength tests depend heavily on motivation, and to elicit maximal effort, considerable encouragement of elderly persons may be necessary.

Body composition. Body composition can be gauged by reference to actuarial tables, by measuring the thickness of skinfolds, or by hydrostatic

weighing. Specialized laboratories also offer more sophisticated methods to determine lean tissue and bone density.[129]

Actuarial tables. One problem in using actuarial "norms" is that the "ideal" weight for height thus specified applies to survival from the age when insurance was purchased, commonly as a young adult. However, the value does not necessarily reflect the prognosis for healthy elderly persons, and, indeed, the "optimal" body mass seems to increase slightly with age.[4]

Furthermore, a progressive loss of both lean tissue and bone mineral occurs during adult life, but because these changes may be masked by an equivalent accumulation of body fat, an apparently "normal" total body mass can reflect an unsatisfactory body composition.

Skinfold measurements. The technique of skinfold measurement is now well established, and the principles of data collection are similar for the young and for the healthy older person. However, the overlying skin, 2 to 3 mm of the total fold in a young person, becomes thinner and more compressible with aging. The ratio of deep to superficial fat is also greater in elderly persons.[142] A given skinfold reading thus implies a substantially greater proportion of body fat in an older person. To predict body density or total body fat from skinfold readings, age-specific formulas are needed. Alternatively the skinfold data may be interpreted in their own right, but again, age-specific norms are required. Particular attention has recently been directed to the relative amounts of fat distributed over the chest and the hips; if the ratio is high (the so-called masculine pattern of fat distribution), the risk of ischemic heart disease is increased.[13]

Underwater weighing. For a long time, underwater weighing was regarded as the "gold standard" against which other methods of measuring body composition were to be evaluated.[129] However, a progressive loss of bone mineral reduces the density of "lean" tissue in elderly persons, so unless age and sex-specific densities are assumed for the lean compartment, the hydrostatic data become quite questionable in older persons.[94]

Determinations of lean tissue. Body potassium determinations[94] require access to a whole-body counter, but minimal cooperation is needed from the patient. Account must be taken of the reduced potassium content of lean tissue in older persons[152] and of the screening of ^{40}K emissions by an increased thickness of the subcutaneous fat layer. Likewise, the use of deuterated or tritiated water is complicated by changes in tissue water content.[129]

Whole-body impedance can be determined relatively simply,[23] but if body composition is to be predicted, some major assumptions are needed regarding the reactance of tissue membranes, the electrical conductivity of lean tissue, and the geometry of the body parts relative to the measuring electrodes. In an older person these assumptions become compromised by differences in the amount and distribution of body water and the thickness of fascial sheaths; reasonably accurate estimates of lean mass are obtained, but there are large errors in the estimated percentages of body fat.

Flexibility. Flexibility becomes an increasingly important determinant of function as age increases.[126] Although aging causes a general deterioration of collagen,[151] the loss of flexibility becomes increasingly joint specific in older persons[133] because the effects of general changes in collagen structure and the impact of inherited local anatomic peculiarities are compounded by local arthritic change.

The standard sit-and-reach test[48,155] provides a stable, reproducible measure of spinal flexibility. The range of movement at other joints can be assessed by a simple goniometer but the results are inherently unreliable,[133] since the observed range of motion depends largely on success in aligning the goniometer with the axis of rotation of the joint.

Balance. Laboratory determinations of balance can be based on stabilometer scores[121] or, more precisely, on movements of the center of gravity as observed when standing on a force plate. Approximate data can be obtained in the field by timing the ability to stand on one leg with and without the eyes closed.

EXERCISE PRESCRIPTION FOR HEALTHY ELDERLY PERSONS

We now consider general principles of exercise prescription for healthy elderly persons, including an appropriate intensity, frequency, and duration of activity and methods of sustaining motivation.

Principles

Occasionally elderly patients may still wish to prepare for Masters' age-class competition, stressing themselves to the limit of their potential,[70,99,112] but most older persons wish to participate in milder forms of exercise that are perceived as appropriate to their age group.[100] Essentially they seek a prescription that will maintain a reasonable level of physical condition and improve their general health.

Until recently it was assumed that training sessions had to be quite intense either to restore function or to ensure health benefit. However, this dogma is now coming under increasing scrutiny, particularly with respect to elderly persons.[39] Physicians are realizing that even modest increases of regular physical activity will improve the functional capacity and health of elderly patients who have become quite sedentary. Moreover, gains in endurance performance may outstrip the gains in maximal oxygen intake, as observed in the laboratory.[91] However, realization of the individual's full training potential depends on continuing compliance and on a regular upward adjustment of the exercise prescription. As in younger individuals, a large part of the gains obtained from training are dissipated by 2 or 3 weeks of detraining or bed rest for some intercurrent illness.[27,95]

Intensity. Based largely on the early experiments of Karvonen, Kentala, and Mustala[66] it was long argued that endurance training required 30- to 60-minute sessions of a large muscle exercise such as jogging, cycling, or vigorous swimming that was pursued on at least alternate days at an initial 60% to 70% of maximal oxygen intake. It was further assumed that to maximize the training response, there should be a progression to between

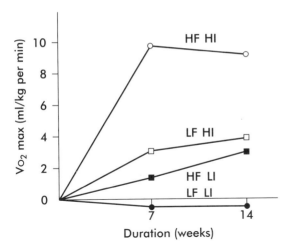

Fig. 11-9 Response of 65-year-old persons to various self-selected patterns of training. *HF,* High frequency; *HI,* high intensity; *LF,* low frequency; *LI,* low intensity. (From Sidney KH, Shephard RJ: *Med Sci Sports* 10:125, 1978.)

70% and 80% of maximal oxygen intake as soon as the patient's condition permitted.

However, the initial fitness of the individual relative to the intensity and frequency of the prescribed activity is also an important consideration. In older persons some cardiorespiratory training develops in response to relatively low intensities of effort. Thomas et al.[148] suggested that the intensity and frequency of exercise explained only 10% of the training-induced gains of performance in older age groups.

Sidney and Shephard[138] noted that the largest increase in maximal oxygen intake (a dramatic 33% increment during 7 weeks of conditioning) occurred in healthy persons who averaged 3.3 training sessions per week at an intensity increasing from 60% to 80% of maximal oxygen intake. Nevertheless, a slower but useful increment of aerobic power (10% increase during 14 weeks) occurred in persons who exercised frequently at no more than 60% of maximal oxygen intake (Fig. 11-9). Others have confirmed that elderly persons show some improvement in cardiovascular endurance in response to a low-intensity exercise pre-

scription. Badenhop et al.[6] found almost equal gains of maximal oxygen intake with training at 30% to 45% and 60% to 75% of the maximal heart rate reserve. Seals et al.[118] found some response to 6 months of training at 40% of the heart rate reserve, although larger gains developed at 75% to 80% of the heart rate reserve. Such observations have considerable practical importance for elderly individuals, who often lack the motivation to exercise for long periods at 70% or 80% of maximal endurance.

Low-intensity exercise also carries a lower risk of musculoskeletal and cardiorespiratory injuries.[76] Thus recent biomechanical studies have indicated that the impact stress on the knee joint is three to six times higher during jogging than during walking, even at an equivalent oxygen consumption.[107,113] Likewise, the chances of a cardiovascular emergency (although low with all patterns of physical activity)[120] are particularly low if training is restricted to moderate rather than strenuous exercise.[153]

If a specific advantage is to be gained from intensive training, this benefit is focused on an improvement of myocardial performance. In contrast, the consumption of fat is greater with prolonged bouts of moderate exercise than with short periods of intensive effort, since fat cannot be metabolized during anaerobic conditions.[121] Thus if a major objective of the training program is to control body fat, it is more effective to prescribe long periods of moderate activity than to prescribe short but intensive training sessions.

Frequency and Duration of Effort

The beneficial effects of exercise on longevity are realized if a critical volume of training is undertaken regularly every week. Paffenbarger et al.[102] suggested that the longevity of healthy adults was increased by an added leisure energy expenditure of 2.2 megajoules (500 kcal) per week, and that benefit was maximized with an added expenditure of 8.8 megajoules (2000 kcal) per week. In contrast, little increase in life span was obtained from irregular or seasonal bursts of activity.[89]

Recovery processes such as the replenishment of glycogen stores and the repair of microtraumata proceed more slowly in elderly persons than in younger persons, taking as long as 2 days to complete. The optimal frequency of exercise for older persons may thus be three sessions of vigorous exercise per week, with light walking on intervening days.

The optimal duration of cardiovascular training per session is probably at least 30 minutes; indeed, an hour is preferable if a moderate intensity of exercise is to be adopted. To optimize the serum lipid profile,[90,161] a leisure energy expenditure equivalent to walking 18 to 20 km per week is needed.[39,72,158] This expenditure could be accomplished by covering 6 km during 1 hour three times per week or by walking for 40 minutes at a similar pace three times per week, with 20 minutes of walking on relaxation days.

Other aspects of training, such as strengthening specific muscles[56] or increasing joint flexibility, may require relatively brief periods of isotonic and stretching activity per session. Many early exercise prescriptions neglected muscle building exercises because of fears of provoking an excessive rise in blood pressure. However, the rise in blood pressure at any given fraction of maximal voluntary force is no greater in an elderly person than that observed in a young person. Thus it is particularly desirable to supplement fast walking or jogging with some upper-body exercises so that muscles in this part of the body do not atrophy. A full range of isotonic, isometric, and circuit training exercises can be used to develop muscle force. However, individual contractions should not be held for more than a few seconds, and the recovery interval between contractions must be sufficient to allow the removal of blood pressure–stimulating metabolites.[46,74]

The voluntarily selected leisure activities of the senior citizen are unlikely to take all the major joints through their full range of motion each day; thus function can be improved through a combination of flexibility exercises and dance-type movements.[83] Dance sessions are valuable from a social and a motivational point of view, but violent twisting movements may provoke injuries. Gentle stretching at the extremes of motion is also helpful, using either body weight or a partner as the propelling force, but jerking movements, again, can cause injury.

The best pattern of exercise for reversing osteoporosis is still under investigation.[117] However, the loss of bone mineral in astronauts suggests that gravitational forces normally provide an important stimulus to calcium deposition. Walking should strengthen the bones of the lower limbs, hips, and spine, but some baggage (for example, a bag of groceries, a briefcase, or weights) must be carried if the arms are to receive adequate stimulation. Studies of swimmers have sometimes suggested that they are less vulnerable to osteoporosis than are sedentary persons, but in most instances it has not been clearly demonstrated that swimming was the only pursuit of the active group.

Any group pursuit (whether active or passive) provides mood-elevating social contacts. Most types of exercise also offer arousing proprioceptive stimulation. However, an elderly person is unwise to seek and unlikely to attain the sustained bouts of high-intensity exercise associated with an increased secretion of β endorphins.[59]

It is worth emphasizing that some objectives of the exercise participant (such as an increase in social contacts) may be satisfied merely by attending an exercise program, without active involvement in training sessions.

EXTENT OF TRAINING RESPONSE IN HEALTHY ELDERLY PERSONS
Qualitative Changes

Regulatory responses. In the elderly individual the qualitative response to training is much like that in a younger person. The earliest adjustments are regulatory. Habituation and learning have already been discussed. There is an increase in total blood volume, and the impact of this increase upon preloading of the heart is enhanced by an increase in peripheral vascular tone.[62] These changes lead to an increase in end-diastolic filling and thus (because of the Frank Starling relationship) to an increase in stroke volume at rest and during exercise of submaximal intensity. Partly because of the enhanced stroke volume and partly because of an altered balance of parasympathetic and sympathetic activity, the heart rate is slowed both at rest and during submaximal effort. The altered autonomic balance is associated with a small (5 to 10 mm Hg) reduction in resting blood pressure,[58,118] and (because of a lesser secretion of catecholamines and greater muscle strength), there is a larger reduction in blood pressure during exercise.[47] The combination of a slower heart rate and a lower systolic pressure reduces the cardiac work rate, and a lengthening of the diastolic phase of the cardiac cycle further improves the relative oxygen supply to the heart muscle. The result of all these changes is a larger peak oxygen transport.

In skeletal muscle a combination of greater relaxation of antagonists, better synchronization of neural discharge, and involvement of a larger motoneuron pool can lead to a substantial increase in peak voluntary force,[97] whereas the regular use of joints can lead to an increase in the water content and thus the thickness of articular cartilage.[121]

Training induces changes in many of the endocrine systems. For example, the output of fat-mobilizing growth hormone is better sustained during exercise, and secretion of catecholamines is decreased at any given intensity of effort.

Social contacts, proprioceptive stimulation, and a secretion of catecholamines contribute to an enhanced mood state.

Morphologic changes. If training is both rigorous and prolonged, morphologic changes may be anticipated, including hypertrophy of ventricular muscle, hypertrophy of skeletal muscle,[52,78] strengthening of the ligaments about major joints, breakdown of collagen cross-linkages with a resultant increase in joint flexibility, and a reversal of osteoporotic change in bones supporting body mass or withstanding vigorous muscle contractions.

In the first few months of rehabilitation a high-intensity program seemingly has little advantage over a less vigorous regimen.[15,108] On the other hand, if training is continued for a year or more, intensive activity induces a continuing increase in maximal oxygen intake[120] and an associated increase in stroke volume, whereas light exercise merely improves peripheral circulation.[42,108]

Currently no evidence exists that many years of regular nontraumatic exercise increases the risk of osteoarthritis,[77,104,105] but an overvigorous program can apparently aggravate existing osteoarthritic disease.

Quantitative response. On theoretic grounds it might be anticipated that training would be less easily accomplished as a person becomes older. Functional adaptations to many other types of stress (such as heat and cold) are less successful in elderly persons, and slower rates of protein synthesis could reduce the likelihood of morphologic adaptations such as hypertrophy of cardiac or skeletal muscle. On the other hand, given the low initial level of fitness in many senior citizens, the physiologic gap between current status and the potential condition of an active individual may be larger than in a younger person.[126] Although the old person may move more slowly from a sedentary to a trained state, the ultimate potential of the conditioning response is not greatly altered by aging.

It is difficult to make formal comparisons of trainability in young and older adults since the low initial fitness level exaggerates the training response (as in the observations of Kasch et al.[68]). The ideal experiment would compare responses in persons who are of different ages but who are at the same level of physical condition relative to their age-matched peers. When such a comparison has been made, 65-year-old persons seem to have at least the same long-term percentage of gain in fitness as younger individuals have,[6,57,138] although in the short term (14 weeks) absolute responses in the elderly age group are smaller than in a younger sample.[138] Certainly training can do much to maximize residual function with respect to both oxygen transport and muscle strength while increasing flexibility and countering osteoporosis.

Exercise Programming in Frail Elderly Persons

Preliminary screening. Preexercise assessment is a particularly controversial issue in training for frail elderly persons. Because they are frail and often have one or more chronic diseases or disorders, the risk of death is substantially increased; indeed, some gerontologists have characterized aging as an increased probability of death.[49] Thus physicians are cautious about challenging the body in any manner, and complicated laboratory testing is sometimes seen as a useful form of defensive medicine, even if interpretation of the test results is obscure. Typical advice that emerges from a several-hundred-dollar "work-up" is to "be careful" and "take it easy."

A formal exercise test itself can be hazardous, since it requires substantially more vigorous activity than is customary for frail elderly individuals and the test is performed in a strange, sometimes forbidding environment under the eye of a doctor who often appears to be nervous. Many frail elderly persons have resting electrocardiographic abnormalities that would contraindicate vigorous exercise in a younger person,[137] so it becomes difficult to decide whether to initiate or to proceed with a test. During the Canada Fitness Survey, 19% of persons in the 60- to 69-year-old category saw themselves as unable to perform a simple submaximal-intensity step test that was carried to 70% of maximal aerobic power, and 55% of potential participants in the same age category were "screened out" by anxious health professionals who conducted the tests.[21,125] Laboratory stress tests are often halted far short of maximal effort because symptoms or electrocardiographic findings that appear dangerous to the supervising physician have developed. Although the score from such a "symptom-limited" test may still find some application in diagnosis, prognosis, exercise prescription, and program assessment, it inevitably lacks scientific precision.

Simple submaximal-intensity tests are further compromised by changes in the oxygen cost of many standardized activities. For example, when walking on a treadmill, frail elderly persons adopt an awkward posture and move with hesitant steps, in part because of fear of falling. Practice at the test reduces these fears, and a large habituation response is evident. The gait also becomes more

normal after the patient has had opportunity to practice the test, and such task learning adds to a spurious impression of training. Likewise, a frail order person often makes clumsy initial attempts to climb a staircase or to operate a cycle ergometer, and the oxygen cost decreases as these tasks are relearned.

Orthopedic problems are a common reason for refusing a test. The knee joints tend to become unstable as a result of both muscle weakness and a degeneration of the articular surface. A light hand support is thus welcomed by an older person, both for treadmill walking and for stepping. The use of such a support necessarily has a large effect on the energy cost of movement. Thus the oxygen consumption must be measured directly rather than predicted from the supposed intensity of exercise, as is sometimes done when the Bruce protocol or a simple step test is used. When stepping is used, it is helpful to reduce the height of the risers to no more than 30 or 35 cm, high enough to elicit maximal effort from frail elderly persons and to prevent problems caused by a limited range of motion at the hip joint. Jogging in place has been suggested as a simple alternative method of exercising for those who remain reasonably fit.[106] Again, for such a test to have any diagnostic or prescriptive value, a measurement of oxygen consumption is needed. The cycle ergometer has been recommended for those with unstable knees or a history of back problems, but when frail elderly persons undertake cycle exercise, maximal effort tends to be seriously limited by quadriceps weakness. Electrocardiogram leads make it difficult to dismount from a cycle ergometer in an emergency, and in some older men a varicoele or prostatic problems are further obstacles to satisfactory completion of the test.

Most predictions of aerobic power based on exercise of submaximal intensity exploit a supposedly linear heart rate–oxygen consumption line. In frail elderly persons the heart rate may be irregular. Further, a failing stroke volume makes linearity of the heart rate–oxygen consumption relationship less likely and the peak heart rate is reduced by a weakness of skeletal muscles, myocardial is-chemia, and aging. Another important variable is medication. Frail elderly persons consume a wide variety of prescribed and nonprescribed drugs. Some agents, particularly the β blockers, impair the heart rate response to a given intensity of exercise, precluding both the use of standard procedures for the prediction of maximal oxygen intake and exercise prescriptions that are based on heart rate readings. Possible alternatives are a determination of ventilatory threshold[154] (although this may be distorted by muscle weakness) or a rating of perceived exertion[12,16] (which can be distorted by lack of recent exercise as a reference criterion).

Alternatives to the usual laboratory physical assessment avoid the risk and the potential criticism that testing has provoked a cardiac catastrophe, circumventing some of the technical problems previously discussed. Options are (1) to observe the range of normal daily activities,[80] (2) to measure the normal rate of walking,[10,19,31,32] and (3) to determine the heart rate that is developed at a moderate walking speed such as 1.3 m per second.[9,31] The coefficient of correlation between walking speed and maximal oxygen intake (r = 0.25) does not allow the observer to characterize the aerobic fitness of an individual patient, as has sometimes been claimed. In the study of Cunningham et al.[32] the correlation with maximal oxygen intake was, indeed, only slightly greater than that with age itself (-0.13). Bassey et al.[9] noted that the walking speed was also influenced by the strength of the calf muscles. In persons over the age of 65 years, the authors found that correlation coefficients of 0.41 and 0.36 linked strength and walking speed in men and women, respectively.

In those who are very frail, it is difficult to carry out any type of testing that requires standing. Smith and Gilligan[144] suggested that such patients could perform a progressive step test while seated in a straight-backed chair; this procedure augmented metabolism from an initial figure of 2.3 metabolic equivalents of oxygen consumption (METS) to a peak of 3.9 METS (ratios to basal metabolic rate). The mechanical efficiency is quite

variable for seated exercise, since results are affected by such factors as habitual posture and thigh length. Direct measurements of oxygen consumption are needed when such an approach is used. A lack of teeth hampers the attempts of frail elderly persons to use a mouthpiece, and hollowed cheeks limit the effectiveness of gas collection by means of a face mask. Nevertheless, the peak METS value that a patient can reach gives some indication of the potential to initiate an exercise program, the type of activities that should be recommended, and the likely prognosis.

A final method of evaluating aerobic fitness is to assess the range of activities of daily living.[80] The tasks that are accomplished depend greatly on the determination of the individual; however, an inventory of this sort allows a simple ranking of aerobic fitness and provides some indication of activities that the individual is likely to undertake.

Electrocardiographic Changes

The problem of abnormal ECG readings, which was discussed earlier for healthy elderly persons, becomes more marked in those who are frail. Many such patients are taking diuretics on a regular basis, and the resultant potassium excretion can influence both ECG appearances and vulnerability to an abnormal cardiac rhythm. The use of other medications such as β blockers also influences the extent of ST depression by altering exercise heart rate, by modifying myocardial contractibility, or by both means. A high percentage of "abnormalities" become evident, but many of these are false-positive findings with respect to the patient's remaining anticipation of life and the contemplated intensity of exercise.[137] Certainly it would seem inappropriate to restrict the activity of frail elderly persons on the basis of a supposed ECG abnormality if the patient is asymptomatic. Why persuade either an 80-year-old man who can still enjoy a weekly game of golf or an 85-year-old woman who still likes to putter in the garden that it would be "safer" to give up such habits? What social good would be served if these patients lived 5 years longer but spent 4 of those years paralyzed as a result of a severe stroke or suffering from senile dementia? Clues to a more cautious approach include a history of multiple cardiac risk factors, dangerous abnormalities of heart rhythm such as multiple, early polyphasic premature ventricular contractions, a low peak heart rate, failure of the blood pressure to show the anticipated rise with increase of effort,[51] severe, increasing chest pain, severe exercise-induced breathlessness, and a low peak power output or maximal oxygen intake.

Continuous monitoring. Motivation to perform regular, progressive physical activity is particularly difficult in frail elderly persons. Thus it remains counterproductive to suggest that physical activity necessitates detailed minute-by-minute electronic surveillance, even if laboratory tests suggest an adverse prognosis. The general use of ambulatory electrocardiographic monitoring is plainly an unnecessary luxury. DeBusk et al.[35] arranged home exercise programs for patients with cardiac disease who were up to 70 years of age. The only instrumental regulation of exercise was the provision of pulse rate monitors and twice-weekly telephonic transmission of the ECG signal to the supervising clinic. None of the group had any cardiovascular complications during 26 weeks of vigorous progressive exercise, although, admittedly, some high-risk patients with congestive heart failure or unstable angina were excluded from the program.

Blood Pressure

Because of declining cardiac function (myocardial fibrosis, relative ischemia, decreased responsiveness to catecholamines) and increasing afterload (arterial rigidity), peak blood pressure is lower in frail elderly persons than in younger individuals, although the elderly person may also have a greater hypertensive reaction to submaximal effort.

Frail elderly persons are further vulnerable to a sharp decrease in blood pressure after exercise. Causes include "drop" attacks associated with arthritic compression of a vertebral artery,[101] a substantial rise in core temperature because of obesity and impaired temperature regulation, loss of

venous tone while swimming (with a slow readjustment to a normal gravitational field), and failure to sit down after vigorous exercise. If the patient has a history of arrhythmia or myocardial infarction, there is some possibility that the patient may die in an overheated, humid shower area immediately after vigorous exercise.[92,120]

If the patient describes a history of fainting, a tilt-tolerance test may be worthwhile. If cardiovascular reflexes are well preserved, a small increase in systemic blood pressure occurs in response to sudden assumption of the upright position, but in "very old" persons the blood pressure frequently falls. When responses of frail elderly individuals are examined, it is important to obtain full details of any continuing medication, since many commonly prescribed drugs modify blood pressure during and after exercise.

Muscle Function

A lack of normal values and poor motivation to all-out effort make assessments of muscle force of limited value in frail elderly persons. Results for simple tests such as grip strength are impaired if overall weakness precludes obtaining measurements with the patient in a standing position.[147] Performance may be restricted because of joint pain, and any testing should be preceded by inquiry about musculoskeletal disorders affecting the joints under investigation. When the patient has a history of back problems, rapid spinal movements such as timed sit-ups are probably unwise, and when signs of osteoporosis, such as a "dowager's hump," are present, there is a risk that overvigorous muscular efforts could cause a fracture.

DeVries[36] has suggested that problems of motivation, physical injury, and hypertension can all be avoided by use of submaximal-intensity tests. In his approach force is related to the corresponding level of electromyographic activity; the stronger individual can develop a greater force for a given electromyographic signal. Functional capacity also provides some guide to muscle strength. For example, strength in the triceps surae shows a modest correlation ($r = 0.4$) with walking pace.[9] In older and more frail patients further information can be garnered from an inventory of the activities of daily living. For example, is the quadriceps muscle strong enough to lift the body mass from a chair or a toilet seat?[126]

Body Composition

Actuarial tables. The following specific difficulties arise when actuarial norms of body mass are applied to frail elderly persons:

1. Special weighing devices are needed if the patient has difficulty in standing.[24] Alternatively, body mass (M) can be estimated from determinations of calf circumference (C), arm circumference (AC), knee height (K), and subscapular skinfold thickness (SS),[24] as shown in the following equations:

For men

$$M = 0.98C + 1.16K + 1.73AC + 0.37SS(cm) - 81.69$$

For women

$$M = 1.27C + 0.87K + 0.98AC + 0.40SS(cm) - 62.35$$

2. Identification of an appropriate "ideal weight" is complicated because stature is often decreased by kyphosis and vertebral collapse; in such cases, overall stature (H) can be estimated from determinations of knee height and age (A),[25] as shown in the following equations:

For men

$$H = 2.20K(cm) - 0.04A(yr) + 64.19$$

For women

$$H = 1.83K(cm) - 0.24A(yr) + 84.88$$

3. Other problems are the same as those discussed for healthy elderly persons.

Skinfold measurements. Frail elderly individuals are sometimes reluctant to shed the layers of clothing necessary for skinfold measurements. In any event, the undressing of a frail elderly person is a tedious, time-consuming operation. Measurement errors tend to occur because the skin moves independently of subcutaneous fat when the fold is pinched from the underlying muscle. The problem of thin, compressible skin also increases as age advances.

Underwater weighing. Frail elderly persons are understandably nervous about total immersion. There may be a history of blackouts or hypotensive episodes on emerging from the water, and a danger exists that the person may slip on a wet deck, particularly if balance is impaired.[126]

A high probability exists for the presence of chronic chest disease and a variable deterioration of lung function. Thus it is no longer possible to assume the residual gas volume or to predict it from vital capacity, as is possible in younger individuals. Chronic chest disease also slows expulsion of air from the lungs while the person is under water, and a combination of uneven gas distribution and frank bronchospasm delays the equilibration of helium or oxygen when estimating residual gas volume. The use of a closed-circuit breathing apparatus is further complicated by poorly fitting dentures, which cause mouthpiece leakage. One helpful possibility is to measure the residual gas volume when the patient's head is out of the water.[37]

Flexibility. No special precautions are necessary when testing joint flexibility. However, because deterioration of the joints varies widely from one articulation to another, joint function must be evaluated by testing all major articulations and inquiring about related functional difficulties.

IDEAL PROGRAM
General Considerations

Exercise prescription plainly must be tailored carefully to both the physical and the medical condition of the individual patient. In essence the search is for a recommendation that remains safe but is also effective and sufficiently motivating to provide a good chance of sustained compliance.

Specific aims are to check the continuing deterioration of cardiovascular function and muscular strength, to maintain reasonable flexibility of the major joints, to counter osteoporosis and thus avoid life-threatening fractures, and to exploit the social and mood-elevating functions of exercise.

Cardiovascular Function

Cardiovascular function is improved by any training program that involves a substantial fraction of the body musculature.[2] If the patient is no longer able to stand, a considerable cardiovascular stimulus can still be developed by using the muscles of the arms and shoulder girdle.[126,127] For instance, several arm and wheelchair ergometers are now available[130]; McNamara, Otto, and Smith[93] have described chair exercises that mimic both cycling and rowing.

Many elderly patients have undertaken almost no activity for many years. In such individuals some cardiovascular stimulus initially results from heart rates in the range of 110 to 120 beats/minute, although gains in condition quickly reach a plateau unless the intensity of exercise is increased as fitness improves.

Because of such factors as unstable heart rhythms, tremor, loss of tactile sensitivity, and difficulty in reading watches, it is often difficult for the frail elderly patient to count the pulse rate accurately. Other potential indications of an appropriate intensity of effort are a level of activity that is perceived as "somewhat hard," a level that causes sweating, and a level that induces some breathlessness while allowing conversation to continue. Initially, individual exercise bouts may be for periods of 10 to 15 minutes, but if possible, the patient should be encouraged to extend the duration of each session to 30 to 60 minutes as condition improves. The optimal duration of cardiovascular training per session can be related to the prescribed intensity of effort in METS by means of using the following formula, as suggested by Barry[8]:

Duration (min) = 218 per metabolic equivalent − 60

For example, if an intensity of 2 METS is selected, the optimal recommendation for an improvement in cardiovascular function would be to undertake 49 minutes of exercise per day. When physical activity is first renewed, a frail elderly person would lack the strength needed to continue a bout of conditioning for 49 minutes; thus the best plan might be to break the exercise prescription into several feasible segments, alternating periods of rest and light activity. Some authors have found a good response to a circuit training plan in which 1- to 2-minute periods of light activity are interspersed with 5-minute bouts of performing five or six different tasks.[159]

An optimal recommendation for frail elderly persons is probably three sessions per week of deliberate exercise and light activity on intervening days. If intensity, frequency, and duration are well planned, the patient is likely to have nothing more than pleasant tiredness on the day after a vigorous exercise session.

Muscle Function

Frontera et al.[52] have demonstrated that "very old" persons are surprisingly tolerant of muscle strengthening programs. The key to safety is the avoidance of prolonged straining against a closed glottis. Even if mobility is very limited, muscle function can still be improved by tensing one muscle group against another or by pressing periodically against the back of a chair or a bed board. Also, weights such as books can be secured to a short plank, which is balanced on the ankles. Raising of this weight then provides a valuable stimulus to the leg muscles.

Flexibility. Era[44] has argued that when exercise is prescribed for elderly individuals, particular attention should be paid to balance, coordination, agility, and joint flexibility. Balance, coordination, and flexibility can be developed by walking on a narrow board and by jumping a short distance onto the floor. Flexibility is improved by a combination of active movements and passive stretching that is designed to take a joint through its full range of movements.

If individual joints have become painful or unstable, weight-supported activities in a heated swimming pool provide a useful component of training.[75,79,124]

Osteoporosis. The ideal exercise for preventing osteoporosis of the femur and hip continues to be walking, but Smith, Reddan, and Smith[144] have claimed that 80-year-old persons gained some pro-tection against this disorder by performing chair exercises at an intensity of 1.5 to 3.0 METS. Water-supported gymnastics seem unlikely to provide a stimulus adequate to strengthen the bones.

Mood elevation. Anxiety and depression are common problems in frail elderly patients. Whether such patients can perform sufficient exercise to improve mood state is less clear.[132]

Some proprioceptive stimulation certainly occurs if movements are made while sitting in bed. Other potential sources of elevated mood state are increased opportunities for social contacts (some types of group exercise), a pleasant esthetic or relaxing experience (for example, a walk in the country), and improvements of self-image associated with increased independence. Together, these several factors seem likely to yield some relief of anxiety and depression.[64]

EXTENT OF TRAINING RESPONSES IN FRAIL ELDERLY PERSONS

Training responses in frail elderly persons are qualitatively similar to those seen in healthy elderly individuals, provided that the threshold intensity for a training response can be reached. However, disease may preclude this goal. For example, because severe dyspnea prevents effective cardiorespiratory training in the patient with severe chronic obstructive lung disease, there is no improvement in cardiac or respiratory function, even after several months of training. Nevertheless, the patient reports feeling better and is able to do more. Some of the observed benefit is undoubtedly a placebo effect. A second factor is an increase in mechanical efficiency, which permits the patient to make better use of available function. Some muscle strengthening may occur, raising the ventilatory threshold. Also, bones are recalcified.[22,143] In addition, persuading the patient to resume activity breaks the vicious cycle of fear, inactivity, loss of function, worsening symptoms, and increased anxiety.

In some cases the functional gain may be quite small; nevertheless, it may have a major impact on the quality of life. For example, a strengthening of the leg muscles may permit the patient to rise un-

aided from a toilet seat or take a few paces around a room.

The beneficial impact of training on the cardiovascular system[14,82] and thus on cardiac mortality seems to be less marked in very old persons than in younger individuals, possibly because those elderly persons most at risk for sudden death may already have died.[102,103,109] The gain in longevity associated with an active life-style decreases from about 2.5 years at 35 years of age to only 0.4 years at 75 years of age.[102] However, the length of life alone is probably an inappropriate criterion to apply to frail elderly persons; the quality of the remaining years is much more important. Thus it is worth emphasizing that although progressive training has little impact on the intrinsic rate of aging, such training in elderly persons can increase both cardiovascular and muscle function until function matches the standard function anticipated for a person 10 to 20 years younger.[126,128] *There seems to be no other simple, safe, pleasant treatment that can match such dramatic benefits, and on this basis regular exercise should be strongly recommended to frail elderly individuals.*

REFERENCES

1. American College of Sports Medicine: *Guidelines for graded exercise testing and prescription,* Philadelphia, 1986, Lea & Febiger.
2. American College of Sports Medicine: The recommended quantity and quality of exercise for developing and maintaining cardiorespiratory and muscle fitness in healthy adults, *Med Sci Sports Exerc* 22:265,1990.
3. Andersen, KL et al: *Fundamentals of exercise testing,* Geneva, 1971, World Health Organization.
4. Andres R: Mortality and obesity: the rationale for age-specific height-weight tables. In Andres R, Bierman EL, Hazzard WR, editors: *Principles of geriatric medicine,* New York, 1985, McGraw-Hill.
5. Åstrand PO: Exercise physiology of the mature athlete. In Sutton J, Brock RM, editors: *Sports medicine for the mature athlete,* Indianapolis, 1988, Benchmark.
6. Badenhop, DJ et al: Physiological adjustments to higher or lower intensity exercise in elders, *Med Sci Sports Exerc* 15:496, 1983.
7. Bailey DA, Shephard RJ, Mirwald RL: Validation of a self-administered home test of cardiorespiratory fitness, *Can J Appl Sport Sci* 1:67, 1976.

8. Barry HC: Exercise prescription for the elderly, *Geriatrics* 34:155, 1986.

9. Bassey EJ, Bendall MJ, Pearson M: Muscle strength in the triceps surae and objectively measured customary walking activity in men and women over 65 years of age, *Clin Sci* 74:85, 1988.

10. Bassey EJ et al: Self-paced walking as a method for exercise testing in elderly and young men, *Clin Sci Mol Med* 51:609, 1976.

11. Bender A: Trainability of old men, *Acta Med Scand* 178:321, 1965.

12. Birk T, Birk C: Use of ratings of perceived exertion for exercise prescription, *J Sports Med* 4:1, 1987.

13. Björntorp P: Physiological and clinical aspects of exercise in obese persons, *Exerc Sport Sci Rev* 11:159, 1983.

14. Blair S et al: Physical fitness and all-cause mortality: a prospective study of healthy men and women, *J Am Med Assoc* 262:2395, 1989.

15. Blumenthal JA et al: Comparison of high- and low-intensity exercise training early after acute myocardial infarction, *Am J Cardiol* 61:26, 1988.

16. Borg G: The perception of physical performance. In Shephard RJ, editor: *Frontiers of fitness,* Springfield, Ill, 1971, Charles C Thomas.

17. Brown JR, Shephard RJ: Some measurements of fitness in older female employees of a Toronto department store, *Can Med Assoc J* 97:1208, 1967.

18. Buskirk ER, Hodgson J: Age and aerobic power: the rate of change in men and women, *Fed Proc* 46:1824.

19. Butland RJA et al: Two-, 6- and 12-minute walking tests in respiratory disease, *Br Med J* 284:1607, 1982.

20. *Canada Health Survey,* Ottawa, 1982, Health and Welfare, Canada.

21. Canada Fitness Survey: *Fitness and lifestyle in Canada,* Ottawa, 1983, Canadian Fitness and Lifestyle Research Institute.

22. Chow RK et al: The effect of exercise on bone mass of osteoporotic patients on fluoride treatment, *Clin Invest Med* 10:59, 1987.

23. Chumlea WC, Baumgartner RN: Bioelectrical impedance methods for the estimation of body composition, *Can J Sport Sci* 15:172, 1990.

24. Chumlea WC, Roche A, Mukherjee D: *Nutritional assessment of the elderly through anthropometry,* Columbus, Ohio, 1987, Ross Laboratories.

25. Chumlea WC, Roche A, Steinbaugh ML: Estimating stature from knee height for persons 60 to 90 years of age, *J Am Geriatr Soc* 33:116, 1985.

26. Comfort A: Test battery to measure ageing rate in man, *Lancet* 2:411, 1969.

27. Convertino V et al: Cardiovascular responses to exercise in middle-aged men after 10 days of bed rest, *Circulation* 65:134, 1982.

28. Cooper KH: Guidelines in the management of the exercising patient, *J Am Med Assoc* 211:1663, 1970.

29. Cumming GR, Borysyk LM: Criteria for maximum oxygen intake in men over 40 in a population survey, *Med Sci Sports* 4:18, 1972.

30. Cummings S et al: Epidemiology of osteoporosis and osteoporotic fractures, *Epidemiol Rev* 7:178, 1985.

31. Cunningham DA, Rechnitzer PA, Donner AP: Exercise training and the speed of self-selected walking pace in retirement, *Can J Aging* 5:19, 1986.

32. Cunningham DA et al: Determinants of self-selected walking pace across ages 19 to 66, *J Gerontol* 37:560, 1982.

33. Dambrink JHA, Wieling W: Circulatory response to postural change in healthy male subjects in relation to age, *Clin Sci* 72:335, 1987.

34. Davies CTM, White MJ: Effects of dynamic exercise on muscle function in elderly men aged 70 years, *Gerontology* 1:26, 1983.

35. DeBusk RF et al: Exercise training soon after myocardial infarction, *Am J Cardiol* 44:1223, 1979.

36. DeVries HA: Physiology of exercise, ed 4, Dubuque, Iowa, 1986, WC Brown.

37. Donnelly JE, Sintek SS: Hydrostatic weighing without head submersion. In Day, JAP editor: *Perspectives in kinanthropometry,* Champaign, Ill, 1986, Human Kinetics.

38. Drake V et al: Fitness performance tests and their relationship to maximum oxygen uptake, *Can Med Assoc J* 99:844, 1968.

39. Drygas W, Jegler A, Kunski H: Study on threshold dose of physical activity in coronary heart disease prevention. I. Relationship between leisure time physical activity and coronary risk factors, *Int J Sports Med* 9:275, 1988.

40. Dummer GM et al: Age-related differences in muscular strength and muscular endurance among female Masters swimmers, *Res* 56:97, 1985.

41. Dustan H: Atherosclerosis complicating chronic hypertension, *Circulation* 50:871, 1985.

42. Ehsani AA et al: Cardiac effects of prolonged and intense training in patients with coronary artery disease, *Am J Cardiol* 50:246, 1982.

43. Elwood PC: Epidemiological aspects of iron deficiency in the elderly, *Gerontol Clin* 13:2, 1971.

44. Era P: Sensory, psychomotor, and motor functions in men of different age, *Scand J Soc Med Suppl* 39:1, 1987.

45. Fisher MB, Birren JE: Age and strength, *J Appl Psychol* 31:490, 1947.

46. Franklin BA et al: Exercise prescriptions for the myocardial infarction patient, *J Cardiopulm Rehabil* 6:62, 1986.

47. Franz IW: Blood pressure response to exercise in normotensives and hypertensives, *Can J Sport Sci* (in press).

48. Frekany G, Leslie D: Effects of an exercise program on selected flexibility measures of senior citizens, *Gerontologist* 15:182, 1975.

49. Fries JF: Aging, natural death, and the compression of morbidity, *New Engl J Med* 303:130, 1980.

50. Froelicher VF: Exercise testing and training, St Louis, 1983, Mosby.

51. Froelicher VF et al: Application of meta-analysis using an electronic spread sheet to exercise testing in patients after myocardial infarction, *Am J Med* 83:1045, 1987.

52. Frontera W et al: Strength conditioning in older men: skeletal muscle hypertrophy and improved function, *J Appl Physiol* 64:1038, 1988.

53. Gandee R et al: The influence of age upon isokinetic leg strength of adult males, In Harris R, Harris S, editors: *Physical activity, aging and sports,* Albany, NY, 1989, Center for Study of Aging.

54. Garden NF et al: Assessment of a geriatric exercise programme using ambulatory electrocardiography, *South Afr Med J* 64:169, 1983.

55. Godin G, Shephard RJ: Body weight and the energy cost of activity, *Arch Environ Health* 27:289, 1973.

56. Grimby G et al: Muscle morphology and function in 67 to 81-year-old men and women, *Med Sci Sports* 12:95, 1980.

57. Haber P et al: Effects in elderly people of 67 to 76 years of age of 3 months' endurance training on a bicycle ergometer, *Eur Heart J* 5:37, 1984.

58. Hagberg J, Seals D: Exercise training and hypertension, *Acta Med Scand Suppl* 711:131, 1986.

59. Harber VJ, Sutton J: Endorphins and exercise, *Sports Med* 1:154, 1984.

60. Heikkinen E: Normal aging: definitions, problems, and relation to physical activity. In Orimo H, et al, editors: *Recent advances in gerontology,* Amsterdam, 1979, Excerpta Medica.

61. Hollander W: Role of hypertension in atherosclerosis and cardiovascular disease, *Am J Cardiol* 38:786, 1976.

62. Holmgren A: Cardiopulmonary determinants of cardiovascular fitness, *Can Med Assoc J* 96:697, 1967.

63. Hughes AL, Goldman RF: Energy cost of hard work, *J Appl Physiol* 29:570, 1970.

64. Ingebtretsen R: The relationship between physical activity and mental factors in the elderly, *Scand J Soc Med* 29:153, 1982.

65. Irion G et al: The effect of age on the hemodynamic response to thermal stress during exercise. In Cristafalo V et al, editors: *Altered endocrine states during aging,* New York, 1984 HA Liss.

66. Karvonen M, Kentala E, Mustala O: The effects of training on heart rate: a "longitudinal" study, *Ann Med Exp Fenn* 35:307, 1957.

67. Kasch F, Kulberg J: Physiological variables during 15 years of endurance exercise, *Scand J Sports Sci* 3:59, 1981.

68. Kasch F, Wallace JP, Van Camp SP: Effects of 18 years of endurance exercise on the physical work capacity of older men, *J Cardiopulm Rehabil* 5:308, 1985.

69. Katz S et al: Active life expectancy, *New Engl J Med* 309:1218, 1983.

70. Kavanagh T, Shephard RJ: The effects of continued training on the aging process, *Ann N Y Acad Sci* 301:455, 1977.

71. Kavanagh T, Shephard RJ: Can regular sports participation slow the aging process? Some further data on Masters athletes, *Phys Sportsmed* 18(6):94, 1990.

72. Kavanagh T et al: Influence of exercise and lifestyle variables upon high-density lipoprotein cholesterol after myocardial infarction, *Arteriosclerosis* 3:249, 1983.

73. Kay C, Shephard RJ: On muscle strength and the threshold of anaerobic work, *Int Z Angew Physiol* 27:311, 1969.

74. Keber RE, Miller RA, Najjar SM: Myocardial ischemic effects of isometric and combined exercise in coronary artery disease, *Chest* 67:388, 1975.

75. Koszuta LE: From sweats to swimsuits: is water exercise the wave of the future? *Phys Sportsmed* 17(4):203, 1989.

76. Lampman R: Evaluating and prescribing exercise for elderly patients, *Geriatrics* 42:63, 1987.

77. Lane NE et al: Long-distance running, bone density and osteoarthritis, *J Am Med Assoc* 255:1147, 1986.

78. Larsson L: Physical training effects on muscle morphology in sedentary males at different ages, *Med Sci Sports Exerc* 14:203, 1982.

79. Lawrence G: *Aquafitness for women,* Toronto, 1981, Personal Library.

80. Lee TH et al: Estimation of maximum oxygen uptake from clinical data: performance of the specific activity scale, *Am Heart J* 115:203, 1988.

81. Lenfant C, Wittenberg CK: Exercise and cardiopulmonary health. In Harris R, Harris S, editors: *Physical activity, aging and sports,* Albany, NY, 1989, Center for Study of Aging.

82. Leon A: Physical activity and coronary heart disease, *Med Clin North Am* 69:3, 1985.

83. Levarlet-Joye H, Simon M: Study of statics and litheness of aged persons, *J Sports Med Phys Fitness* 23:8, 1983.

84. Lewis S et al: Role of muscle mass and mode of contraction in circulatory responses to exercise, *J Appl Physiol* 58:146, 1985.

85. Lind AR, McNicol JW: Muscular factors which determine the cardiovascular responses to sustained and rhythmic exercise, *Can Med Assoc J* 96:706, 1967.

86. Lipsitz LA, Wei JY, Rowe JW: Syncope in an elderly institutionalized population: prevalence, incidence, and associated risk: *Q J Med* 55:45, 1985.

87. MacDougall J et al: Arterial blood pressure responses to heavy resistance exercise, *J Appl Physiol* 58:785, 1985.

88. Reference deleted in proofs.

89. Magnus K, Matroos A, Strackee J: Walking, cycling, or gardening with or without seasonal interruption in relation to acute coronary events, *Am J Epidemiol* 110:724, 1979.

90. Matter S, Stanford BA, Weltman A: Age, diet, maximal aerobic capacity, and serum lipids, *J Gerontol* 35:332, 1980.

91. Mazzeo RS, Brooks GA, Horvath SM: Effects of age on metabolic responses to endurance training in rats, *J Appl Physiol* 57:1369, 1984.

92. McDonough J, Bruce RA: Maximal exercise testing in assessing cardiovascular function. Proceedings of

National Conference on Exercise in the prevention, in the evaluation, and in the treatment of heart disease, *J South Carolina Med Assoc* 65(suppl)1:26, 1969.

93. McNamara PS, Otto RM, Smith TK: The acute response of simulated bicycle and rowing exercise on the elderly population, *Med Sci Sports Exerc* 17(abstract):266, 1985.

94. Mernagh JR et al: Composition of lean tissue in healthy volunteers for nutritional studies in health and disease, *Nutr Res* 6:499, 1986.

95. Miyashita M, Haga S, Mizuta T: Training and detraining effects on aerobic power in middle-aged and older men, *J Sports Med Phys Fitness* 18:131, 1978.

96. Montoye HJ: *Physical activity and health: an epidemiological study of an entire community,* Englewood Cliffs, NJ, 1975, Prentice Hall.

97. Moritani T, DeVries HA: Potential for gross muscle hypertrophy in older men, *J Gerontol* 35:672, 1980.

98. Niinimaa V, Shephard RJ: Training and oxygen conductance in the elderly. II. The cardiovascular system, *J Gerontol* 33:362, 1978.

99. Oja P et al: Cardiorespiratory strain of middle-aged men in mass events of long-distance cycling, rowing, jogging and skiing, *Int J Sports Med* 9:45, 1988.

100. Ostrow AC: *Physical activity and the older adult,* Princeton, NJ, 1984, Princeton Book.

101. Overstall PW et al: Falls in the elderly related to postural imbalance, *Br Med J* 1:261, 1977.

102. Paffenbarger RS et al: Physical activity, all-cause mortality, and longevity of college alumni, *New Engl J Med* 314:605, 1986.

103. Palmore ED: Exercise and longevity: a review of the epidemiological evidence. In Harris R, Harris S, editors: *Physical activity, aging and sports,* Albany, NY, 1989, Center for Study of Aging.

104. Panush RS, Brown DG: Exercise and arthritis, *Sports Med* 4:54, 1987.

105. Panush RS et al: Is running associated with degenerative joint disease? *J Am Med Assoc* 255:1147, 1986.

106. Papazoglou NM et al: Jogging in place: a valid alternative to multistage exercise testing, *Am J Cardiol* 61:1146, 1988.

107. Pascale M, Grana WA: Does running cause osteoarthritis? *Phys Sportsmed* 17(3):157, 1989.

108. Paterson DH et al: Effects of physical training on cardiovascular function after myocardial infarction, *J Appl Physiol* 47:482, 1979.

109. Pekkanen J et al: Reduction of premature mortality by high physical activity: a 20-year follow-up of middle-aged Finnish men, *Lancet* 1(8548):1473, 1987.

110. Pickering T, Gribbin B, Oliver D: Baroreflex sensitivity in patients on long-term hemodialysis, *Clin Sci* 43:645, 1972.

111. Pollock M, Wilmore J: *Exercise in health and disease: evaluation and prescription for prevention and rehabilitation,* ed 2, Philadelphia, 1990, WB Saunders.

112. Pollock ML et al: Effect of age and training on aerobic capacity and body composition of Master athletes, *J Appl Physiol* 62:725, 1987.

113. Pollock M et al: Injuries and adherence to aerobic and strength training exercise programs for the elderly, *Med Sci Sports Exerc* 21:S88, 1989.

114. Rabbit PMA: Age and discrimination between complex stimuli. In Welford AT, Birren, JE, editors: *Behavior, aging and the nervous system,* Springfield, Ill, 1973, Charles C Thomas.

115. Sagiv M, Grodjinovsky A: Influence of age on mean arterial blood pressure (MABP) response to upright isometric exercise. In Harris R, Harris S, editors: *Physical activity, aging and sports,* Albany, NY, 1989, Center for Study of Aging.

116. Saltin B: Oxygen transport by the circulatory system during exercise. In Keul J, editor: *Limiting factors of physical performance,* Stuttgart, 1973, Georg Thieme.

117. Schoutens A et al: Effects of inactivity and exercise in bone, *Sports Med* 7:71, 1989.

118. Seals JR et al: Endurance training in older men and women. I. Cardiovascular responses to exercise, *J Appl Physiol* 57:1024, 1984.

119. Shephard RJ: *Endurance fitness,* ed 2, Toronto, 1977, University of Toronto.

120. Shephard RJ: *Ischemic heart disease and exercise,* London, 1981, Croom Helm.

121. Shephard RJ: *Physiology and biochemistry of exercise,* New York, 1982, Praeger.

122. Shephard RJ: Prognostic value of exercise testing for ischaemic heart disease, *Br J Sports Med* 16:220, 1982.

123. Shephard RJ: Can the exercise ECG indicate prognosis? *J Cardiovasc Pulm Med* 12:29, 1984.

124. Shephard RJ: Physical activity for the senior: a role for pool exercises? *CAHPER J* 50:(6):2, 20, 1985.

125. Shephard RJ: Fitness of a nation: lessons from the Canada Fitness Survey, Basel, 1986, S Karger.

126. Shephard RJ: *Physical activity and aging,* ed 2, London, 1987, Croom Helm.

127. Shephard RJ: Physiology of aging and adapted physical activity. In Berridge M, Ward G, editors: *International perspectives on adapted physical activity,* Champaign, Ill, 1987, Human Kinetics.

128. Shephard RJ: The aging of cardiovascular function. In Eckert H, Spirduso W, editors: *The academy papers,* Champaign, Ill, 1988, Human Kinetics.

129. Shephard RJ: *Body composition,* London, 1990, Cambridge University.

130. Shephard RJ: *Fitness of special populations,* Champaign, Ill, 1990, Human Kinetics.

131. Shephard RJ: Metaphors of health and aging. In Kenyon GS, editor: *Metaphors of aging in science and the humanities,* Fredericton, Canada, 1991, University of New Brunswick.

132. Shephard RJ, Leith L: Physical activity and the cognitive change with aging. In Howe ML, editor: *Cognitive change and aging,* New York, 1989, Springer-Verlag.

133. Shephard RJ, Montelpare W, Berridge M: On the generality of the sit-and-reach test, *Res Q* 61:326, 1990.

134. Shephard RJ et al: Marathon jogging in post-myocardial infarction patients, *J Cardiac Rehabil* 3:321, 1983.

135. Shock NW: Physical activity and the rate of ageing, *Can Med Assoc J* 96:836, 1967.

136. Sidney KH, Shephard RJ: Maximum and submaximum exercise tests in men and women in the seventh, eighth, and ninth decades of life, *J Appl Physiol* 43:280, 1977.

137. Sidney KH, Shephard RJ: Training and ECG abnormalities in the elderly, *Br Heart J* 39:1114, 1977.

138. Sidney KH, Shephard RJ: Frequency and intensity of exercise training for elderly subjects, *Med Sci Sports* 10:125, 1978.

139. Sidney KH, Shephard RJ, Harrison J: Endurance training and body composition of the elderly, *Am J Clin Nutr* 30:326, 1977.

140. Simmons R, Shephard RJ: Measurement of cardiac output in maximum exercise: application of acetylene rebreathing method to arm and leg exercise, *Int Z Angew Physiol* 29:159, 1971.

141. Siscovick DS, Laporte RE, Newman JM: The disease-specific benefits and risks of physical activity and exercise, *Public Health Rep* 100:180, 1985.

142. Skerlj B: Age changes in fat distribution in the female body, *Acta Anatomica* 38:56, 1958.

143. Smith EL, Reddan W, Smith PE: Physical activity and calcium modalities for bone mineral increase in aged women, *Med Sci Sports Exerc* 13:60, 1981.

144. Smith EL, Gilligan C: Physical activity prescription for older adults, *Phys Sportsmed* 11 (8):91, 1983.

145. Suominen H, Heikkinen E, Parkatti T: Effect of 8 weeks' physical training on muscle and connective tissue of the m. vastus lateralis in 69-year-old men and women, *J Gerontol* 32:33, 1977.

146. Templeton G et al: Influence of aging on left ventricular hemodynamics and stiffness in beagles, *Circ Res* 44:189, 1979.

147. Teraoka T: Studies on the peculiarity of grip strength in relation to body positions and aging, *Kobe J Med* 25:1, 1979.

148. Thomas SG et al: Determinants of the training response in elderly men, *Med Sci Sports Exerc* 17:667, 1985.

149. Thomas SG et al: Protocols and reliability of maximal oxygen uptake in the elderly, *Can J Sport Sci* 12:144, 1987.

150. Van Camp SP, Peterson RA: Cardiovascular complications of outpatient cardiac rehabilitation programs, *J Am Med Assoc* 256:1160, 1986.

151. Viidik A: Experimental evaluation of the tensile strength of isolated rabbit tendons, Biomed Eng 2:64, 1967.

152. Von Kriegl W, Airsherl W: Zur Wirkung von Aldosteron und Corticosteron auf den Elektrolyt- und Wassergehalt-bindegewbuger Organe der Ratte, *Acta Endocrinol* 46:47, 1964.

153. Vuori I, Suurnakki L, Suurnakki T: Risk of sudden cardiovascular death (SCVD) in exercise, *Med Sci Sports Exerc* 14:114, 1982.

154. Wasserman K, Beaver WL, Whipp BJ: Mechanisms and patterns of blood lactate increase during exercise in man, *Med Sci Sports Exerc* 18:344, 1986.

155. Wells KF, Dillon EK: The sit-and-reach test: a test of back and leg flexibility, *Res Q* 23:115, 1952.

156. Weisfeldt ML: Left ventricular function. In Weisfeldt ML, editor: *The aging heart,* New York, 1981, Raven.

157. Weisfeldt ML, Gerstenblith ML, Lakatta EG: Alterations in circulatory function. In Andres R, Bierman EL, Hazzard WR, editors: *Principles of geriatric medicine,* New York, 1985, McGraw-Hill.

158. Williams PT et al: The effects of running mileage and duration on plasma lipoprotein levels, *J Am Med Assoc* 247:2672, 1982.

159. Wolfel EE, Hossack KF: Guidelines for the exercise training of elderly healthy individuals and elderly patients with cardiac disease, *J Cardiopulm Rehabil* 9:40, 1989.

160. Wright GR, Shephard RJ: Brake reaction time: effects of age, sex, and carbon monoxide, *Arch Environ Health* 33:141, 1978.

161. Yano K et al: Biological and dietary correlates of plasma lipids and lipoproteins among elderly Japanese men in Hawaii, *Arteriosclerosis* 6:422, 1986.

STUDY QUESTIONS

■ Describe the effects of aging on cardiorespiratory function and the impact of endurance training.

■ Describe the effects of aging on neuromuscular function and the impact of endurance and strength training.

■ How does exercise prescription vary for healthy and frail elderly persons from that for healthy adults?

■ Describe the effects of aging on joints and flexibility and the impact of exercise training.

■ Describe the psychologic and sociologic implications of physical activity programming for elderly persons.

CHAPTER 12

TRAINING CONSIDERATIONS FOR CHILDREN AND ADOLESCENTS WITH CHRONIC DISEASE

Oded Bar-Or

Although children's physiologic and clinical responses to training are similar to those of adults, training of individuals during their years of growth merits special considerations. These reflect growth- and maturation-related differences in trainability, spontaneous physical activity, ability to understand principles of training dosage, temperament, and attention span. Additional consideration should be given to children and adolescents with chronic diseases. Such patients may differ from their healthy peers in the level and pattern of spontaneous physical activities, physical abilities, attitudes towards exercise and sports, and motivation for changing life-style.

The intent of this chapter is to review the principles that govern the responses to training in children and adolescents with chronic diseases, highlighting the previously mentioned considerations. An attempt is made to provide information that has been generated by research. When scientific evidence is not available, however, my own clinical experience is described. For easier readability I use the word *children* to represent the entire spectrum of childhood and adolescence (including prepubescence, pubescence, and postpubescence) unless a specific reference to the developmental stage is indicated. The word *therapist* refers to any profes-

sional who prescribes or conducts an activity program. *Trainability* denotes measurable physiologic changes in a body system or an organ that are induced by training.

FACTORS THAT LIMIT EXERCISE TOLERANCE

To prescribe an effective training program, the practitioner must first understand the pathophysiologic factors that limit the physical performance of the patient. These often differ among diseases and individuals. In this section the notion of disease-specific limiting factors is briefly explained. Bar-Or's reviews of the literature[6,7] provide a more detailed profile.

Although low maximal aerobic power limits ability to perform many physical activities, fitness components other than maximal aerobic power may be deficient. Furthermore, each fitness component depends on one or more physiologic functions, each of which may be deficient in pediatric disease. Table 12-1 groups the relevant diseases according to the physiologic function(s) that may be a limiting factor in exercise tolerance. The following discussions of anemia, cerebral palsy, and cystic fibrosis illustrate the notion of disease-specific limiting factors.

Table 12-1 Physiologic functions that limit physical performance and exercise tolerance of children and adolescents with chronic diseases

Function	Diseases
Low maximal heart rate	β Blockers, congenital complete atrioventricular block, anorexia nervosa, artificial pacemakers (fixed and variable rate), postsurgical period after Mustard operation for transposition of the great arteries
Low maximal stroke volume	Aortic stenosis, cardiomyopathy, detraining, Ebstein's anomaly of the tricuspid valve (also postoperatively), severe hypoydration, pulmonary stenosis, tetralogy of Fallot (also postoperatively), postsurgical period after Mustard operation for transposition of the great arteries, ventricular septal defect
Low oxygen-carrying capacity of arterial blood	Anemia, cyanotic heart defects, hemoglobinopathies, 2, 3-diphosphoglycerate deficiency
Low peripheral oxygen extraction	Detraining, severe malnutrition, muscle atrophies and dystrophies, spina bifida, 2, 3-diphosphoglycerate deficiency
Low lung diffusion capacity	Cystic fibrosis
Low maximal alveolar ventilation	Cystic fibrosis, muscle atrophies and dystrophies, extreme obesity, advanced kyphoscoliosis
High submaximal oxygen cost	Arthritis, cerebral palsy, muscle atrophies and dystrophies, advanced obesity, leg prosthetics (e.g., after amputation)
Low muscle strength	Cerebral palsy, muscle atrophies and dystrophies, storage diseases, Prader-Willi syndrome
Low muscle endurance and peak power	Advanced anorexia, advanced cystic fibrosis, cerebral palsy, McArdle's disease, muscle atrophies and dystrophies

Anemia

Regardless of its cause, anemia limits the child's ability to sustain exercise at moderate to high intensities.[68] A low hemoglobin concentration (or an abnormal hemoglobin value) interferes with the oxygen-carrying capacity of the blood and as a result interferes with maximal oxygen uptake ($\dot{V}O_2max$). This interference has been evident in diseases such as chronic renal failure,[93] iron deficiency,[95] and sickle cell anemia.[26] At low exercise intensities the low oxygen-carrying capacity is compensated by a high cardiac output (through an increase in heart rate) and by a high extraction of oxygen from the blood. At high intensities, however, these compensatory mechanisms reach a ceiling, and the child's ability to exercise is diminished. As a rule, the more severe the anemia, the lower the maximal aerobic power. For example, at a maximal cardiac output of 12 L per minute the $\dot{V}O_2max$ of a child with a hemoglobin concentration of 140 g per L is 1.6 L per minute, as compared with a $\dot{V}O_2max$ 1.2 L per minute when hemoglobin level is 100 g per L and a $\dot{V}O_2max$ of 0.8 L per minute when hemoglobin concentration is 70 g per L.[4]

Cerebral Palsy

In cerebral palsy the function that limits the patient's performance is not necessarily maximal aerobic power. Although $\dot{V}O_2max$ is low in such patients,[11,15] their local muscle endurance and peak muscle power are often three to four standard deviations below mean for age.[7] Muscle endurance and peak mechanical power in patients with cerebral palsy and other neuromuscular diseases have been assessed by means of the Wingate anaerobic test.[8] This test has been found feasible for and highly reliable in patients with moderate to severe cerebral palsy and muscle dystrophies and atrophies.[92]

A factor other than low muscle endurance and peak muscle power that limits the exercise capacity of children with cerebral palsy is a high metabolic cost of movement. The oxygen cost of cycling in patients with cerebral palsy can be twice as high as that in healthy persons.[56] This abnormality depends on the degree of spasticity.

Cystic Fibrosis

In the multisystem disease of cystic fibrosis the lungs are affected most severely, and pulmonary insufficiency is often the cause of death. The function traditionally described as limiting the child's exercise capability is oxygen diffusion capacity.[41,101] The low diffusion capacity and the damage to lung parenchyma induce an abnormal increase in the physiologic and the anatomic dead spaces.[24,39,41] The results are arterial oxygen desaturation during intense activity[24,27] and a gradual reduction in lung volumes.

Less appreciated is the possible effect of malnutrition (that accompanies cystic fibrosis) on exercise capacity. Abnormally low calorie and protein nutrition has been shown to reduce muscle strength and power.[47] Parenteral nutrition supplementation for 1 month induced an increase in inspiratory and expiratory pressures in patients with cystic fibrosis. A group of scientists at McMaster University is currently studying the effects of undernutrition and of nutritional enrichment in children with cystic fibrosis on their respiratory and skeletal muscle strength and on skeletal muscle endurance, power, and contractile properties. Individual data obtained for patients with cystic fibrosis in our clinic at the Children's Exercise and Nutrition Centre indeed suggest that those with a poor nutritional status also have low muscle endurance and power, as determined by the Wingate anaerobic test.

PRINCIPLES OF EXERCISE PRESCRIPTION

Components of an exercise prescription for children, as for adults, include *type, intensity, frequency, duration of each session,* and *duration of the whole program.* Likewise the physiologic principles of specificity, gradual increase in dosage, and overload are valid for all ages. *The differences in prescribing exercise for children and adults are in the manner by which the prescribed activities are presented to the child (or the parent) and in the expected outcomes. Executing a prescription under the watchful eyes of a therapist is much easier than performing the activities at home or in a community center.* The following discussion assumes a scenario in which the therapist prescribes activities during a clinic visit that are to be performed away from the clinic.

Prescribing Exercise Intensity

When given an exercise prescription, a child can usually grasp the notions of type (for example, soccer versus swimming), frequency of sessions, duration of each session, and duration of the whole program. In contrast, it is expected that children will find it more difficult to pace themselves so that they perform an activity at a required physiologic intensity. Concepts such as "run at 75% of your maximal speed" may be clear to an athlete but not to a sedentary patient.

Several physiologic functions reflect a person's metabolic level, hence, the exercise intensity. Among these, heart rate is linear with oxygen uptake ($\dot{V}o_2$) at a wide range of intensities and is potentially a good tool for self-estimation of activity level. Adults who take part in exercise rehabilitation programs are often taught to palpate the carotid or radial pulse and use the rate as an index of effort. We have tried this method with 8- to 10-year-old schoolchildren* and have used electrocardiographic telemetry as a reference. While jogging, the children found it extremely hard to palpate the pulse. Palpation became easier to perform

---

*Unpublished observations from the Wingate Institute, Israel.

after the run, but then the timing of measurement became crucial: a deviation of as little as 5 seconds from the planned time of measurement yielded major underestimates or overestimates of heart rate. We concluded that it is unrealistic to expect children to obtain valid pulse rates by palpation during or after an exercise bout. With the advent of miniaturized heart rate monitors it may become feasible to use self-monitoring of heart rate as a technique for prescribing exercise intensity for children. It has yet to be shown, however, that this approach can be useful as part of a training program outside the laboratory.

Some success has been achieved by conveying to children the notion of "walk (or run) as fast as you can but not so fast that you cannot talk." An implied objective in using this principle is that the child should not overexert himself or herself. This approach has been used in rehabilitation after operation for congenital cardiac defects, as reviewed by Ruttenberg et al.[81] The authors stated that at the previously described intensity heart rate is equivalent to 60% to 80% of maximal heart rate. I am not aware of studies that have assessed the reliability and validity of the "walk and talk" approach. Another limitation is that it produces only one intensity.

An attempt has been made in our laboratory at McMaster University to prescribe exercise intensities by using the Borg[19] 6 to 20 scale for rating of perceived exertion (RPE). This attempt was based on previous findings[4,12] that children as young as 9 years of age can rate exercise intensities in a reliable and accurate manner by using this scale. "Accuracy" was determined by correlating the rating with the respective heart rate. In one study[97] 9- to 15-year-old obese (30% to 38% body fat) girls and boys practiced rating their exercise intensities while cycling on an ergometer. In subsequent visits they were asked to select either walking or running tasks or cycling tasks that corresponded to ratings of 7, 10, 13, and 16 on the RPE scale. Heart rate was monitored during each of the four tasks. As shown in Table 12-2, the patients managed to produce four distinct intensities while performing the prescribed cycling tasks but did less well when producing the walking or running tasks. When compared with heart rates during the learning phase of the study, heart rates at the patients' choices of intensities for all track tasks and the two light (RPE, 7 and 10) cycling tasks demonstrated that their choices were exaggerated. Their choice of intensity for the moderate cycling task (RPE, 13) was accurate, but they selected intensities that were too low when prescribed the most intense (RPE, 16) cycling task. In another study[13] wheelchair-bound children and adults were taught the RPE scale and then (using an arm crank ergometer) practiced repeatedly their perception at near highest and near lowest intensities (that is, at ratings of 19 and 7, respectively). They were subsequently requested to wheel their chairs on an indoor track at each of four intensities equivalent to ratings of 7, 10, 13, and 16. Both the children and the adults were capable of producing four distinct wheeling velocities, which yielded distinct heart rate ranges. As expected, the ability to reproduce the prescribed tasks was better among the trained participants than among the sedentary ones, regardless of age, but most persons chose wheeling velocities that were higher than expected.

The two studies[13,97] just described included children as young as 9 years of age. Whether prescription of exercise intensity by means of RPE is also feasible with younger children has yet to be shown. Although further research is necessary to optimize the methods of learning and practicing the RPE scale, the prescription of exercise intensity by means of RPE is a promising approach.

Caloric Equivalents of Exercise

In some training programs it is important to consider the caloric equivalents of the activities. For example, in obesity the energy expended by the child has a direct effect on the energy balance, which in turn may determine the success of a weight control program. Likewise in diabetes mellitus the calories expended during an activity, especially if prolonged, must be offset by changes in calorie intake or insulin dose, or both, to prevent hypoglycemia.

Table 12-2 Heart rate, percentage of peak mechanical power, and walking or running speed* of 9- to 15-year-old obese girls and boys who perform tasks prescribed to them as rating numbers on the Borg rating of perceived exertion (RPE) scale

Prescribed exercise intensity (RPE scale)	Cycling		Walking or running	
	Heart rate (beats per min)	Peak mechanical power (%)	Heart rate (beats per min)	Speed (m per sec)
7	142.6	36.8	173.3	2.2
10	150.6	45.7	186.6	2.5
13	162.8	58.3	194.7	2.9
16	171.2	68.7	197.3	3.1

*Differences among the cycling heart rates and percentages of peak mechanical power are all significant. Walking or running heart rate at an RPE of 7 is different from all other values. Speeds at an RPE of 7 and an RPE of 10 are different from those at higher intensities.

Whether a structured training program (such as for 1 hour per day) would affect the *spontaneous* activity of the child remains a question. For example, it is possible that the child will compensate for the structured program by reducing his or her activities during the rest of the day. The total caloric value of the program would then be less than anticipated. A study recently completed with prepubescent obese boys[18] showed that based on the calculated expenditure during the training sessions the net caloric value of daily sessions was *higher* than that expected.

Marked fluctuations in daily energy expenditure may disrupt the metabolic control of the child with insulin-dependent diabetes mellitus. Ideally when planning a program for such a child, one should attempt to maintain an equicalorie expenditure from one day to the next. It is impractical, however, to expect a child to perform the same menu of activities every day. An alternative is to prescribe a variety of activities that are equivalent to each other in total caloric demand.

One approach that I have suggested[4,10] is the use of "exercise exchanges," which are analogous to the "food exchanges" that have been advocated in the dietary education of diabetics. One exercise exchange equals 100 kcal (420 kJ). When the average caloric contribution of carbohydrates during exercise is 60%, 60 kcal, or 15 g, carbohydrates would be expended in performing one exercise ex-

change. This exchange is identical to one "sugar exchange" in the diet. The greater the child's body mass, the less time the child needs to expend one exercise exchange during any given activity, as summarized in Table 12-3.

Characteristics of a Pediatric Exercise Program

The characteristics of an optimal exercise program may differ among diseases and children. However, certain issues should be considered in the planning and execution of each pediatric training program. These are summarized in the box on p. 271.

Indications. As a rule, enhanced activity can benefit any pediatric patient who is sedentary. However, disease-specific indications should also be formulated before enrolling the young patient in a training program. These determine the contents and expectations of the program. For some patients training is indicated as a means of controlling body adiposity; for others it is aimed at strengthening a muscle group, lowering the arterial blood pressure, increasing range of motion, enhancing mucus clearance from the airways, or increasing self-esteem. The general and disease-specific benefits of training are discussed later in this chapter.

Risks and contraindications. Exertion is rarely detrimental to the pediatric patient's health. Therefore only rarely is enhanced activity contraindicated. However, as with other therapeutic

Table 12-3 Duration (in minutes) of physical activities that are equivalent to one "exercise exchange"* in children of various body weights

Activity	Speed (km per hr)	Duration (min)		
		At 20 kg	At 40 kg	At 60 kg
Cycling	10	65	40	25
	15	45	25	18
Running	8	25	15	10
	10	20	12	8
Sitting or quiet play	—	90	65	50
Cross-country skiing (leisure)	—	40	20	15
Snowshoeing	—	30	15	10
Walking	4	60	40	30
	6	40	30	25

From Bar-Or O: *Pediatr Exerc Sci* 2:384, 1990; adapted from Bar-Or O: *Pediatric sports medicine for the practitioner: from physiologic principles to clinical applications,* New York, 1983, Springer-Verlag.
*100 kcal or 420 kJ.

> **ISSUES TO BE CONSIDERED IN AN INDIVIDUALIZED PEDIATRIC TRAINING PROGRAM**
>
> Are there clear indications for training?
> Does enhanced activity entail risk?
> Are the objectives clear to the child and parent?
> Are the interim and final goals feasible?
> Is the program compatible with other ongoing therapeutic modalities?
> Have intrinsic and extrinsic motivators been considered?
> Will this child accept group activities (with healthy peers or with other patients)?
> Do program components include sufficient recreation and fun?
> Have evaluation of progress and feedback to the patient been incorporated?

modalities, risks and side effects exist. These should be recognized and considered.

The notion of "side effects" of exercise in children is not commonly recognized. It commonly occurs that an adult patient with peripheral vascular disease (with no other symptoms of atherosclerosis) may develop angina pectoris as a result of training. This condition reflects the patient's performance of increased levels of exercise, which in turn induces a greater metabolic demand by the myocardium and exertional chest pain. The pediatric equivalent of the preceding situation is an obese girl with asthma who develops exercise-induced bronchoconstriction after starting a training program. Evidently her level of activity before the program was so low that exercise-induced bronchoconstriction had not been provoked.

Clarity of objectives. *Exercise therapy is different from most therapeutic modalities in that it cannot be executed without parental support and full and active participation by the patient. In a sense the child is not only the recipient of the therapy but also its effector.* It is therefore not sufficient that the therapist has defined objectives for a training program. These should also be conveyed clearly to the child and the parents. In our clinic we have found that children 8 to 9 years of age and older (with normal mental capacity) better adhere to an exercise program if they are made partners within the decision-making process. The adherence of less mature children depends more on the ability of their parents to motivate them. Stated differently, it is unlikely that a child older than 9 years of age will succeed in the program unless he or she has become convinced of its importance.

Clear understanding of the role of exercise in the management of obesity is a case in point. It has been common knowledge that changes in eating habits are necessary for weight control. In contrast, the relevance of exercise (see the discussion later in this chapter of benefits of training for children with obesity) is little recognized. Unless the patient and parent appreciate the caloric value of activity (and, in the case of the more mature patient, additional subtle effects of exercise), it is unlikely that the child will have the motivation to increase his or her activity.

Feasibility of goals. *Many of the patients who need an exercise program are not only sedentary but also lack confidence in their ability to exercise. This often puts them in a vicious cycle of hypoactivity-low fitness-lack of confidence-further hypoactivity. The first stage in a program for such a child should aim at breaking this vicious cycle. Assuming that "there is no success like success itself," it is important that the patient attain a perceptible success right from the start of the program. To achieve such success, initial goals that are not too demanding should be set.* For some children who hitherto have had a sedentary life-style the mere ability to engage in some activities is perceived as success, even in the absence of any physiologic improvement. Only when such a child (and the parents) becomes more self-confident can the demands be increased so that physiologic benefits are gained.

The ultimate goal of any program should be realistic. For example, a prepubertal patient may have hypotonic muscles. The child and, in particular, the parents may express their hope that the muscles become "stronger and bigger." Although resistance training can, indeed, strengthen muscles of prepubescents, these muscles usually do not increase in size (unlike in adolescents and adults, whose muscle bulk increases as they become stronger).[73] The onus, therefore, is on the therapist to tone down the patient's expectations for such a program.

Compatibility with concurrent ongoing therapies. Many patients with a chronic disease are receiving other therapies while taking part in a training program. It is extremely important that a possible interaction between these therapeutic modalities be anticipated.

One interaction is that exercise may be antagonistic to or synergistic with a certain drug. For example, a child with insulin-dependent diabetes mellitus may start a training program. Because exercise and insulin are synergistic, in this child hypoglycemia is now more likely to develop,[31] unless both insulin and calories are adjusted.

Corticosteroid therapy may conflict with training in a child who is participating in a weight control program. Among other effects the medication of corticosteroid therapy often improves appetite and enhances obesity, which are antagonistic to the effects of exercise. Another potential effect of corticosteroid therapy, although uncommon in children, is an increase in arterial blood pressure. A patient who is receiving corticosteroid therapy and wishes to start training should be given a maximal aerobic test, to ensure that her or his blood pressure does not rise excessively during exercise. Another potential problem may occur in a patient with adrenal insufficiency who needs full replacement of corticosteroids. Although the dosage originally prescribed is sufficient to cover the child's needs while practicing a sedentary life-style, the dosage may have to be increased once he or she becomes more active.

Another incompatibility occurs when other therapies interfere with the child's ability to train. For example, a patient who has had middle-ear surgery may be required to refrain from swimming, or a child with kyphoscoliosis who had a rod inserted for spinal stability may be required to avoid weight-bearing activities.

Motivational approaches. *In general healthy children are sufficiently motivated to be physically active, but those with chronic diseases may need an extra motivation to alter their sedentary lifestyles. Seldom does intrinsic motivation (that is, wishing to become active for the sake of activity itself) induce greater activity in the young patient. Extrinsic motivators such as token prizes are usually more effective and should be considered.*

One approach that seems nonproductive is the use of "better health" and "prevention of future disease" as motivators. As shown in other programs that require changes in life-style (for example, antismoking campaigns), most children and adolescents seem oblivious to their future health. They are reluctant to change their activity or eating patterns just because such changes may reduce the risk for a heart attack or for hypertension 30 years hence. *Motivational approaches that do seem to work are those related to the* immediate *appearance or performance of the child. For example, an obese boy may be willing to increase his activity so that he can "be selected to the football team." For some obese girls the chance of fitting into age-appropriate clothing is a powerful motivator.*

Maintenance of a high level of motivation is an ongoing challenge throughout any pediatric exercise program. In addition to a token award policy (usually given by the parents), the therapist can conduct campaigns that may induce better adherence. We have found the use of "frequent jogger" games (the child accumulates points for each mile, while competing with other patients) to be effective. Other successful campaigns have been nature hikes and charity runs, in which children obtained pledges for the distance they logged, as well as "special event" evenings that included games and contests of low exercise intensity.

Individual versus group activities. Although some rehabilitation programs require a one-on-one approach, there is much advantage to conducting group-based programs. These allow the child to exercise in a playlike atmosphere while socializing with peers. Group-based programs are also more cost-effective.

*Some patients function well within a group. Others, especially those who lack confidence in their physical prowess, feel inhibited and are reluctant to work out with other children. In our experience children with a "visible" defect (such as kyphoscoliosis, cerebral palsy, obesity, or short stature) often decline to exercise with their healthy peers but gladly join a program with other children who have a similar condi-*tion*. Some children insist on starting to exercise on their own but agree to join a group once they gain confidence. A therapist should be sensitive to this issue and not impose an activity framework within which the child does not feel comfortable.*

Children who will not join a group can become more active at home by performing daily routines that are not necessarily sports or structured exercise, such as doing household and garden chores and taking the dog for a walk. The parents should understand that, for example, work on the farm and swimming in a club may induce similar physiologic benefits.

Recreation and fun. From the preceding discussion it is apparent that, *to obtain compliance and adherence and to make a training program an overall positive experience, fun and a playlike atmosphere are important ingredients in any pediatric training program. This point cannot be overemphasized. Recreation and fun should be included, even if the program becomes less than optimal from a physiologic point of view.* For most patients therapy by exercise should be a spark for a more active life-style long after the program itself has been concluded. Little is known about the best way of achieving this long-range goal, but it seems that those children who take part in nonregimented programs are more likely to sustain an active life-style than are those who attend more structured programs.[34]

Evaluation and feedback. As with any other therapy, the response of the patient to training should be evaluated periodically and findings relayed to the child and the parents. Evaluation can include exercise testing (in the laboratory and in the field) and assessment of body composition, lung functions, serum lipoprotein profile, and any other relevant physiologic function. In addition, questionnaires and interviews regarding such issues as state of depression, self-efficacy, and attitudes towards physical activity and health can be administered.

Most of our young patients seem eager to improve their scores, particularly on the fitness tests.

Reporting the findings to them can become an important tool in sustaining their motivation. Some patients improve their adherence to an exercise program just by knowing that a test will be performed on their next clinic visit.

GENERAL BENEFITS OF TRAINING

Physical training can induce nonspecific changes in physiologic function, physical performance, and psychosocial variables. Although the degree of trainability differs among individuals, persons of all ages are trainable. As I have recently reviewed,[9] muscle strength, peak anaerobic power, and muscle endurance are as trainable in healthy prepubescents as they are in pubescents, postpubescents, and adults. Aerobic power is also trainable in prepubescents but to a somewhat lower extent than in more mature groups.[4,79]

One problem in assessing trainability of the growing child and adolescent is that many of the physiologic functions are affected not only by training but also by growth and maturation. For example, heart rate at submaximal exercise intensity drops with aerobic training and with growth, as do the energy cost of walking and running and the ventilatory equivalent for oxygen and for carbon dioxide. Stroke volume increases with training and with growth, as do Vo_2max (L per minute), peak anaerobic power, muscle endurance, and sweating rate. Other physiologic functions respond to growth and training in opposite directions. For example, anaerobic threshold (expressed as a percentage of Vo_2max) increases with growth and decreases with aerobic training, as does arterial blood pressure.

One implication of the preceding data is that training studies of children must include controls who do not train. Although this is usually feasible in studies of healthy children, it sometimes may be impractical in studies with patients, whether for ethical reasons or because of the small pool of available participants.

DISEASE-SPECIFIC BENEFITS OF TRAINING

In recent years an increasing number of publications have claimed disease-specific benefits that are induced by training. For reviews of this topic see Bar-Or[4,5,10] and Rowland.[80] Most of the studies in this area are lacking in their design (absence of properly selected controls), and their findings cannot be considered definitive.[10] Therefore the following information should be treated accordingly. Table 12-4 lists some of the common pediatric diseases for which exercise has been prescribed and the presumed disease-specific benefits of training.

Asthma

There is no doubt that aerobic training can induce improvement in maximal aerobic power and endurance performance in persons with asthma, since a large number of world-class athletes have asthma.[96] However, whether training can reduce the intensity and frequency of exercise-induced bronchoconstriction or the clinical severity of the disease is controversial. Some authors have reported no effect on exercise-induced bronchoconstriction.* Others have described a training-induced decrease in the severity or frequency, or both, of exercise-induced bronchoconstriction[42,45,65,89] and a reduced need for medication.[50] One study suggested an improvement in the clinical severity of the asthma after a 5-month swimming program.[37] In another study, which included a randomly selected "placebo" control group (patients who were given relaxation and mild physical activities, as compared with the intense calisthenics given in the experimental group), both groups had a decrease in exercise-induced bronchoconstriction.[90] Regardless of the long-term effects of training, the therapist is often called on to suggest means by which the acute deleterious effects of exercise can be prevented. With the use of currently available drug and other therapies the great majority of persons with asthma should be able to exercise with little or no exercise-induced bronchoconstriction. The use of inhaled bronchodilators (mostly β_2 sympathomimetics) with or without other medication is most efficacious. Several additional strategies are available to the therapist, as summarized in the box on p. 275.

---

*References 36, 37, 50, 54, 60, and 64

Table 12-4   Disease-specific benefits attributed to training in chronic pediatric diseases

Disease	Suggested training-induced benefits
Asthma	Lower intensity and frequency of exercise-induced bronchoconstriction, reduced need for medication
Cerebral palsy	Increased range of motion, enhanced ambulation, reduction in the energy cost of exercise and in spasticity
Cystic fibrosis	Enhanced clearance of bronchial mucus, higher lung volumes and endurance of the respiratory muscles
Diabetes mellitus	Increased sensitivity of insulin receptors, better diabetic control
Hypertension	Reduction of arterial blood pressure at rest
Muscle atrophies and dystrophies	Strengthening of residual muscle fibers, prolongation of ambulation status, prevention of contractures, weight control
Obesity	Weight and fatness control, improved lipoprotein profile, enhanced socialization and self-esteem

From Bar-Or O: *Pediatr Exerc Sci* 2:384, 1990.

NONPHARMACOLOGIC MEANS FOR THE PREVENTION OR REDUCTION OF EXERCISE-INDUCED BRONCHOCONSTRICTION DURING OR AFTER A BOUT OF EXERCISE IN THE CHILD WITH ASTHMA

1. Emphasize activities that are least asthmogenic (swimming, water-based games, low-intensity prolonged activities, and short sprints).
2. Warm up by performing prolonged low-intensity exercise or by running several short sprints (for example, 4 to 5 seconds in duration).
3. On a cold day reduce exercise intensity, attempt nasal inhalation, or cover mouth and nose with a scarf

---

Cerebral Palsy

Children with cerebral palsy respond to aerobic training with an improvement in physical performance (that is, speed of walking and other motor skills) and in several physiologic functions.[11,14,32,83,85] The improvement in walking ability can be achieved with little or no increase in maximal aerobic power.[11] No published studies have measured changes in peak anaerobic power or local muscle endurance, but measurements in our laboratory suggest that training regimens that include stretching and strengthening improve peak power and the endurance of the upper and the lower limbs, as measured by the Wingate anaerobic test.

As stated earlier, a high metabolic cost of moving the limbs is a main reason for the low exercise tolerance of children with cerebral palsy. In one study[32] a 10-week program of three-per-week sessions of high-intensity judo, swimming, and games resulted in a 10% decrease in oxygen cost of cycling. Four months later the V_{O_2} returned to its preprogram levels. Such changes in oxygen cost suggest that training might induce a reduction in muscle spasticity.[84] However, a 2-year intervention study of adolescents with cerebral palsy could not show any decrease in spasticity as assessed by the ratio between the Hoffman reflex (also called H-reflex) and the motor action potential of the muscle elicited by direct stimulation,[85] nor did monitoring of the integrated electromyogram as an index of spasticity before and after a 1-year program with 6- to 18-year-old patients disclose any changes.[78]

Cystic Fibrosis

The aerobic fitness of children with cystic fibrosis is trainable.[3,63,87] Because of the progression of disease, however, it is sometimes hard to gauge the extent of training-induced changes. The three suggested disease-specific benefits of training are an increase in some lung volumes and flows at rest, improved endurance of the respiratory muscles, and enhanced clearance of mucus from the bronchi. For reviews see Cerny and Armitage,[23] Orenstein,[62] and Stanghelle.[86]

A training-induced increase in vital capacity and bronchial indices such as forced expiratory volume in 1 second has been claimed by some authors[46,99,100] but not by others.[63] Respiratory muscle endurance as measured by the time period during which the patient can sustain all-out isocapnic ventilation has been shown to increase after such "aerobic" programs as prone immersion in water,[25] canoeing, swimming and respiratory muscle strengthening (maximal normocapnic hyperpnea),[49] and distance running.[63] None of the studies that examined changes in respiratory functions had a randomly selected control group.

Enhancement of the drainage of bronchial mucus is one of the main objectives of therapy in persons with cystic fibrosis. This objective has traditionally been achieved by forceful percussion of the chest either manually or by means of an apparatus while the child is lying at different postures. Two laboratories have reported increased volumes of sputum on days when children with cystic fibrosis were exercising, which was taken to represent enhanced clearance of bronchial mucus.[63,99,100] Because of crude methodology, these data, although encouraging, cannot be considered definitive. Further research that makes use of a technique such as technetium 99 clearance rate[61,77] is indicated to determine whether exercise, indeed, enhances mucus clearance and whether the effect is only acute or is also long-standing.

Insulin-Dependent Diabetes Mellitus

Patients with insulin-dependent diabetes mellitus are trainable and can reach athletic excellence. Training-induced biochemical changes include enhanced sensitivity of insulin receptors, a decrease in fasting blood glucose level, and an improved lipoprotein profile. For a review see Dorchy and Poortmans.[31]

An important practical and theoretic question is whether training improves overall diabetic control. Some authors have shown that the frequency of glycosuria[16,53] and the blood level of hemoglobin A_1[16,22,28,40] are lower in active patients than in sedentary ones, which suggests a beneficial effect of training. Other studies, however, could not find such differences.[2,53] Poortmans et al.[72] have reported a higher maximal aerobic power in adolescents with good diabetic control (hemoglobin A_1 blood level lower than 8.5%) than in those with poor control. Of interest are the longitudinal works by Campaigne et al.[22] and Landt et al.[52] who included randomly assigned controls. The combined message of these studies was that training did improve the diabetic control of prepubescents but not of older adolescents, as reflected in their blood levels of hemoglobin A_1.

Another effect of training is on renal function. Poortmans[70] reported a lower degree of exercise-induced proteinuria in trained diabetics than in sedentary diabetics. In a 2-week training study 11- to 18-year-old patients had a 50% reduction in their exercise-induced albuminuria and β_2 microglobulinuria as compared with the pretraining values.[71] An as yet unanswered question is whether physical training has any effect on the risk for diabetic neuropathy.

Hypertension

A training-induced reduction in the resting blood pressure is of practical importance, mostly for patients with borderline or mild hypertension. A reduction of 10 to 15 mm Hg may be the difference between the need for medication and a medication-free regimen. Such an effect of training has been shown for adults, as reviewed by Tipton.[91] A similar pattern in adolescents with hypertension was also found in some[43,44] but not all[35,51,55] studies.

Although an intense static exercise such as weight lifting causes a dramatic rise in arterial blood pressure in young adults,[58] no data exist on the acute effect of weight training on the blood pressure of children with hypertension. Of interest is the study by Hagberg et al.,[44] who administered a 5-month weight training program to adolescents with hypertension. These patients had just completed a 6-month jogging program. The resting systolic and diastolic pressures decreased by 8 and 5 mm Hg, respectively, during the jogging phase and decreased further during the weight training phase.

Muscle Atrophies and Dystrophies

Although the various pediatric muscle atrophies and dystrophies are distinct entities, they are discussed together here. A close link exists between the functional ability of a patient with these diseases and the deficiency in muscle endurance, strength, and peak power[7]: hence the rationale for using training as a therapeutic modality. There are several limitations to studying the effects of training in children with muscle atrophies and dystrophies. One is the scarcity of available subjects. Another is the progressive nature of diseases such as Duchenne's dystrophy or spinal muscle atrophy, which makes it hard to assess the *extent* of any training-induced changes.[38] Special study designs are needed to overcome these constraints.[20]

Both muscle strength[48] and aerobic power[57] are trainable in adults with myopathies. In children with Duchenne's dystrophy, changes in strength were found to be minimal.[1,29,82,94] As stated previously, the progressive nature of this disease may mask any training-induced changes. One methodologic solution is to train only one limb, using the contralateral limb as control. This was done in one study,[29] in which a training effect was reported. In our clinic we have had success with some patients with Duchenne's and Becker's dystrophies and central core and other myopathies; peak muscle power, muscle endurance, and strength increased as the children increased their activity levels. Nonetheless, more research is necessary to determine the extent of trainability, if any, in children with a specific muscle atrophy or a myopathy.

One potential use of training in patients with atrophies or dystrophies is related to prevention of obesity. Excess weight, even mild excess, in a child with weak muscles may be a major functional handicap. A low-calorie diet can be efficacious in inducing weight and fat loss in children and adolescents with a dystrophy. However, such a loss is sometimes accompanied by a negative nitrogen balance.[33] A loss of fat-free body mass has been shown in able-bodied obese children who were exposed to a diet extremely low in calories.[17] In the same children a 4-week training program increased the fat-free body mass.[18] Therefore it is possible that the inclusion of exercise in a weight control program for the child with a muscle disease might prevent the loss of lean tissue, even in the absence of increase in strength.

Obesity

Obesity is the most prevalent pediatric chronic disease in North America. Its reported prevalence is 10% to 25%,[75] and it seems to be on the rise.[76] Because obesity "tracks well" from childhood to adolescence and from adolescence to adulthood,[30] its prevention at a young age is a major public health challenge.

Because many weight control studies have combined training with nutritional changes and behavior modification, it is hard to tease out those changes that are specific to training. The main benefits of enhanced physical activity with or without other therapies are a decrease (or slowing down of an increase) in body weight,[21,34,66] decreases in body fat[59,66] and resting blood pressure,[21,74] increases in body-image and self-image,[88] self-esteem and the ability to function with peers,[69] and, possibly, an improved profile of blood lipids.[98] As recently suggested by Blaak et al.,[18] physical training induces an increase in fat-free body mass of obese prepubescent boys, whereas a decrease follows a low-calorie diet.[17] For a recent review of the physiologic benefits see Parker and Bar-Or.[67]

Whether training can induce *long-lasting* changes in body composition once the program has been completed remains unresolved. Current evidence suggests that unless dietary changes and behavior modification (of the child and the parents) are included, training *per se* is not likely to induce a long-lasting effect.[34]

REFERENCES

1. Abramson AS, Rogoff J: *Physical treatment in muscular dystrophy* (abstract), Proceedings of the Second Medical Conference of the Muscular Dystrophy Association of America, 1952.
2. Akerblom, HK, Koivukangas T, Ilkka J: Experiences from a winter camp for teenage diabetics, *Acta Paediatr Scand Suppl* 283:50, 1980.
3. Andreasson B et al: Long-term effects of physical exercise on working capacity and pulmonary function in cystic fibrosis, *Acta Paediatr Scand* 76:70, 1987.
4. Bar-Or O: *Pediatric sports medicine for the practitioner: from physiologic principles to clinical applications,* New York, 1983, Springer-Verlag.
5. Bar-Or O: Response to physical conditioning in children with cardiopulmonary disease, *Exerc Sport Sci Rev* 13:305, 1985.
6. Bar-Or O: Exercise in pediatric assessment and diagnosis, *Scand J Sports Sci* 18:276, 1986.
7. Bar-Or O: Pathophysiological factors which limit the exercise capacity of the sick child, *Med Sci Sports Exerc* 18:276, 1986.
8. Bar-Or O: The Wingate anaerobic test: an update on methodology, reliability, and validity, *Sport Med* 4:381, 1987.
9. Bar-Or O: Trainability of the prepubescent child, *Physician Sportsmed* 17(5):65, 1989.
10. Bar-Or O: Disease-specific benefits of training in the child with a chronic disease: what is the evidence? *Pediatr Sports Sci* 2:384, 1990.
11. Bar-Or O, Inbar O, Spira R: Physiological effects of a sports rehabilitation program on cerebral palsied and postpoliomyelitic adolescents, *Med Sci Sports* 8:157, 1976.
12. Bar-Or O, Ward DS: Rating of perceived exertion in children. In Bar-Or O, editor: *Advances in pediatric exercise sciences,* vol 3, Champaign, Ill, 1989, Human Kinetics.
13. Bar-Or O, Ward DS, Longmuir P: Use of the RPE scale for exercise prescription with wheelchair-bound children and adults (abstract), *Med Sci Sports Exerc* 22:S2, 1989.
14. Berg K: Adaptation in cerebral palsy of body composition, nutrition, and physical working capacity at school age: *Acta Paediatr Scand Suppl* 204, 1970.
15. Berg K, Bjure J: Methods for evaluation of physical working capacity of school children with cerebral palsy, *Acta Paediatr Scand Suppl* 204:15, 1970.
16. Bergstad I et al: The effect of intensive physical training in young insulin dependent diabetic patients (abstract), *Diabetologia* 19:257, 1980.
17. Blaak EE et al: Effect of VLCD on daily energy expenditure and body composition in obese boys (abstract), *Int J Obes* 14(suppl 2):86, 1990.
18. Blaak EE et al: Effect of training on total energy expenditure and spontaneous activity in obese boys (abstract), *Int J Obes* 14(suppl 2):118, 1990.
19. Borg G: Perceived exertion as an indicator of somatic stress, *Scand J Rehabil* 2, 3:92, 1970.
20. Brooke MH et al: Clinical investigation in Duchenne dystrophy. II. Determination of the "power" of therapeutic trials based on the natural history, *Muscle Nerve* 6:91, 1983.
21. Brownell KD, Kelman JH, Stunkard AJ: Treatment of obese children with and without their mothers: changes in weight and blood pressure, *Pediatrics* 71:515, 1983.
22. Campaigne BN et al: Effects of a physical activity program on metabolic control and cardiovascular fitness in children with insulin-dependent diabetes mellitus, *Diabetes Care* 7:57, 1984.
23. Cerny FJ, Armitage LM: Exercise and cystic fibrosis: a review, *Pediatr Exerc Sci* 1:116, 1989.
24. Cerny FJ, Pullano TP, Cropp GJA: Cardiorespiratory adaptations to exercise in cystic fibrosis, *Am Rev Respir Dis* 126:217, 1982.
25. Clement M, Jankowski LW, Beaudry PH: Prone immersion physical therapy in three children with cystic fibrosis: a pilot study, *Nurs Res* 28:325, 1979.
26. Covitz W et al: Exercise-induced cardiac dysfunction in sickle cell anemia, *Am J Cardiol* 51:570, 1983.
27. Cropp GJ et al: Exercise tolerance and cardiorespiratory adjustments at peak work capacity in cystic fibrosis, *Am Rev Respir Dis* 126:211, 1982.
28. Dahl-Jorgensen K et al: The effect of exercise on diabetic control and hemoglobin A_1 (HbA_1) in children, *Acta Paediatr Scand Suppl* 283:53, 1980.
29. de Lateur BJ, Giaconi RM: Effect on maximal strength of submaximal exercise in Duchenne muscular dystrophy, *Am J Phys Med* 6, 1979.
30. Despres J, Bouchard C, Malina RM: Physical activity and coronary heart disease risk factors during childhood and adolescence, *Exerc Sport Sci Rev* 18:243, 1990.
31. Dorchy H, Poortmans J: Sport and the diabetic child, *Sports Med* 7:248, 1989.
32. Dresen MHW et al: Aerobic energy expenditure of handicapped children after training, *Arch Med Rehabil* 66:301, 1985.
33. Edwards RHT et al: Weight reduction in boys with muscular dystrophy, *Dev Med Child Neurol* 26:384, 1984.
34. Epstein LH et al: A comparison of lifestyle change and programmed aerobic exercise on weight and fitness changes in obese children, *Behav Ther* 13:651, 1982.
35. Fisher AG, Brown M: The effects of diet and exercise on selected coronary risk factors in children (abstract), *Med Sci Sport Exerc* 14:171, 1982.
36. Fitch KD, Blivitch JD, Morton AR: The effect of running training on exercise-induced asthma, *Ann Allergy* 57:90, 1986.
37. Fitch KD, Morton AR, Blanksby BA: Effects of swimming training on children with asthma, *Arch Dis Child* 51:190, 1976.
38. Fowler WM Jr, Taylor M: Rehabilitation management of muscular dystrophy and related disorders. I. The role of exercise, *Arch Phys Med Rehabil* 63:319, 1982.

39. Germann K, Orenstein D, Horowitz J: Changes in oxygenation during exercise in cystic fibrosis (abstract), *Med Sci Sports Exerc* 12:105, 1980.

40. Ginsberg-Fellner F, Witt ME: The effects of exercise on hemoglobin A₁C and blood lipids in diabetic children (abstract), *Diabetes* 27:436, 1978.

41. Godfrey S, Mearns M: Pulmonary function and response to exercise in cystic fibrosis, *Arch Dis Child* 46:144, 1971.

42. Grilliat JP et al: Rehabilitation of asthmatic patients to effort (in French), *Rev Fr Mal Resp* 5:431, 1977.

43. Hagberg JM et al: Effect of exercise training on the blood pressure and hemodynamic features of hypertensive adolescents, *Am J Cardiol* 52:763, 1983.

44. Hagberg JM et al: Effect of weight training on blood pressure and hemodynamics in hypertensive adolescents, *Pediatrics* 104:147, 1984.

45. Henriksen JM, Nielsen T: Effect of physical training on exercise-induced bronchoconstriction, *Acta Paediatr Scand* 72:31, 1983.

46. Jankowski LW: Exercise testing and exercise prescription for individuals with cystic fibrosis. In Skinner JS, editor: *Exercise testing and exercise prescription for special cases,* Philadelphia, 1987, Lea & Febiger.

47. Jeejeebhoy KN: Muscle function and nutrition, *Gut* 27(suppl 1):25, 1986.

48. Kawazoe Y et al: Effects of therapeutic exercise on masticatory function in patients with progressive muscular dystrophy, *J Neurol Neurosurg Psychiatr* 45:343, 1982.

49. Keens TG et al: Ventilatory muscle endurance training in normal subjects and patients with cystic fibrosis, *Am Rev Resp Dis* 116:853, 1977.

50. King MJ, Noakes TD, Weinberg EG: Physiological effects of a physical training program in children with exercise-induced asthma, *Pediatr Exerc Sci* 1:137, 1989.

51. Laird WP, Fixler DE, Swanbom CD: Effect of chronic weight lifting on the blood pressure in hypertensive adolescents (abstract), *Prevent Med* 8:184, 1979.

52. Landt KW et al: Effects of exercise training on insulin sensitivity in adolescents with type 1 diabetes, *Diabetes Care* 8:461, 1985.

53. Larson Y et al: Effects of exercise on blood lipids in juvenile diabetes, *Lancet* 1:350, 1964.

54. Leisti S, Finnila M-J, Kiura E: Effects of physical training on hormonal responses to exercise in asthmatic children, *Arch Dis Child* 54:524, 1979.

55. Linder CW, DuRant RH, Mahoney OM: The effect of physical conditioning on serum lipids and lipoproteins in white male adolescents, *Med Sci Sports Exerc* 15:232, 1983.

56. Lundberg A: Oxygen consumption in relation to work load in students with cerebral palsy, *J Appl Physiol* 40:873, 1976.

57. McCartney N et al: The effects of strength training in patients with selected neuromuscular disorders, *Med Sci Sports Exerc* 20:362, 1988.

58. MacDougall JD et al: Arterial blood pressure response to heavy resistance exercise, *J Appl Physiol* 58:785, 1985.

59. Moody DL et al: The effects of a jogging program on the body composition of normal and obese high school girls, *Med Sci Sports* 4:210, 1972.

60. Nickerson BG et al: Distance running improves fitness in asthmatic children without pulmonary complications or changes in exercise-induced bronchospasm, *Pediatrics* 71:147, 1983.

61. Oldenburg FA et al: Effects of postural drainage, exercise, and cough on mucus clearance in chronic bronchitis, *Am Rev Resp Dis* 120:739, 1979.

62. Orenstein DM: Research in exercise and cystic fibrosis: new directions, *Scand J Sports Sci* 7:29, 1985.

63. Orenstein DM et al: Exercise conditioning and cardiopulmonary fitness in cystic fibrosis: the effects of a 3-month supervised running program, *Chest* 80:392, 1981.

64. Orenstein DM et al: Exercise conditioning in children with asthma, *J Pediatr* 106:556, 1985.

65. Oseid S, Haaland K: Exercise studies on asthmatic children before and after regular physical training. In Eeiksson BO, Ferberg B, editors: *Swimming Medicine,* vol 4, Baltimore, 1978, University Park.

66. Parizkova J, Vamberova M: Body composition as a criterion of the suitability of reducing regimens in obese children, *Dev Med Child Neurol* 9:202, 1967.

67. Parker DF, Bar-Or O: Physiological effects of enhanced physical activity on obese children and adolescents: a selective review, *Physician Sportsmed* 19(6):113-125, 1991.

68. Parsons CG, Wright FH: Circulatory function in the anemias of children. I. Effect of anemia on exercise tolerance and vital capacity, *Am J Dis Child* 57:15, 1939.

69. Peckos PS, Spargo JA, Heald FP: Program and results of a camp for obese adolescent girls, *Postgrad Med* 27:527, 1960.

70. Poortmans JR: Exercise and renal function, *Sports Med* 1:125, 1984.

71. Poortmans JR, Waterlot B, Dorchy H: Training effect on postexercise microproteinuria in type 1 diabetic adolescents, *Pediatr Adolesc Endocr* 17:166, 1988.

72. Poortmans JR et al: Influence of the degree of metabolic control on physical fitness in type 1 diabetic adolescents, *Int J Sports Med* 7:232, 1986.

73. Ramsey JA et al: Strength training effects in prepubescent boys, *Med Sci Sports Exerc* 22:605, 1990.

74. Rocchini AP et al: Blood pressure in obese adolescents: effect of weight loss, *Pediatrics* 82:16, 1988.

75. Rosenbaum M, Leibel RL: Obesity in childhood, *Pediatr Rev* 11:43, 1989.

76. Ross JG, Gilbert GG: The National Children and Youth Fitness Study. *J Phys Ed Recr Dance* 56:45, 1985.

77. Rossman CM et al: Effect of chest physiotherapy on the removal of mucus in patients with cystic fibrosis, *Am Rev Respir Dis* 126:131, 1982.

78. Rotzinger H, Stoboy H: Comparison between clinical judgement and electromyographic investigation of the effect of special training program for CP children, *Acta Paediatr Belg* 28 (suppl):121, 1974.

79. Rowland TW: Aerobic response to endurance training in prepubescent children: a critical analysis, *Med Sci Sports Exerc* 17:493, 1985.

80. Rowland TW: *Exercise and Children's Health,* Champaign, Ill, 1990, Human Kinetics.

81. Ruttenberg HD et al: Recommended guidelines for graded exercise testing and exercise prescription for children with heart disease, *J Cardiol Rehabil* 4:10, 1984.

82. Scott OM et al: Effect of exercise in Duchenne muscular dystrophy, *Physiotherapy* 67:174, 1981.

83. Sommer M: Improvement of motor skills and adaptation of the circulatory system in wheelchair-bound children with cerebral palsy: lecture No 11. In Simri U, editor: *Sports as a means of rehabilitation,* Netanya, Israel, 1971, Wingate Institute.

84. Spira R: Contribution of the H reflex to the study of spasticity in adolescents, *Dev Med Child Neurol* 16:150, 1974.

85. Spira R, Bar-Or O: *An investigation of the ambulation problems associated with severe paralysis in adolescents: influence of physical conditioning and adapted sports activities.* Final report, project No 19-P-58065-F01 Tel Aviv, Washington, DC, 1975, U.S. Department of Health, Education and Welfare.

86. Stanghelle JK: Physical exercise for patients with cystic fibrosis: a review, *Int J Sports Med* 9(suppl):6, 1988.

87. Stanghelle JK, Michalsen H, Skyberg D: Five-year follow-up of pulmonary function and peak oxygen uptake in 16-year-old boys with cystic fibrosis, with special regard to the influence of regular physical exercise, *Int J Sports Med* 9:19, 1988.

88. Stanley EJ et al: Overcoming obesity in adolescents: a description of a promising endeavor to improve management, *Clin Pediatr* 9:29, 1970.

89. Svenoniu E, Kautto R, Arborelius M Jr: Improvement after training of children with exercise-induced asthma, *Acta Paediatr Scand* 72:23, 1983.

90. Swann IL, Hanson CA: Double-blind prospective study of the effect of physical training on childhood asthma. In Oseid S, Edwards AM, editors: *The asthmatic child in play and sport,* Bath, England, 1983, Putnam.

91. Tipton CM: Exercise, training, and hypertension, *Exerc Sport Sci Rev* 12:245, 1984.

92. Tirosh E, Bar-Or O, Rosenbaum P: New muscle power test in neuromuscular disease: feasibility and reliability, *Am J Dis Child* 144:1983, 1990.

93. Ulmer HE et al: Cardiovascular impairment and physical working capacity in children with chronic renal failure, *Acta Paediatr Scand* 67:43, 1978.

94. Vignos PJ, Watkins MP: The effect of exercise in muscle dystrophy, *J Am Med Assoc* 197:843, 1966.

95. Viteri FE, Torun B: Anaemia and physical working capacity, *Clin Haematol* 3:609, 1974.

96. Voy RO: The U.S. Olympic Committee experience with exercise-induced bronchospasm: 1984, *Med Sci Sports Exerc* 18:328, 1986.

97. Ward DS, Bar-Or O: Use of the Borg scale in exercise prescription for overweight youth, *Can J Sport Sci* 15:120, 1990.

98. Widhalm K, Maxa E, Zyman H: Effect of diet and exercise upon the cholesterol and triglyceride content of plasma lipoproteins in overweight children, *Eur J Pediatr* 127:121, 1978.

99. Zach M, Oberwaldner B, Hauslen F: Cystic fibrosis: physical exercise versus chest physiotherapy, *Arch Dis Child* 57:587, 1982.

100. Zach M, Purrer B, Oberwalder B: Effect of swimming on forced expiration and sputum clearance in cystic fibrosis, *Lancet* 2:1201, 1981.

101. Zelkowitz PS, Giammona ST: Effects of gravity and exercise on the pulmonary capacity in children with cystic fibrosis, *J Pediatr* 74:393, 1969.

STUDY QUESTIONS

■ Describe the factors that may limit the exercise tolerance of a child with chronic disease.

■ How is an exercise prescription for a child different from that for an adult?

■ Describe the effect of exercise training on children with asthma and cystic fibrosis.

■ Describe the effect of exercise training on children with cerebral palsy and muscular dystrophy.

■ Describe the effect of exercise training on children with diabetes, obesity, and hypertension.

INDEX